Diagnostic Testing of Allergic Disease

CLINICAL ALLERGY AND IMMUNOLOGY

Series Editor

MICHAEL A. KALINER, M.D.
Medical Director
Institute for Asthma and Allergy
Washington, D.C.

1. Sinusitis: Pathophysiology and Treatment, *edited by Howard M. Druce*
2. Eosinophils in Allergy and Inflammation, *edited by Gerald J. Gleich and A. Barry Kay*
3. Molecular and Cellular Biology of the Allergic Response, *edited by Arnold I. Levinson and Yvonne Paterson*
4. Neuropeptides in Respiratory Medicine, *edited by Michael A. Kaliner, Peter J. Barnes, Gert H. H. Kunkel, and James N. Baraniuk*
5. Provocation Testing in Clinical Practice, *edited by Sheldon L. Spector*
6. Mast Cell Proteases in Immunology and Biology, *edited by George H. Caughey*
7. Histamine and H_1-Receptor Antagonists in Allergic Disease, *edited by F. Estelle R. Simons*
8. Immunopharmacology of Allergic Diseases, *edited by Robert G. Townley and Devendra K. Agrawal*
9. Indoor Air Pollution and Health, *edited by Emil J. Bardana, Jr., and Anthony Montanaro*
10. Genetics of Allergy and Asthma: Methods for Investigative Studies, *edited by Malcolm N. Blumenthal and Bengt Björkstén*
11. Allergic and Respiratory Disease in Sports Medicine, *edited by John M. Weiler*
12. Allergens and Allergen Immunotherapy: Second Edition, Revised and Expanded, *edited by Richard F. Lockey and Samuel C. Bukantz*
13. Emergency Asthma, *edited by Barry E. Brenner*
14. Food Hypersensitivity and Adverse Reactions: A Practical Guide for Diagnosis and Management, *edited by Marianne Frieri and Brett Kettelhut*
15. Diagnostic Testing of Allergic Disease, *edited by Stephen F. Kemp and Richard F. Lockey*

ADDITIONAL VOLUMES IN PREPARATION

Diagnostic Testing of Allergic Disease

edited by

Stephen F. Kemp
University of Mississippi Medical Center
Jackson, Mississippi

Richard F. Lockey
University of South Florida
Tampa, Florida

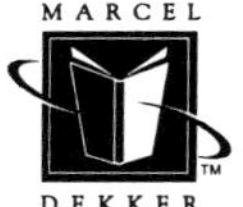

MARCEL DEKKER, INC. NEW YORK • BASEL

ISBN: 0-8247-0303-0

This book is printed on acid-free paper.

Headquarters
Marcel Dekker, Inc.
270 Madison Avenue, New York, NY 10016
tel: 212-696-9000; fax: 212-685-4540

Eastern Hemisphere Distribution
Marcel Dekker AG
Hutgasse 4, Postfach 812, CH-4001 Basel, Switzerland
tel: 41-61-261-8482; fax: 41-61-261-8896

World Wide Web
http://www.dekker.com

The publisher offers discounts on this book when ordered in bulk quantities. For more information, write to Special Sales/Professional Marketing at the headquarters address above.

Current printing (last digit):
10 9 8 7 6 5 4 3 2 1

PRINTED IN THE UNITED STATES OF AMERICA

Introduction

Each of the allergic diseases—allergic rhinitis, asthma, sinusitis, urticaria, food allergy, eczema—is increasing in prevalence and becoming more widely recognized by both the medical and lay communities. Unfortunately, the formal education of physicians and other health-care providers in allergy and its diagnosis is being emphasized less and less. Medical schools and residency programs continue to focus on the hospitalized patient and rare or unusual diseases rather than the common everyday problems that allergy represents. Moreover, the number of allergy training programs is also falling, resulting in fewer academic teachers capable of instructing students and residents in the principles and practice of allergy. We can therefore predict a time in the near future when the medical community will have to learn about allergic diseases through postgraduate education involving books and seminars.

This fine book, created by Richard Lockey and Stephen Kemp, will serve two excellent purposes. It will provide the specialist with a very important and timely reference on a number of clinically important diagnostic tests. This book will also help the nonallergist with the diagnosis of allergy and may provide an important reference on who to treat and who to refer. Thus, for the 20% (or more) of the population suffering from one of the allergic diseases, this book will help keep physicians up to date or may help ease the gap in knowledge between the specialist and the generalist in regard to diagnostic testing. I found this text to be very helpful to my practice and will recommend it to my colleagues, most of whom are nonspecialists.

Michael Kaliner

Preface

An estimated 35 million or more Americans have allergic diseases, such as allergic asthma and rhinitis, insect and food allergy, urticaria, drug allergy, and many others. Allergic diseases account for approximately one in nine outpatient visits. However, most physicians have only a rudimentary knowledge of allergic and immunological diseases and the tests that are essential for their diagnosis and treatment, primarily because physicians receive inadequate training in medical schools and during residency.

Knowledge about and scientific exploration of primary immunodeficiency diseases and immunology have led to a better understanding of the immune system. Such information has permitted successful bone marrow and solid organ transplantation and rapid progress in the understanding and treatment of immunologically based diseases, including AIDS. Many of these and other discoveries have also advanced the understanding and treatment of allergic diseases.

At the same time these great advancements were taking place, some physicians and lay individuals came to view the immune system in a naive manner, which led to the conception of allegedly new illnesses such as ''multiple chemical sensitivity,'' ''candida hypersensitivity syndrome,'' and others; the existence of these illnesses, however, is not supported by controlled objective studies. News reports often heighten public expectations that previously unexplained symptoms have a yet to be discovered allergic or immunological basis that will be substantiated if only the ''proper'' immunological or allergic test is performed.

Diagnostic Testing of Allergic Disease outlines a rational approach for the use and interpretation of the most important laboratory and clinical tests that not only confirm the presence of allergic diseases but also help guide therapy. Chapters contain discussions on many topics, including the preparation and storage of diagnostic allergens; skin testing and in vitro diagnostic tests for immediate (IgE-mediated) hypersensitivity; delayed hypersensitivity tests; and diagnostic tests for certain kinds of urticaria and angioedema, ocular allergic diseases, otitis media, drug allergy, allergic lung diseases and asthma, nasal and paranasal diseases, and food allergy. Radiographic imaging of the sinuses, fiberoptic rhinolaryngoscopy, spirometry, food challenges, bronchoprovocation, intranasal provocation, drug challenge/desensitization, and patch testing for contact dermatitis also are discussed. Unconventional and unproven tests are included to enable the physician to better understand them and help patients who are convinced they are affected by an illness that has no logical medical or scientific basis.

This book will be an invaluable reference for physicians who wish to gain a better understanding of the indications, benefits, and limitations of current diagnostic tests and procedures used to care for patients with allergic diseases.

We thank the authors for their excellent contributions to this book. We are also grateful for the assistance of our secretary associates, Mary Hagaman, Peggy Hales, and Geeta Gehi.

Stephen F. Kemp
Richard F. Lockey

Contents

Contributors

John A. Arrington, M.D. University of South Florida College of Medicine, Tampa, Florida

Leonard Bielory, M.D. Associate Professor of Medicine, Pediatrics, and Ophthalmology, Department of Medicine, UMDNJ–New Jersey Medical School, Newark, New Jersey

Ronald R. Brancaccio, M.D. Clinical Professor of Dermatology, Ronald O. Perelman Department of Dermatology, New York University School of Medicine, New York, New York

A. Wesley Burks, Jr., M.D. Professor of Pediatrics, Department of Allergy and Immunology, University of Arkansas for Medical Sciences and Arkansas Children's Hospital, Little Rock, Arkansas

David E. Cohen, M.D., M.P.H. Ronald O. Perelman Department of Dermatology, New York University School of Medicine, New York, New York

Marc Dinowitz, M.D. Department of Ophthalmology, UMDNJ–New Jersey Medical School, Newark, New Jersey

Howard M. Druce, M.D., F.A.C.P. Clinical Associate Professor of Medicine, Division of Allergy and Immunology, UMDNJ–New Jersey Medical School, Newark, New Jersey

Donnie P. Dunagan, M.D. Assistant Professor of Medicine, Section of Allergy, Pulmonary and Critical Care Medicine, Department of Internal Medicine, Wake Forest University, Winston-Salem, North Carolina

Philip Fireman, M.D. Professor of Pediatrics and Internal Medicine, Division of Allergy, Department of Pediatrics, Immunology, and Infectious Diseases, University of Pittsburgh School of Medicine and Children's Hospital of Pittsburgh, Pittsburgh, Pennsylvania

John W. Georgitis, M.D. Department of Pediatrics, Wake Forest University, Winston-Salem, North Carolina

Robert G. Hamilton, Ph.D., D.ABMLI Associate Professor, Johns Hopkins Asthma and Allergy Center, Johns Hopkins University School of Medicine, Baltimore, Maryland

John M. James, M.D. Colorado Allergy and Asthma Centers, P.C., Ft. Collins, Colorado

Anne Kagey-Sobotka, Ph.D. Johns Hopkins Asthma and Allergy Center, Johns Hopkins University School of Medicine, Baltimore, Maryland

Phillip H. Kaleida, M.D. Professor, Division of General Academic Pediatrics, Department of Pediatrics, University of Pittsburgh School of Medicine, and Children's Hospital of Pittsburgh, Pittsburgh, Pennsylvania

Allen P. Kaplan, M.D. Professor, Department of Medicine, Medical University of South Carolina, Charleston, South Carolina

Stephen F. Kemp, M.D. Department of Medicine, University of Mississippi Medical Center, Jackson, Mississippi

Jørgen Nedergaard Larsen, Ph.D. Scientific Secretary, Research Department, ALK-Abelló A/S, Hørsholm, Denmark

Dennis K. Ledford, M.D. Associate Professor of Medicine and Director, Clinical and Laboratory Immunology Training Program, Division of Allergy and Clinical Immunology, Department of Internal Medicine, University of South Florida College of Medicine and the James A. Haley Veterans Hospital, Tampa, Florida

Phillip L. Lieberman, M.D. Divisions of Allergy and Immunology, University of Tennessee College of Medicine, Memphis, Tennessee

Richard F. Lockey, M.D. Division of Allergy and Immunology, University of South Florida, Tampa, Florida

Henning Løwenstein, D.Sc., Ph.D. Executive Vice President, Research, ALK-Abelló A/S, Hørsholm, Denmark

Gailen D. Marshall, Jr., M.D., Ph.D., F.A.C.P. Associate Professor and Director, Division of Allergy and Clinical Immunology, University of Texas Medical School, Houston, Texas

Ronald Rescigno, M.D. Director, Uveitis Service, Department of Ophthalmology, UMDNJ–New Jersey Medical School, Newark, New Jersey

Nicholas A. Soter, M.D. Professor, Ronald O. Perelman Department of Dermatology, New York University School of Medicine, New York, New York

Sheldon L. Spector, M.D. Professor, Department of Medicine, University of California Medical Center, and Director, California Allergy and Asthma Medical Group, Los Angeles, California

Ricardo A. Tan, M.D. California Allergy and Asthma Medical Group, Los Angeles, California

Abba I. Terr, M.D. Clinical Professor of Medicine, Department of Medicine, Stanford University Medical Center, Stanford, California

Paul C. Turkeltaub, M.D. Associate Director, Division of Allergic Products and Parasitology, Center for Biologics Evaluation and Research, Food and Drug Administration, Rockville, Maryland

1

Allergen Vaccines for Specific Diagnosis

Jørgen Nedergaard Larsen and Henning Løwenstein
ALK-Abelló A/S, Hørsholm, Denmark

I. INTRODUCTION

Being an immunological disease, the characteristics of allergy are those of specificity and memory. Regardless of whether the clinical manifestation is rhinoconjunctivitis, rhinitis, or asthma, the underlying immunological disorder is based on the adverse reactions of cells in the immune system upon contact with allergens. These cells are specific for epitopes that are structural parts of allergens present in the allergenic source material. Two types of cells (i.e., T-cells and B-cells) produce receptor molecules (i.e., T-cell receptors and immunoglobulin [IgE] antibodies) that, through high-affinity interactions with the allergen, efficiently catalyze the presence of even minute amounts of allergens into clinical symptoms, the extreme consequence of which may be life-threatening to the patient.

Allergens are molecules with the capacity to elicit specific IgE responses in humans. Allergens are proteins, readily soluble in water, and may be found on airborne particles of a certain size. These characteristics are compatible with a notion that the particle carrying the allergen is inhaled and extracted on the mucosal surface of the respiratory tract followed by stimulation of the immune system of the individual. Thus, an allergen is defined by the specific response of the immune system of the individual patient.

Accordingly, any immunogenic protein (that is, any antigen) in the allergenic source material has allergenic potential. Even though most allergic patients have IgE specific for a relatively limited number of ''major'' allergens, when larger numbers of patients are investigated, still more proteins are found that bind IgE. Thus, the number of allergens in a given source material converges toward the total number of antigens, and any antigen has the potential to elicit an IgE response.

Aqueous extraction of organic source materials is an old and well-established pharmaceutical technique. However, the procedures to obtain and control vaccines that retain all potential allergens and exclude irrelevant materials under conditions that preserve biological activity are not straightforward and require standardization. Standardization, however, is not an absolute concept. Dependent on technical feasibility, the practical level of standardization advances with the progress in biochemical methodology. The minimum requirements for a contemporary standardization procedure are threefold: (1) the securing of an optimal complexity; (2) the control of individual major allergens; and (3) reproducible overall allergenic potency.

Our understanding of the interaction between allergens and the human immune system has improved dramatically in recent years, not least by virtue of the application of the versatile techniques of molecular biology. Today, the genes of all important allergens have been cloned and, although often refractory, the conversion into recombinant allergens is progressing rapidly. Specific allergy diagnosis based on recombinant allergens has been shown to be almost as efficient as when natural allergen vaccines are used. However, the potential for qualitative improvement may be associated with increased specificity and the possibility of determining ''disease-relevant IgE'' based on epitope engineering. Theoretically, it may be possible with these advanced methods to determine the sensitizing grass species or identify a pollen allergy possibly causing allergenic cross-reactivity with foods. Furthermore, it might be possible to avoid confusing diagnoses caused by clinically irrelevant IgE to carbohydrate moieties.

The following chapter will describe general aspects of selection of source materials, vaccine preparation and standardization, and specific aspects of important allergen vaccines. Although recombinant allergens will be mentioned, the emphasis of the chapter will be on naturally occurring allergens inasmuch as they are the basis of current allergen-specific diagnostic testing.

II. GENERAL ASPECTS OF VACCINE PREPARATION

A. Source Materials

Source materials are those raw materials from which active allergenic substances can be derived. The natural source is the material to which patients are exposed under normal conditions. In some cases, the source of the active allergenic material is very clear (for instance, insect venoms), but in others it may still be debated. The source materials should be selected with attention to the need for specificity on the one hand and for inclusion of all relevant allergens in sufficient amounts on the other hand (1). Furthermore, safety is a prime concern. Source materials should be selected in order to minimize the risk of including infectious agents.

Highly qualified personnel should collect the source materials, and reasonable measures must be used by the producer of allergenic vaccines to assure that collector qualification and collection procedures are appropriate to verify the identity and quality of the source materials. This means that only specifically identified allergenic source materials that do not contain foreign substances should be used in the manufacture of allergenic vaccines. Means of identification and limits of foreign materials should meet established acceptance criteria for each source material. When identity and purity cannot be determined by direct examination of the source material, other appropriate methods should be applied to trace the material from its origin. This includes complete identity labeling and certification from competent collectors. The processing and storage of source materials should be done to ensure that no microorganisms are introduced into the material. When possible, fresh source materials should be used, or source materials should be stored in a manner to prevent deterioration. Records should describe source materials in as much detail as possible, including the particulars of collection and storage.

1. Pollens

Pollens are the natural sources of allergens inhaled from plants. These may be obtained naturally or from cultivated fields or greenhouses. Several collection methods may be used, such as vacuum collection or drying and grinding the flower heads. Furthermore, the pollen may be cleaned by flotation or filtration through sieves of different mesh sizes. Finally the pollens are dried under controlled conditions and stored in sealed containers at 4 °C or −20 °C. The maximum level of accepted contamination with pollen from other species is 0.5% by number. The pollen should be free from flower and plant debris originating from the same species within the limit of 5% by weight. Pollens may show large variation in composition depending on season and location of growth. They should be pooled for the production of allergen vaccines to achieve relatively constant composition harvests from different years and sites of collection.

2. Acarids

For the production of allergen vaccines of domestic (house dust) mites, the mites are grown in pure cultures containing only one species. Source materials for mite allergen vaccines are either pure mite bodies (PMB) or whole mite cultures (WMC). An advantage of the WMC vaccine is that it contains all the material to which a mite allergic patient is exposed under natural conditions, whereas an advantage of the PMB vaccine is the avoidance of contamination with debris from the culture medium. The WMC vaccine includes material from mite bodies, eggs, larvae, and fecal particles, as well as mite decomposition material and contaminants from the culture medium, which should be shown not to be allergenic. The PMB vaccine contains only material extracted from the mite bodies, including eggs and fecal particles. The relative concentration of group 1 and 2 allergens is dependent on the source materials, but clinical trials comparing vaccines based on WMC and PMB have demonstrated that the two types of vaccines have similar clinical effects in specific allergy vaccination (2).

3. Animal Emanations

Allergens of mammalian origin may emanate from various sources (for example, hair, dander, serum, saliva, or urine). The allergens to which humans are exposed depend on the normal behavior of the animal. Therefore, the optimal source of allergens from mammals cannot be generalized, and in many cases is still debated. However, most allergens are present in the pelt, whether derived from dander or deposited from body fluids. Safety considerations demand that source materials must be collected only from animals that are declared healthy by a veterinarian at the time of collection. Furthermore, the risk of infection is minimized by excluding the use of internal parts of mammals. When sacrificed animals are used, storage conditions should minimize post mortem decomposition until the source materials can be collected. The source materials should be free from visible traces of blood, serum, or other extractable materials. The optimal source material is often dander. Hair proteins are insoluble, and thus it is not practical to use hair alone in the manufacture of mammalian allergen vaccines.

Due to the quantitative differences in the yield of allergens from various dog breeds, use of a minimum of five different breeds as source materials has been recommended.

4. Insects

The optimal source for insect allergens depends on the natural route of exposure (inhalation, bite, or sting). When whole insects or insect debris are inhaled, the whole insect body is selected as the allergen source. In the cases of a biting or stinging insect, saliva or venom is the proper allergen source. As is the case for sources of mammalian allergens, avoidance of infectious agents is a primary concern. Selection of source materials should aim for pure insects devoid of microorganisms.

5. Fungi

Raw materials are obtained by growing the fungi under controlled conditions. The harvested raw materials should consist of mycelia and spores. Because of the difficulties involved in maintaining a constant composition of fungal cultures, it is recommended that a vaccine be derived from at least five independent cultures of the same species. Production of the source material should be conducted under aseptic conditions to reduce the risk of contamination by microorganisms or other fungi. The inoculum should be obtained from established fungal culture banks [such as American Type Culture Collection (ATCC) or Central Bureau Schimmelcultures (CBS)]. The cultivation medium should be synthetic or at least devoid of antigenic constituents (that is, proteins). If the culture is slain prior to extraction, care should be taken not to disturb the conformation of the proteins. Controls performed in fungal allergen vaccine production must include tests for known toxins.

6. Foods

Foods constitute a diversified area for allergen characterization, and the market for standardized allergen vaccines is scarce. Foods are often derived from various subspecies, grown under a broad variety of conditions reflecting geographical regions worldwide. In addition, foods are often cooked prior to ingestion, and the cooking procedures are not at all standardized. Consequently, the allergen composition, qualitative as well as quantitative, is highly variable (3).

Ideally, source materials for food allergen vaccines should reflect local subspecies, conditions, and habits for the cultivation, harvesting, storing, and cooking of the foods. However, ingested foods are increasingly derived from distant parts of the world. The best solution to these problems may be to combine source materials from as many places as possible, reflecting variation in as many parameters as possible.

A further problem in food allergen vaccine production is the frequent presence of natural or microbial toxins, pesticides, antibiotics, preservatives, and other additives that may be concentrated during the manufacturing process. The use of ecological source material is therefore preferred.

B. Preparation of Allergen Vaccines

The production of allergen vaccines imposes a number of constraints on both the selection of source materials and the physicochemical conditions used during the extraction procedure. The process must neither denature the proteins (allergens) nor alter their composition significantly, including the quantitative ratio between the individual components. The extraction should be performed under conditions (pH and ionic strength) both resembling the physiological conditions and suppressing possible proteolytic degradation and microbial growth. Thus the extraction should be performed at low temperatures and possibly in the presence of substances suppressing bacterial and fungal growth (4). The most widely used extraction media are aqueous buffer systems of pH 6 to 9 and ionic strength 0.05 to 0.2. In general, nonaqueous solvents should be avoided due to the risk of protein denaturation.

The time needed to obtain a representative vaccine is always a compromise between degradation/denaturation and yield. Furthermore, it is generally preferable to minimize the content of low molecular weight (that is, weight below 5000 Da), nonantigenic material in the final vaccine. Dialysis, ultrafiltration, or size exclusion chromatography can accomplish this task. Any substance excluded from the final vaccine should be verified as nonallergenic material. The production procedure should include assessment of known toxins, viral particles, microorganisms, and free histamine, among others, and verify that their concentrations are below defined thresholds.

The final vaccine should be stored under conditions that maintain allergenic activity. Allergens are decomposed primarily by proteinases in the vaccines or by contaminating microorganisms. Preservation of the allergen vaccine is best performed by lyophilizing the vaccine or by storage at low temperatures (−20 °C–−80 °C), possibly in the presence of stabilizing agents such as 50% glycerol or nonallergenic proteins such as human serum albumin.

C. Standardization

Allergen vaccines are complex mixtures of antigenic components produced by the extraction of naturally occurring source materials, which are known to vary considerably in composition. Without intervention, this variation will be reflected in the final products.

The purpose of standardization is to minimize both qualitative and quantitative variations in composition so that a higher level of safety, efficacy, accuracy, and simplicity in allergy diagnosis and allergy vaccination may be obtained. Standardization of allergen vaccines can never be absolute, but it can be improved progressively as new methodologies and technologies are developed and the understanding of the properties of the allergens and the immune responses of allergic patients is increased. Improved standardization of allergen vaccines enables easier differentiation between allergy and nonallergy and a more precise definition of the specificity and degree of allergy.

Standardization of allergen vaccines is complicated due to the complexity of the allergen vaccines, the allergen molecules, and their epitopes. Raw materials differ in composition due to natural variation, but the cultivation or harvest conditions also may vary. Furthermore, the vaccines are produced by protocols that differ among manufacturers. The allergens themselves also have been shown to be complex mixtures of isoallergens and variants, which differ in amino acid sequence. Some allergens are composed of two or more subunits, the association and dissociation of which will affect IgE binding. In addition, incomplete denaturation or degradation, which may be imposed by the physical or chemical conditions in the production procedure, is difficult to assess and has a significant effect on the IgE-binding activities of the allergens. The IgE-binding B-cell epitopes are largely conformational by disposition, meaning that they will be absent from the vaccine if the allergens are irreversibly denatured.

Another aspect complicating standardization is the complexity of the immune responses of individual patients. Patients respond individually to allergen sources with respect to both specificity and potency. Allergens are proteins, and all proteins are potential allergens. A "major allergen" is statistically defined as an allergen, which is frequently recognized (more than 50%) by patients' serum IgE when a larger panel of patient sera is analyzed. Less frequent IgE-binding allergens (below 50%) are termed "minor allergens" (5). Furthermore, patients respond individually to B- and T-cell epitopes and hence to isoallergens and variants.

A major aspect of allergen vaccine standardization is the assurance of an adequate complexity in composition of the vaccine. Knowledge of all essential allergens is a precondition for ensuring their presence in the final products.

The other important aspect of standardization is the control of the total allergenic potency. The total IgE-binding activity is intimately related to the content of major allergen (6), and control of the content of major allergen is essential for an up-to-date standardization procedure.

A variety of techniques are available for the assessment of allergen vaccine complexity and potency. A majority of these use antibodies as reagents, adding another level of complexity to the standardization procedure. Both human IgE and antibodies generated by the immunization of animals are subject to natural variation and may change over time.

The establishment of reference and control vaccines addresses these problems. International collaboration is necessary to ensure that manufacturers, control authorities, clinicians, and research laboratories worldwide will be able to refer to the same preparations when comparing the results of quality control studies and potency estimates for different allergen vaccines. Ideally, standards for reagents also should be established by international collaboration.

1. The Establishment and Use of International Standards

A subcommittee under the International Union of Immunological Societies (IUIS) for the establishment of international standards (IS) agreed on guidelines in 1980–81. It was assumed that the collaboration and joint authority of the World Health Organization would be essential to achieve acceptance at an international level. In the following years the subcommittee selected, characterized, and produced international standards from several allergenic sources including *Ambrosia artemisiifolia* (short ragweed) (7), *Phleum pratense* (timothy grass) (8), the domestic mite *Dermatophagoides pteronyssinus* (9), *Betula verrucosa* (birch) (10), and *Canis familiaris* (dog) (11). Additional standards were planned for the mold *Alternaria alternata* (12), for the grasses *Cynodon dactylon* (Bermuda grass) (13) and *Lolium perenne* (rye grass) (14), *Felis domesticus* (cat), and the domestic mite *Dermatophagoides farinae*, but this initiative unfortunately seems to have stopped prematurely.

Each of these standard reference vaccines has been thoroughly investigated in collaborative studies in which laboratories and clinics worldwide have participated. The results of the characterization and comparison of several coded vaccines, which were made available voluntarily by allergen manufacturers, as well as the selection of the international standard, have been published and are available to all interested parties. Each international standard has been produced in lyophilized form in 3000 to 4000 glass-sealed ampules and is available for use as a standard for measurements of relative potency. On payment, ampules can be obtained from the National Institute of Biological Science and Control (NIBSC), London, England.

The content of each ampule is defined by the arbitrary assignment of 100,000 IU (international units). This means that each ampule contains 100,000 IU of any included individual allergen and 100,000 IU of potency as measured by any relevant method. Potency estimates will depend on production methods and reagents, which must be stated, whereas IUs are independent of methods and reagents.

It is important to realize that the international standards are only recommended for use as calibrators (that is, standards for measurement of relative potency). They are not recommended for use as prototypes (materials to which a vaccine is to be matched in all respects). The existence and availability of international standards enable the assignment of a relative potency to internal reference vaccines, which is in use in different laboratories of manufacturers, allergen research groups, or control authorities.

2. Strategy for Standardization

An allergen vaccine should include all potential allergens in their appropriate forms, and major allergens should be present in relevant ratios. The allergen vaccine should display a predetermined IgE-binding activity, and all irrelevant material should ideally be absent.

Irrelevant material includes all components that do not act as antigens (that is, potential allergens). All allergens described so far are water-soluble proteins with molecular weights between 5 and 70 kDa and, in fact, only a few allergens of minor importance are of a size less than 10 kDa or larger than 40 kDa. In general, components of low molecular weight may be regarded as irrelevant material, and these components should be removed from the vaccine before standardization.

The standardization procedure requires well-defined standards for comparison. In-house standards are references used to match the vaccines. This process is called the "blueprint principle." However, the in-house standards should be compared to external references available from central control authorities. The external references are used to compare specific activities of vaccines. This process is called the "yardstick principle." In this way, measures from different manufacturers can be compared and consistency in internal standardization can be achieved (15).

The standardization of allergen vaccines uses the following three-step procedure:

1. Determination of allergen composition to ensure the presence of all important allergens
2. Quantification of specific allergens to ensure the presence of essential allergens in constant ratios
3. Quantification of the total allergenic activity to ensure that the overall potency of the vaccine is constant (in vivo and in vitro)

3. Methods for the Assessment of Allergen Vaccine Quality

The quality of an allergen vaccine is a measure of the complexity of the composition, including the concentration of the various constituents. That is, the presence or absence of individual constituents determines the quality. Only selected constituents (i.e., the major allergens or other marker proteins) can be quantified independently. The complexity of the composition of allergen vaccines can be assessed by several techniques. These are standard separation techniques in biochemistry and traditional immunochemistry.

Polyacrylamide gel electrophoresis with sodium dodecylsulphate (SDS-PAGE) (16) is a widely used, high-resolution technique available in rapid and partly automated systems. The proteins are separated according to size but only after denaturation. Densitometric scanning has been reported, but this technique is not quantitative due to differences in staining intensities and should only be used for a qualitative assessment of the allergen vaccine. In combination with electroblotting (17), the proteins can be immobilized on protein-binding membranes, such as nitrocellulose, and stained using a variety of dyes or labeled antibodies (such as immunoblotting), thereby increasing the sensitivity considerably. When used for identification of allergens, the technique is dependent upon the selected patient panel. Furthermore, attention should be drawn to the fact that some allergens lose their ability to bind IgE, totally or partially, upon denaturation (18).

Isoelectric focusing (IEF) (19) is a qualitative electrophoretic technique that separates proteins according to charge (isoelectric points [pI]). However, individual allergens are difficult to identify because several allergens are distributed in many bands due to differences in charge between isoallergens and variants.

Crossed immunoelectrophoresis (CIE) (20) is a technique by which individual antigens are distinguished in the form of bell-shaped antigen-antibody precipitates in agarose gels. The technique is dependent on the availability of broadly reactive polyspecific rabbit antibodies, but the method yields information on the relative concentrations of all important antigens in a single experiment. In crossed radioimmunoelectrophoresis (CRIE) (21), the plates are incubated with patient serum for the identification of allergens.

4. Quantification of Specific Allergens

Having determined an adequate potency and complexity in composition, an allergen vaccine may still be deficient in the content of major allergen (Fig. 1).

Only a few manufacturers of allergen vaccines have acknowledged the importance of controlling individual allergens in the vaccines, but the principle is gaining more acceptance among control authorities and clinicians, both in Europe and in the United States.

Today allergen vaccine manufacturers have access to published purification procedures for most major allergens, and the purified major allergens can be used for the production of antibodies for independent quantification, even in complex mixtures such as allergen vaccines. For this purpose, polyspecific or monospecific polyclonal rabbit antibodies or murine monoclonal antibodies are most often used.

Several immunoelectrophoretic techniques might be applied for the quantitative determination of individual allergens. These techniques are usually referred to as quantitative immunoelectrophoresis (QIE) (20), and they are convenient and reliable for measurements of allergen concentrations relative to an in-house standard. In single radial immunodiffusion (SRID), also known as the Mancini

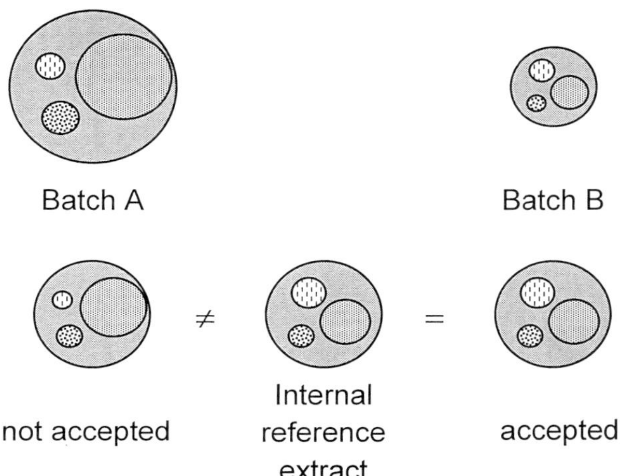

Figure 1 Standardization of allergen vaccines. Complexity of allergen vaccines represented by a model with three major allergens. The area of shaded circles represents the relative potency of individual components. The area of outer circles represents the total allergenic potency of the vaccines. The total allergenic potency of batches A and B may be adjusted by dilution or concentration, but the composition of the vaccines may still vary, accentuating the significance of the measurement of individual components.

technique, the area of a diffusion ring formed by the precipitated antigen in the monospecific antibody-containing gel can be correlated to the amount of antigen applied. In rocket immunoelectrophoresis (RIE) or quantitative CIE the area or the height of the precipitate formed by electrophoresis of the antigen into the agarose gel containing the monospecific antibody is proportional to the antigen concentration. Both SRID and RIE are dependent on monospecific antibodies, whereas CIE is dependent on polyspecific antibodies.

The ELISA (enzyme-linked immunosorbent assay) (22) is a technique in which the allergen is directly bound to a microtiter plate or captured using a monoclonal or polyclonal, monospecific antiserum coated to the plate and subsequently detected using monoclonal or polyclonal, monospecific antiserum. It is very accurate when optimized properly and it offers the possibility of multisample testing and partial automation.

5. Allergen Vaccine Potency

The potency of an allergen vaccine is the total allergen activity (that is, the sum of the contribution to allergenic activity from any individual IgE molecule specific for any epitope on any molecule in the allergen vaccine). It follows that potency measures always will depend on the serum pool or patient panel selected as well as the methodology used. Methods used for the assessment of allergen vaccine potency may be divided into in vitro or in vivo techniques.

The predominant in vitro technique for the estimation of relative allergenic potency is RAST (radioallergosorbent test) inhibition (23) or a related method. A standardized reference vaccine is coupled to a solid phase, which may be paper discs, Sepharose gels, magnetic particles, or others. A serum pool is added, and bound IgE is detected using labeled anti-IgE. In RAST inhibition, the binding of IgE to the solid phase is inhibited by the simultaneous addition of a dilution series of the allergen vaccine subject to testing. The activity is determined relative to the reference vaccine itself. Parallel inhibition curves indicate similar composition, whereas nonparallel curves indicate that the vaccines differ both qualitatively and quantitatively.

The results depend on the patient panel selected. The serum pool is a critical reagent and preferably should contain sera from 20 or more different patients with clinically well-established allergy to the allergen source in question. A large serum pool should be prepared to ensure continuity, and care should be taken when the control serum pool is changed.

Enzyme-linked immunosorbent assay-based inhibition techniques using microtiter plastic trays as solid phase may be applied utilizing the same principles.

Tests of histamine release from washed human leukocytes quantify the histamine liberated from allergic patients' leukocytes upon allergenic stimulation (24). Their dependence on freshly drawn blood samples from a panel of allergic individuals diminishes the practical applicability of these tests in routine extract potency determination.

Direct skin testing of human allergic subjects is the predominant in vivo method for the assessment of allergen vaccine potency (25). For ethical reasons, in vivo testing in humans cannot be used as a routine assay for batch release in production. However, production batches may be compared by suitable in vitro methods to internal reference vaccines for which the in vivo activity has been established. The patient selection criteria are important since all in vivo methods will be dependent on the patient panel.

Skin testing in humans is the method underlying the establishment of biological units of allergen vaccine potency. Several units are in use.

In Europe the potency unit is based on the dose of allergen vaccine resulting in a wheal comparable in size to the wheal produced by a given concentration of histamine. This unit was originally called "histamine equivalent potency," or HEP. The "biological unit," or BU, is also used and is based on the same principle.

In the United States the Food and Drug Administration proposed a unit based on intradermal testing with the allergen vaccine and subsequent measurement of the flare rather than the wheal size. The "intradermal endpoint" is expressed as the number of threefold dilutions producing a summed erythema diameter of 50 mm. The mean value of 15 individuals defines the potency of the allergen extract, which is expressed in ''allergy units,'' AU. More recently the CBER in the United States proposed the ''bioequivalent allergy unit,'' or BAU. The method for assigning BAU is named the $ID_{50}EAL$ method (*i*ntradermal *d*ilution for *50* mm sum of *e*rythema diameters determines bioequivalent *al*lergy units).

D. Allergen Nomenclature

The nomenclature system for allergens officially recommended by the IUIS is applicable to highly purified, well-characterized allergens. The main rules are as follows (5):

1. The first three letters of the genus; space; first letter of the species name; space; an Arabic numeral. For example, Lol p 1 will refer to *Lolium perenne* allergen number one (perennial rye group 1, Rye 1).
2. Structurally homologous (but not necessarily cross-reactive) components from *different* species will be assigned the same numbers (e.g., Der p 1, *Dermatophagoides pteronyssinus* P_1 and Der f 1, *D. farinae* Ag 1).
3. Homologous, immunologically closely related components within the same species (isoallergens) will be designated by two digit suffixes separated by a period (e.g., Amb a 5.01, Ra5A [pI 9.6] and Amb a 5.02, Ra5B[pI 8.5]).

The allergen nomenclature further includes rules for naming allergen-encoding genes, messenger RNAs and cDNAs, and allergenic peptides (5).

III. SPECIFIC ASPECTS OF ALLERGEN VACCINES

A. Pollens

1. Tree Pollens

The pollens from amentiferous trees are the main allergen source in the temperate climate zone in the northern hemisphere during spring months (February through May), and the trees of the Fagales order (alder, birch, hazel, hornbeam, and oak) are the most important tree allergen sources (Table 1) (26).

Aqueous vaccines of alder, birch, hazel, hornbeam, or oak pollen each contain approximately 40 antigens when analyzed by CIE. Only a limited number of these components are allergens (27). Each pollen species contains one predominant allergen existing in several antigenically similar but physicochemically (molecular weight [MW], isoelectric point [pI]) different forms. The majority of

Table 1 Tree Pollen Allergens

Betulaceae			
Alder, *Alnus glutinosa*			
Aln g 1		17	GB:S50892
Aln g 2	Ca-binding protein		EMBL:Y17713
Birch, *Betula verrucosa*			
Bet v 1		17	GB:X15877
Bet v 2	profilin	15	GB:M65179
Bet v 3	calmodulin-like protein		GB:X79267
Bet v 4	Ca-binding protein	8	EMBL:X87153
Hornbeam, *Carpinus betulus*			
Car b 1		17	EMBL:X66932
Hazel, *Corylus avellana*			
Cor a 1		17	EMBL:X70999
Fagaceae			
European chestnut, *Castanea sativa*			
Cas s 1		22	PIR:PC2001
White oak, *Quercus alba*			
Que a 1		17	PIR:D53288
Taxodiaceae			
Japanese cedar, *Cryptomeria japonica*			
Cry j 1		41–45	GB:D34639
Cry j 2		37	GB:D29772
Cupressaceae			
Prickly juniper, *Juniperus oxycedrus*			
Jun o 2	Ca-binding protein, EF-hand	29	GB:AF031471
Mountain cedar, *Juniperus sabinoides*			
Jun s 1		50	
Oleaceae			
Ash, *Fraxinus excelsior*			
Fra e 1	Ole e 1 homologue	20	
Privet, *Ligustrum vulgare*			
Lig v 1	Ole e 1 homologue	20	EMBL:X77787
Olive, *Olea europea*			
Ole e 1		16	GB:S75766
Ole e 2	profilin	15–18	GB:Y12425
Ole e 3	Ca-binding protein	9.2	GB:AF015810
Ole e 4		32	SW:P80741
Ole e 5	superoxide dismutase	16	SW:P80740
Ole e 6		10	GB:U86342
Lilac, *Syringa vulgaris*			
Syr v 1	Ole e 1 homologue	20	

Allergen names are listed according to the official allergen nomenclature (5). Old names may be given in parentheses. Biological function of the allergen is indicated where applicable. The third column lists the molecular weight in kDa as determined by SDS-PAGE. References can be found through the accession numbers provided. The electronic sequence databases are available through the Internet. Abbreviations: GB: GeneBank, http://www.ncbi.nlm.nih.gov/; EMBL: European Molecular Biology Laboratory, http://www.embl-heidelberg.de/; SW: Swis-Prot, http://expasy.hcuge.ch/; PIR: The Protein Information Resource, http://nbrfa.georgetown.edu/pir/.

the proteins in a given vaccine seem to have homologous counterparts in the related species, and only a few, if any, of the extractable proteins are species specific.

The major allergens of alder (Aln g 1), birch (Bet v 1), hazel (Cor a 1), hornbeam (Car b 1), and oak (Que a 1) are very similar, both with respect to physicochemical parameters (mw, pI) and immunochemical properties (28). All of the group 1 tree pollen major allergens except for Que a 1 have been cloned and sequenced, and their amino acid sequences exhibit a high degree of sequence identity (> 70%). A number of isoallergens from each species exhibit distinct amino acid substitutions, and the intraspecies variations seem to be similar to the interspecies sequence differences. The biologic function of the group 1 tree pollen allergens is, however, still unknown.

From IgE absorption experiments it is known that the major allergens contain both common and species-specific antibody binding sites (29). The three-dimensional structure of Bet v 1 substantiates the results obtained from antibody epitope mapping experiments (30). The surface structure seems to harbor at least three conserved surface areas (> = 600 Å^2) where no amino acid substitutions are observed in 63 (5 Aln g 1, 39 Bet v 1, 7 Cor a 1, 12 Car b 1) sequences (Fig. 2). The invariant surface areas readily explain the extensive cross-reaction of patients' IgE with group 1 allergens from various Fagales species.

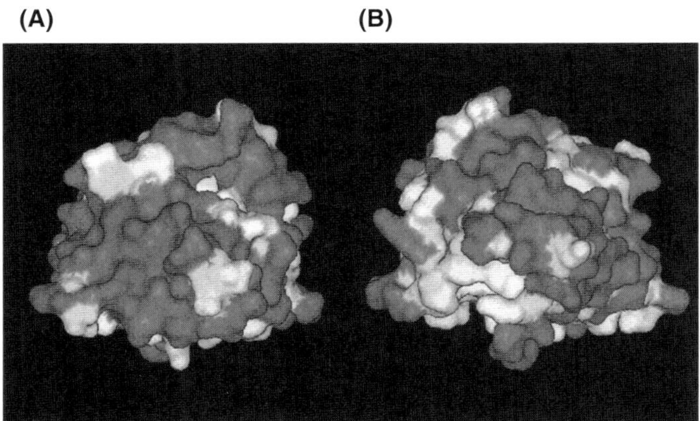

Figure 2 Conserved surface structures on Fagales major allergens. Model of the three-dimensional structure of the major birch allergen, Bet v 1 (30). Darkest shading highlights amino acids conserved (95% identity) among 63 tree pollen group 1 sequences (5 Aln g 1, 39 Bet v 1, 7 Cor a 1, 12 Car b 1). Surface areas large enough to harbor cross-reactive IgE binding epitopes are evident. White areas are variable. Medium-shaded structures represent backbone atoms (CONH) of the amino acid chain conserved in all amino acids. A and B represent the molecule viewed from different angles.

Allergens homologous to the Fagales group 1 allergens have been found in several fruits including apple, pear, and cherry, as well as hazelnut. Conserved surface structures between these molecules may explain the pollen inhalant allergy-related "oral allergy syndrome" (Fig. 3). Furthermore, a more distant homology has been found to a group of pathogenesis-related proteins described in a number of plant species including pea, carrot, and celery.

Birch profilin, Bet v 2, is a second birch allergen that has been described in detail (31). Homologous profilins are likely to exist in all plant species and although they are minor allergens, profilins might account for some cross-reactivity to other pollens and plant foods. Two other birch allergens have been described. Bet v 3 is homologous to calmodulin and other proteins with an affinity for Ca^{2+} ions. Bet v 4 is an allergen with EF-hand calcium binding domains. Similar proteins have been found in several other allergenic source materials.

A number of other tree species, particularly Japanese cedar (32), pecan, walnut, olive (33), and cypress, are important allergen sources in several habitats throughout the world, and the major allergens from Japanese cedar (Cry j 1 and 2) and olive (Ole e 1-6) have been characterized thoroughly. Ole e 2 is a profilin, and Ole e 5 is a superoxide dismutase. Homologous counterparts to the major olive allergen, Ole e 1, have been described in the related species ash (*Fraxinus excelsior*), privet (*Ligustrum vulgare*), and lilac (*Syringa vulgaris*) (34).

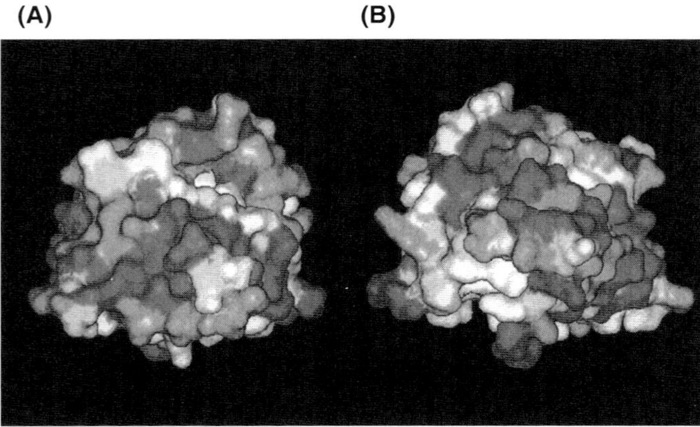

Figure 3 Surface structures conserved between Fagales major allergens and the major allergen from apple, Mal d 1. Depicted on the model of the three-dimensional structure of Bet v 1 are surface-exposed amino acids conserved between the Fagales major allergens and Mal d 1 (dark-shaded), and amino acids conserved among the Fagales major allergens, but not Mal d 1 (medium-gray). Most of the surface structures conserved among the Fagales major allergens are clearly different on the apple allergen. However, some conserved structures exist and provide a molecular basis for the clinical cross-reactivity observed between tree pollen allergy and allergy to ingested fruits, such as apple. (A) and (B) represent the molecule viewed from different angles.

2. Weed Pollens

Pollens originating from weeds are common allergen sources throughout the world (Table 2). Two of the most abundant allergen sources in North America are short and giant ragweed. Mugwort pollen is one of the main allergen sources worldwide. Pollen allergens from different species of *Parietaria* are common in the Mediterranean area.

An aqueous vaccine of short ragweed pollen contains approximately 50 antigens and proteins, of which a substantial number, approximately 20, can be regarded as allergens (35). A number of ragweed allergens have been sequenced either by cDNA cloning or by conventional techniques. The predominant allergen, Amb a 1, has four isoallergens, which exhibit differences with respect to their physicochemical parameters (MW, pI) and amino acid sequence (36). Amb a 2 is homologous to Amb a 1, but the Amb a 2 designation is maintained for historical reasons. The biologic function of Amb a 1 is not known. However, the Amb a 1 sequences are homologous to pectate lyase and to Cry j 1 from Japanese cedar, *Cryptomeria japonica*. Ambrosia group 5, a small 5 kDa minor allergen, has been thoroughly studied, and the three-dimensional structure has been determined by nuclear magnetic resonance (NMR) (37). Amb a 6 is a lipid transfer protein homologous to lipid transfer proteins, which are also described as allergens in other species.

Mugwort pollen contains more than 20 extractable antigens and proteins of which 15 seem to be allergens (38). Art v 1 is a 47 kDa major allergen, and Art v 2 and Art v 3 exist in different isoforms. Both Art v 2 and Art v 3 are glycoproteins containing relatively high amounts of carbohydrate moieties.

Allergy to *Parietaria* pollens is an important problem in the Mediterranean area (39). *Parietaria* pollens contain approximately 30 antigens and proteins of which nine seem to be allergens. The gene encoding the major allergen, Par j 1, from *Parietaria judaica* has been cloned and sequenced. Par j 1 has homology to unspecific lipid transport proteins from several sources, including ragweed and grasses.

3. Grass Pollens

The grasses constitute a large family of closely related genera (Table 3). In fact, the grasses constitute approximately 20% of the earth's vegetation, and during the pollination season their pollens are common in all habitats throughout the world. Grass pollens are responsible for between 10% and 30% of all IgE-mediated allergies in the world.

The allergenic composition of pollen vaccines from different grass species reveals a high degree of immunochemical similarity explaining the fact that sensitivity to pollen from only one grass species has never been observed. Thus, grass pollen-allergic individuals will respond to components from several grasses, including grasses to which they have never been exposed (40).

Table 2 Weed Pollen Allergens

Asteraceae			
Short ragweed, *Ambrosia artemisiifolia*			
Amb a 1.01	(antigen E)	38	GB:M80558
Amb a 1.02	(antigen E)	38	GB:M80559
Amb a 1.03	(antigen E)	38	GB:M80560
Amb a 1.04	(antigen E)	38	GB:M80562
Amb a 2	(antigen K)	38	GB:M80561
Amb a 3	(Ra3)	11	PIR:A00313
Amb a 5	(Ra5)	5	GB:M84987
Amb a 6	(Ra6)	10	GB:U89793
Amb a 7	(Ra7)	12	
Giant ragweed, *Ambrosia trifida*			
Amb t 5	(Ra5G)	4.4	GB:X56279
Western ragweed, *Ambrosia psilostachya*			
Amb p 5			GB:L24465
Mugwort, *Artemisia vulgaris*			
Art v 1		27–29	
Art v 2		35	PIR:A38624
Art v 3			
Sunflower, *Helianthus annuus*			
Hel a 1		34	
Hel a 2	profilin	15.7	
Euphorbiaceae			
Annual mercury, *Mercurialis annua*			
Mer a 1	profilin		EMBL:Y13271
Urticaceae			
Parietaria judaica			
Par j 1			SW:P43217
Parietaria officinalis			
Par o 1			PIR:A53252

Allergen names are listed according to the official allergen nomenclature (5). Old names may be given in parentheses. Biological function of the allergen is indicated where applicable. The third column lists the molecular weight in kDa as determined by SDS-PAGE. References can be found through the accession numbers provided. The electronic sequence databases are available through the Internet. Abbreviations: GB: GeneBank, http://www.ncbi.nlm.nih.gov/; EMBL: European Molecular Biology Laboratory, http://www.embl-heidelberg.de/; SW: Swis-Prot, http://expasy.hcuge.ch/; PIR: The Protein Information Resource, http://nbrfa.georgetown.edu/pir/.

Table 3 Grass Pollen Allergens

Poaceae			
Bent grass, *Agrostis alba*			
Agr a 1		30	PIR:E37396
Sweet verna, *Anthoxanthum odoratum*			
Ant o 1		30	PIR:G37396
Bermuda grass, *Cynodon dactylon*			
Cyn d 1		32	GB:S83343
Cyn d 7	Ca-binding protein		GB:X91256
Cyn d 12	profilin	14	GB:Y08389
Orchard grass, *Dactylis glomerata*			
Dac g 1	(AgDg1)	32	
Dac g 2		11	GB:S45354
Dac g 3			GB:U25343
Dac g 5		31	
Festuca elatior			
Fes e 1			PIR:C37396
Velvet grass, *Holcus lanatus*			
Hol 1 1		34	GB:Z68893
Hol 1 5		30	GB:Z97874
Perennial rye grass, *Lolium perenne*			
Lol p 1		27	GB:M57474
Lol p 2		11	SW:P14947
Lol p 3		11	SW:P14948
Lol p 4		57	PIR:A60737
Lol p 5	(Lol p IX, Lol p Ib)	31/35	GB:M59163
Lol p 10	cytochrome c	12	
Lol p 11	trypsin inhibitor	18	PIR:A54002
Canary grass, *Phalaris aquatica*			
Pha a 1		34	GB:S80654
Pha a 5			SW:P56164
Timothy grass, *Phleum pratense*			
Phl p 1		27	EMBL:X78813
Phl p 2			EMBL:X75925
Phl p 5	(Ag25)	32	GB:X74735
Phl p 6	(Ag19)		GB:Z27082
Phl p 7	Ca-binding protein		EMBL:Y17835
Phl p 12	profilin		GB:X77583
Kentucky bluegrass, *Poa pratensis*			
Poa p 1		33	PIR:A60372
Poa p 5	(Poa p IX)	31/34	SW:P22284
Cultivated rye, *Secale cereale*			
Sec c 5		30	PIR:S38292
	Alpha-amylase inhibitor		GB:167820
Johnson grass, *Sorghum halepense*			
Sor h 1		30	

Allergen names are listed according to the official allergen nomenclature (5). Old names may be given in parentheses. Biological function of the allergen is indicated where applicable. The third column lists the molecular weight in kDa as determined by SDS-PAGE. References can be found through the accession numbers provided. The electronic sequence databases are available through the Internet. Abbreviations: GB: GeneBank, http://www.ncbi.nlm.nih.gov/; EMBL: European Molecular Biology Laboratory, http://www.embl-heidelberg.de/; SW: Swis-Prot, http://expasy.hcuge.ch/; PIR: The Protein Information Resource, http://nbrfa.georgetown.edu/pir/.

The immunochemical similarities are primarily manifested within the grass subfamilies (41). Temperate grasses reveal similar immunochemical properties. Thus, allergens from ryegrass (*L. perenne*), timothy grass (*P. pratense*), Kentucky bluegrass (*Poa pratensis*), and orchard grass (*Dactylis glomerata*) possess similar allergenic characteristics. Despite a high degree of immunochemical similarity, grasses from other subfamilies exhibit measurable differences compared to the temperate grasses (40,42). Hence, Bermuda grass (*Cynodon dactylon*), Bahia grass (*Paspalum notatum*), and Johnson grass (*Sorghum halepense*), all of which are common grasses in subtropical regions of the world, should be regarded as separate allergenic sources and diagnosed separately.

An aqueous vaccine of grass pollen typically contains 30 to 40 components of which 5 to 10 are allergens (40). Historically, the most important grass allergens are classified into groups numbered from 1 to 6 (5). Grass pollen profilin has been designated group 12. Allergens from different grass species, but from the same allergen group, generally exhibit similar physicochemical and immunochemical characteristics. All grass allergens investigated have been shown to contain isoallergens exhibiting closely related immunochemical properties but with minor variations in sequence, molecular weight, or pI.

With respect to IgE-binding prevalence (as observed in SDS-PAGE IgE immunoblotting or CRIE), the two most important allergen groups of grass pollens are the group 1 and the group 5 allergens. The group 1 allergens seem to be present in all grass species studied so far, whereas the group 5 allergens have only been found in the temperate grasses (40).

Several grass pollen allergens have been studied intensively and homologies of cDNA sequences confirm the high degree of similarity between the various allergen groups from different species. The function of the 30 kDa grass group 1 allergens is unknown, but these allergens are homologous to beta-expansin. The 11 kDa group 2 and 3 allergens are homologous to group 1, but they are smaller. The biological function of grass group 4 allergens is unknown. The 29 kDa Phl p 5 is claimed to have RNase activity (43), and Phl p 6 (12 kDa) has homology to group 5. Group 7 allergens are calcium-binding proteins with EF-hand motifs also found in other allergenic source materials. The group 9 designation has been abandoned because these proteins are identical to group 5. Grass group 10 allergens are cytochrome c proteins, and the 18 kDa Lol p 11 is homologous to soybean trypsin inhibitor. Group 12 is profilin, a minor allergen likely to be present in all plants.

B. Acarids

Several genera of mites are found in the environment, and a number of these have been shown to cause allergy (Table 4). The most important species are the domestic mites belonging to the genus *Dermatophagoides* and some species

Table 4 Mite Allergens

Domestic mite, *Dermatophagoides pteronyssinus*			
Der p 1	(antigen P1) cysteine protease	25	GB:U11695
Der p 2		14	SW:P49278
Der p 3	serine protease, trypsin family	28/30	GB:U11719
Der p 4	alpha-amylase	60	SW:P49274
Der p 5		14	GB:S76337
Der p 6	serine protease, chymotrypsin-like	25	SW:P49277
Der p 7		22–28	GB:S80655
Der p 8	glutathione transferase		GB:S75286
Der p 9	collagenolytic serine protease	24	GB:1911659
Der p 10	tropomyosin		GB:Y14906
Domestic mite, *Dermatophagoides microceras*			
Der m 1		25	SW:P16312
Domestic mite, *Dermatophagoides farinae*			
Der f 1	cysteine protease	25	GB:X65196
Der f 2		14	SW:Q00855
Der f 3	serine protease, trypsin family	30	GB:D63858
Der f 6	serine protease, chymotrypsin-like		SW:P49276
Der f 7			SW:Q26456
Der f 10	tropomyosin		SW:Q23939
Euroglyphus maynei			
Eur m 1	cysteine protease		GB:X60073
Tyrophagus putrescentiae			
Tyr p 2			EMBL:Y12690
Lepidoglyphus destructor			
Lep d 2 (Lep d 1)		15	GB:X81399
Blomia tropicalis			
Blo t 1		11–13	
Blo t 5		14	GB:U27702
Blo t 12			GB:U27479
	Fatty acid binding protein		GB:U58106
Acarus siro			
	Fatty acid binding protein		EMBL:AJ006774

Allergen names are listed according to the official allergen nomenclature (5). Old names may be given in parentheses. Biological function of the allergen is indicated where applicable. The third column lists the molecular weight in kDa as determined by SDS-PAGE. References can be found through the accession numbers provided. The electronic sequence databases are available through the Internet. Abbreviations: GB: GeneBank, http://www.ncbi.nlm.nih.gov/; EMBL: European Molecular Biology Laboratory, http://www.embl-heidelberg.de/; SW: Swis-Prot, http://expasy.hcuge.ch/; PIR: The Protein Information Resource, http://nbrfa.georgetown.edu/pir/.

of mites that are primarily found in stored cereals and grain (i.e., storage mites).

1. Domestic Mites

Three species are considered the most important allergen sources: *Dermatophagoides pteronyssinus*, *D. farinae*, and *D. microceras* (44). When analyzed by CIE, vaccines of domestic mites contain more than 50 different antigenic molecules. Thirteen of these antigens have been shown to be allergens (45). The two major allergen groups, 1 and 2, are immunologically cross-reactive between species (46,47). Der p 1, a cysteine protease secreted into the digestive tract of the mite, was the first major allergen to be studied by gene cloning methodology. Mite group 1 allergens are found in several mite species other than *Dermatophagoides*, including *Euroglyphus maynei*. The group 2 allergens are likewise structural homologues that are primarily associated with the somatic parts of the mites, but their biological function is unknown. Der p 2 and Der f 2 are immunologically cross-reactive but also exhibit some species-specific determinants for antibody binding and for reaction with CD4+ human T-cell clones. The three-dimensional structure of Der f 2 has been resolved by NMR (48) but its biological function remains unknown. Interestingly, group 2 mite allergens show 50% homology to proteins secreted from canine epidermis and bovine mammary glands, but the clinical significance of this homology has not been investigated. Group 1 and 2 allergens, depending on patient selection criteria, will react with IgE from 60–100% of mite-sensitive allergic patients (46).

Domestic mite group 3 is trypsin (25 kDa), which is homologous to domestic mite group 6, which is 30 kDa chymotrypsin. Trypsin and chymotrypsin have been found in several other species of mammalian or invertebrate origin. Der p 4 is amylase (56 kDa), whereas the function of 13 kDa Der p 5 and 22 kDa group 7 are unknown. Der p 8 is glutathione transferase, and Der p 9 is a 28 kDa serine protease with homology to groups 3 and 6. Interestingly, domestic mite group 10 is 33 kDa tropomyosin, which may be involved in cross-reactivity to shrimp and other crustaceans. Tropomyosin is a major allergen found in several species of shrimp as well as in the American cockroach, *Periplaneta americana*.

2. Storage Mites and Others

The allergenicity of storage mites is well established (49). Allergen characterization has primarily focused on the species *Lepidoglyphus destructor*, *Tyrophagus putrescentiae*, *Glycyphagus domesticus*, and *Acarus siro*, all of which can be found in stored grain as well as in house dust (50). Major allergens Lep d 2 (formerly Lep d 1) from *L. destructor* and Tyr p 2 from *T. putrescentiae* have been cloned and sequenced and are homologous to domestic mite group 2 allergens. It is likely that standardized vaccines of storage mites will become important in the future as the knowledge on specific sensitization is extended.

Several other species of mites (e.g., *Blomia tropicalis*) have been shown to elicit IgE-responses (51). Some allergens of *Blomia* have been characterized, including an allergen homologous to fatty acid binding proteins characterized in several mammalian species as well as in the storage mite *A. siro*. Blo t 5 is homologous to domestic mite group 5.

C. Animal Emanations

1. Cat

Cat (*Felis domesticus*) allergen vaccines are generally prepared from hair that has been cut close (approximately 1 mm) to the skin surface without severing the skin tissue (Table 5). Several molecules in cat vaccines have been shown to be allergenic including serum albumin (52). The most important allergen clinically, Fel d 1, is a heterotetramer composed of two noncovalently linked disulphide-linked heterodimers of chain 1 and chain 2 (53). Fel d 1 belongs to the uteroglobin family and is secreted into the saliva and the lachrymal fluid. The allergen is found in high concentration in cat hair, where the cat has probably deposited it by licking itself. The molecule has been used to devise antibody-based assays for environmental exposure to cat allergen (54). The nucleotide sequence of the allergen has been determined, and it has been demonstrated that Fel d 1 has epitopes that specifically interact with T-cells from allergic patients (55). Several other molecules in cat vaccine are important elicitors of specific T-cell responses (55). It is conceivable that a good cat vaccine should contain several allergen molecules in addition to Fel d 1 and that the vaccine should be standardized with respect to concentration of Fel d 1. Cat albumin serves as a marker for the content of serum proteins.

2. Dog

Vaccines of dog (*C. familiaris*) hair and dander contain several allergens (56). The clinically most important allergen, Can f 1, is a protein with an apparent molecular weight of 25 kDa by SDS-PAGE. By means of specific antibody-based assays, Can f 1 has been observed to occur at varying concentrations in hair from different individuals within a single dog breed, as well as from one breed to the other (57). The major allergens, Can f 1 and Can f 2, are salivary lipocalin proteins found in high concentration in saliva. Can f 1 has been used as a marker allergen for environmental dog exposure (58). Serum albumin is also an important allergen as judged by CRIE and immunoblotting. There has been some controversy as to whether there are true breed-specific allergens. However, all dog breeds belong to the same species, so it is likely that differences observed among vaccines of different breeds are quantitative rather than qualitative. Until this matter has been thoroughly analyzed, the implications are that a balanced allergenic vaccine of dog should be prepared from a mixture of several breeds.

Table 5 Mammalian Allergens

Cat, *Felis domesticus*			
Fel d 1	uteroglobulin	38	
Fel d 1, Chain 1		8	SW:P30438
Fel d 1, Chain 2		10	SW:P30440
Dog, *Canis familiaris*			
Can f 1	lipocalin	25	GB:AF027177
Can f 2	lipocalin	27	GB:AF027178
Can f 3	albumin	69	GB:S72946
Cow's dander, *Bos domesticus* (see also cow's milk)			
Bos d 1	(Ag1)	25	
Bos d 2	(Ag3, BDA20) Lipocalin	20	SW:Q28133
Bos d 3	(AgIII)	22	
	(BDA11) EF-hand calcium binding protein		SW:Q28050
Horse, *Equus caballus*			
Equ c 1	lipocalin	20	GB:U70823
Equ c 2	lipocalin		SW:P81216
Mouse, *Mus musculus*			
Mus m 1	(MUP) Prealbumin	19	
Mus m 2		16	
	DEC-205	205	GB:1174278
	uteroglobulin		GB:AF008595
Rat, *Rattus norvegicus*			
Rat n 1	prealbumin	21	GB:K03251
Rat n 2	lipocalin	19	
Rat n 3		200	
Guinea pig, *Cavia porcellus*			
Cav p 1	(Ag2)	25	
Cav p 2	(Ag3)	25	
Cav p 3		50	
Rabbit, *Oryctolagus cuniculus*			
Ory c 1		17	

Allergen names are listed according to the official allergen nomenclature (5). Old names may be given in parentheses. Biological function of the allergen is indicated where applicable. The third column lists the molecular weight in kDa as determined by SDS-PAGE. References can be found through the accession numbers provided. The electronic sequence databases are available through the Internet. Abbreviations: GB: GeneBank, http://www.ncbi.nlm.nih.gov/; EMBL: European Molecular Biology Laboratory, http://www.embl-heidelberg.de/; SW: Swis-Prot, http://expasy.hcuge.ch/; PIR: The Protein Information Resource, http://nbrfa.georgetown.edu/pir/.

3. Cow and Horse

Inhalant allergy to horse and to cow is considered occupational. A study of cow hair and dander vaccine identified 18 individual proteins of which 4 were allergens (59). The major allergen, Bos d 2, is a member of the lipocalin family. A calcium ion binding minor allergen with the EF-hand motif has been characterized.

Vaccines of horse hair and dander contain three major allergens, termed Equ c 1, 2, and 3, respectively (60). Equ c 1 and Equ c 2 are members of the lipocalin family and are secreted into saliva and urine.

4. Rodents

Rodents cause occupational allergy to veterinarians and technicians and others exposed to the animals in their daily work. Several species are kept as pets, and therefore nonprofessionals may develop rodent allergy. Prevalence of allergy in persons exposed to rodents in their work has been shown to be up to 13% by skin prick test and 38% by in vitro IgE measurements (61). Rodents have permanent proteinuria and often spray their urine rather than just depositing it. Several of the urinary proteins are subsequently inhaled by humans and can elicit allergic immune responses.

From the mouse, *Mus musculus*, two major allergens have been characterized (62): Mus m 1, which is a prealbumin, has been found in urine as well as in hair follicles. The molecule also has been found in dust obtained from laboratory animal facilities. Mus m 2 is a glycoprotein, which has been shown to reside in hair follicles and on the skin surface. Because both allergens are found in the pelt, it is likely that fur vaccines will provide the best diagnostic tool. Recently a uteroglobulin homologous to Fel d 1 has been described, which is secreted from the salivary glands (63).

The major allergen derived from the rat (*Rattus norvegicus*) is Rat n 1 (64), a thyroid hormone-binding prealbumin (transthyretin) found in the liver and secreted into the urine. The allergen is a homotetramer as determined by X-ray crystallography (65). Another allergen, Rat n 3, with a molecular weight of 200 kDa and of unknown origin has been described. Urinary vaccines are more reliable than epithelial vaccines for skin test and in vitro IgE measurements (66). There appear to be no strain-specific allergens in inbred rats.

Two major allergens have been found in the guinea pig (*Cavia porcellus*), and they are present in urine as well as pelt (67). Both Cav p 1 (Ag 2) and Cav p 2 (Ag 3) are proteins with a molecular weight of approximately 25 kDa. A third urinary allergen (U2) has an apparent molecular weight of 50 to 75 kDa

The major allergen from the rabbit (*Oryctolagus cuniculus*), Ory c 1, is a constituent of saliva and fur but it is present in urine only in low concentrations (68).

Other rodents kept as pets, such as gerbils and hamsters, are likely to have allergens related to those mentioned previously.

D. Insects

1. Stinging Insects

The insects responsible for sting allergy are Hymenoptera, including Vespidae (wasps and hornets), Apidae (honeybees and bumblebees), and Formicidae (fire ants and harvester ants) (Table 6). Commercial wasp and bee allergen vaccines are prepared from pure venom or from whole venom sacs. Ant vaccines are generally whole body vaccines.

The venoms contain a wide array of biogenic amines, enzymes, and small peptides. The clinically important allergens are primarily enzymes (69), but a few of the peptide components have been shown to be allergenic as well (70). The allergens in vespids and bees include group 1 (phospholipases), group 2 (hyaluronidases), group 3 (bee venom melittin), group 4 (trypsin-like serine proteases), and group 5 (vespid antigen 5; unknown function). The majority of allergens from insect venoms have been purified and characterized, and their genes have been cloned. The tertiary structure of Api m 1 from honeybee venom has been determined by x-ray crystallography (71,72).

Fire ants of the genus *Solenopsis* constitute an important allergy problem in the United States and Asia (73). Little or no immunologic cross-reactivity has been observed between allergens from the three taxonomic groups (vespids, bees, and ants) or even within the single allergen group. Specific allergy vaccination is performed with vaccines of all three groups of insects.

2. Insect Inhalant Allergens

Several orders of insects, including Lepidoptera (moths and butterflies), Diptera (mosquitoes, midges, and flies), and Dictyoptera (cockroaches and termites) contain species that cause inhalant allergy (74). Some have local importance, but several species of cockroaches and midges have been shown to cause worldwide allergy. Vaccines of the chironomid midge (*Chironomus thummi thummi*) contain the insect's hemoglobin as a major constituent; this molecule is the major allergen Chi t 1. The molecule has been purified, and its three-dimensional structure has been determined (75). Other allergenic components are found in chironomid vaccines, but their characteristics are not known in detail.

Several cockroaches, such as the American (*Periplaneta americana*) and the German (*Blattella germanica*), are widespread indoor pests. Whole-body vaccines of the two species contain up to 56 antigens, and up to 18 allergenic molecules have been demonstrated, depending on analysis and patient selection criteria (76). Two important allergens have been purified from *B. germanica* (i.e., Bla g 1 and Bla g 2) and both are constituents of house dust (77). From DNA sequencing studies, homologies have been found between several cockroach allergens and proteins of known function. Bla g 2 is a 36 kDa aspartic protease,

Bla g 4 is a 21 kDa calycin belonging to the lipocalin family, Bla g 5 is glutathione transferase, and Bla g 6 is troponin C. Furthermore, a 90 kDa allergen has been characterized. An important allergen, Per a 1, has been purified from *P. americana* and is contained in dust obtained from cockroach-infested environments (78). Per a 3 is a larvae storage protein and Per a 7 is tropomyosin, which is also found in several species of shrimp, as well as in domestic mites. Allergenic activity has been found in vaccines of whole bodies, as well as cast skins, fecal pellets, and egg capsules (79).

3. Biting Insects

Insects belonging to Reduviidae, the kissing bugs, are known to cause allergic reactions. Several species of kissing bugs from the genus *Triatoma* have been investigated. Their allergens are derived primarily from the salivary glands, and allergic sensitization to a large extent is species-specific (80,81). Other biting insects, including fleas, also cause allergic reactions (82). Extracts should probably be obtained from salivary glands to achieve sufficient potency, but it is questionable if the clinical importance of allergy to biting insects justifies the resource-consuming work involved.

E. Fungi

Several fungal species, usually molds, cause allergic reactions (83) (Table 7). Most of the molds of interest in allergy belong to the taxonomic group, ''Fungi Imperfectii,'' usually asexual stages of Ascomycetes, with *Alternaria*, *Cladosporium*, and *Aspergillus* spp. as the most common and best-described allergen sources. However, *Basidiomycetes* species (i.e., mushrooms and puffballs) and yeast-like *Candida albicans* have also been described as important allergen sources.

Alternaria and *Cladosporium* spp. are common in the outdoor environment all over the world, with *Alternaria* predominating in dry, warm climates and *Cladosporium* in the temperate climate zones. Airborne spores and mycelial debris of *Alternaria* and *Cladosporium* are present during spring, summer, and especially autumn because of the degradation of leaves and other organic material. Indoor environments contain other mold species, such as *Aspergillus* and *Penicillium* spp., which have less characteristic seasonal changes.

Patients (often children) suffering from mold allergy usually experience asthma because the small-sized fungal debris (particularly spores) are able to penetrate all the way to the lungs. Immunotherapy of mold-allergic patients has demonstrable efficacy, but it generally is hindered by the problems of preparing mold vaccines with well-defined composition and allergenic potency.

Apart from the problems concerning source materials and cultivation techniques, different extraction conditions introduce vaccine variability. The rather

Table 6 Insect Allergens

1. **Hymenoptera**			
Bees, Apoidea			
Honey bee, *Apis mellifera*			
Api m 1	phospholipase A2	16	GB:X16709
Api m 2	hyaluronidase	44	GB:L10710
Api m 4	melittin	3	GB:X02007
Bumblebee, *Bombus pennsylvanicus*			
Bom p 1	phospholipase	16	PIR:B56338
Bom p 4	serine protease		PIR:A56338
Wasps, Vespoidea			
White face hornet, *Dolichovespula maculata*			
Dol m 1	phospholipase A1	35	GB:X66869
Dol m 2	hyaluronidase	44	GB:L34548
Dol m 5	antigen 5	23	GB:J03601
Yellow hornet, *Dolichovespula arenaria*			
Dol a 5	antigen 5	23	GB:M98859
Wasp, *Polistes annularies*			
Pol a 1	phospholipase A1	35	
Pol a 2	hyaluronidase	44	
Pol a 5	antigen 5	23	GB:M98857
Mediterranean paper wasp, *Polistes dominulus*			
Pol d 4	serine protease	32–34	
Wasp, *Polistes exclamans*			
Pol e 1	phospholipase A1	34	
Pol e 5	antigen 5	23	SW:P35759
Wasp, *Polistes fuscatus*			
Pol f 5	antigen 5	23	SW:P35780
Wasp, *Polistes metricus*			
Pol m 5	antigen 5	23	
European hornet, *Vespa crabo*			
Vesp c 1	phospholipase	34	
Vesp c 5	antigen 5	23	SW:P35781
Yellowjacket, *Vespula flavopilosa*			
Ves f 5	antigen 5	23	SW:P35783
Yellowjacket, *Vespula germanica*			
Ves g 5	antigen 5	23	SW:P35784
Yellowjacket, *Vespula maculifrons*			
Ves m 1	phospholipase A1	33.5	SW:P51528
Ves m 2	hyaluronidase	44	
Ves m 5	antigen 5	23	SW:P35760
Yellowjacket, *Vespula pennsylvanica*			
Ves p 5	antigen 5	23	SW:P35785
Yellowjacket, *Vespula squamosa*			
Ves s 5	antigen 5	23	SW:P35786
Wasp, *Vespula vidua*			
Ves vi 5	antigen 5	23	SW:P35787
Yellowjacket, *Vespula vulgaris*			
Ves v 1	phospholipase A1	35	GB:L43561

Table 6 Continued

Ves v 2	hyaluronidase	44	GB:L43562
Ves v 5	antigen 5	23	GB:M98858
Ants, Formicoidea			
Australian jumper ant, *Myrmecia pilosula*			
Myr p 1			GB:X70256
Myr p 2			GB:S81785
Red imported fire ant, *Solenopsis invicta*			
Sol i 1			GB:1336809
Sol i 2		13	SW:L09560
Sol i 3		24	SW:P35778
Sol i 4		13	SW:P35777
Fire ant, *Solenopsis richteri*			
Sol r 2			SW:P35776
Sol r 3			SW:P35779
2. **Dictyoptera**			
German cockroach, *Blattella germanica*			
Bla g 1		20–25	
Bla g 2	aspartic protease	36	GB:U28863
Bla g 4	calycin	21	GB:U40767
Bla g 5	glutathione transferase	22	GB:U92412
Bla g 6	troponin C	27	
	Bd90k	90	GB:L47595
American cockroach, *Periplaneta americana*			
Per a 1	(Cr-PII)	20–25	
Per a 3	(Cr-PI)	72–78	GB:L40818
Per a 7	tropomyosin	37	
3. **Diptera**			
Midges, *Chironomus thummi thummi*			
Chi t 1.01	hemoglobin, component III	16	SW:P02229
Chi t 1.02	hemoglobin, component IV	16	SW:P02230
Chi t 2.0101	hemoglobin, component I	16	SW:P02221
Chi t 2.0102	hemoglobin, component IA	16	SW:P02221
Chi t 3	hemoglobin, component II-beta	16	SW:P02222
Chi t 4	hemoglobin, component IIIA	16	SW:P02231
Chi t 5	hemoglobin, component VI	16	SW:P02224
Chi t 6.01	hemoglobin, component VIIA	16	SW:P02226
Chi t 6.02	hemoglobin, component IX	16	SW:P02223
Chi t 7	hemoglobin, component VIIB	16	SW:P02225
Chi t 8	hemoglobin, component VIII	16	SW:P02227
Chi t 9	hemoglobin, component X	16	SW:P02228

Allergen names are listed according to the official allergen nomenclature (5). Old names may be given in parentheses. Biological function of the allergen is indicated where applicable. The third column lists the molecular weight in kDa as determined by SDS-PAGE. References can be found through the accession numbers provided. The electronic sequence databases are available through the Internet. Abbreviations: GB: GeneBank, http://www.ncbi.nlm.nih.gov/; EMBL: European Molecular Biology Laboratory, http://www.embl-heidelberg.de/; SW: Swis-Prot, http://expasy.hcuge.ch/; PIR: The Protein Information Resource, http://nbrfa.georgetown.edu/pir/.

Table 7 Fungal Allergens

Alternaria alternata			
Alt a 1		28	GB:U62097
Alt a 2		25	
Alt a 3	heat shock protein 70		GB:U87807
Alt a 6	60S acidic ribosomal protein P2	11	EMBL:X78222
Alt a 7		22	EMBL:X78225
Alt a 10	aldehyde dehydrogenase (NAD+)	53	EMBL:X78227
Alt a 12	60S acidic ribosomal protein P1		GB:U87806
	ribosomal protein P1		EMBL:X84216
	proteinsulfidisomerase		EMBL:X84217
Aspergillus fumigatus			
Asp f 1		18	GB:S39330
Asp f 2		37	GB:U56938
Asp f 3	peroxisomal-like protein	19	GB:U20722
Asp f 4		30	EMBL:AJ001732
Asp f 5	metalloprotease	42	EMBL:Z30424
Asp f 6	manganese superoxide dismutase	26.5	GB:U53561
Asp f 7		12	GB:AJ223315
Asp f 8	ribosomal protein P2	11	
Asp f 9		34	EMBL:AJ223327
Asp f 10	aspartic protease, aspergillopepsin	34	EMBL:X85092
Asp f 11	peptidyl-prolyl isomerase	24	
Asp f 12	heat shock protein P90	90	
Asp f 13		16	EMBL:AJ002026
Aspergillus niger			
Asp n 14	beta-xylosidase	85	EMBL:Z84377
Aspergillus oryzae			
Asp o 21	TAKA-amylase A	53	EMBL:M33218
Asp o 13	alkaline serine protease	34	EMBL:X17561
Candida albicans			
Cand a 1	alcohol dehydrogenase	40	EMBL:X81694
Candida boidinii			
Cand b 2	peroxisomal membrane protein	20	GB:J04984
Cladosporium herbarum			
Cla h 1		13	
Cla h 2		19	
Cla h 3	aldehyde dehydrogenase	53	GB:X78228
Cla h 4	60S acidic ribosomal protein P2	11	GB:X78223
Cla h 5		22	GB:X78224
Cla h 6	enolase	46	GB:X78226
Cla h 12	60S acidic ribosomal protein P1	12	GB:X85180
Malassezia furfur			
Mal f 1			EMBL:X96486
Mal f 2	(MF1) peroxisomal membrane protein	21	GB:AB011804
Mal f 3	(MF2) peroxisomal membrane protein	20	GB:AB011805
Mal f 4		35	
Penicillium citrinum			
	Heat shock protein 70		GB:U64207

Table 7 Continued

Penicillium notatum		
(68 kDa)	68	GB:S77837
Rhizopus nigricans		
(Rhiz IIIb)	12	
(Rhiz VIb)	14	
Saccharomyces cerevisiae		
(40 kDa) alcohol dehydrogenase	37	
(48 kDa) enolase	47	
Trichophyton tonsurans		
Tri t 1	30	SW:P80514

Allergen names are listed according to the official allergen nomenclature (5). Old names may be given in parentheses. Biological function of the allergen is indicated where applicable. The third column lists the molecular weight in kDa as determined by SDS-PAGE. References can be found through the accession numbers provided. The electronic sequence databases are available through the Internet. Abbreviations: GB: GeneBank, http://www.ncbi.nlm.nih.gov/; EMBL: European Molecular Biology Laboratory, http://www.embl-heidelberg.de/; SW: Swis-Prot, http://expasy.hcuge.ch/; PIR: The Protein Information Resource, http://nbrfa.georgetown.edu/pir/.

special composition of the mold raw material (mycelium with spores versus pure spores), the low amount of protein, the high amount of carbohydrates, and the common presence of active proteolytic enzymes, all cause extraction of mold raw material to be very troublesome. For this reason a high level of standardization is important to ensure the presence of all important allergens (84).

Moreover, the fungal taxonomy and the identification of molds and strains of molds can be very complicated (85). Sometimes obsolete names, omitted by the taxonomists, are still used for some important commercial preparations. For example, *Hormodendrum* must now be named *Cladosporium*, *Alternaria tenuis* is now *Alternaria alternata*, and *Monilia albicans* is now *Candida albicans*.

Several mold allergens have been characterized by gene cloning, and sequence analyses in many cases determine the biological functions of the allergens. The best-described species are *A. alternata*, *A. fumigatus*, and *Cladosporium herbarum*. Allergens also have been described for *Asp. niger*, *Asp. oryzae*, *C. albicans*, *C. boidinii*, *Malassezia furfur*, *P. notatum*, *S. cerevisiae* (baker's yeast), *T. tonsurans*, and others. The biological functions of the major allergens Alt a 1, Cla h 1, and Cla h 2 are unknown. Asp f 1 is a ribonuclease that cleaves 28S RNA in eukaryotic ribosomes and thereby exerts an inhibitory effect on protein biosynthesis. Asp f 1 has been used to assess environmental exposure to *Aspergillus*. In general, mold vaccines seem to contain many antigens. For example, more than 70 antigens have been identified in *C. herbarum*, several of which are allergens (86).

Interspecies similarities have been reported between some mold species (for example, between the closely related genera *Alternaria* and *Stemphyllium*, and between *Pityrosporum orbiculare* and *C. albicans*). However, no immunochemical similarities were detected between the major allergens of these species when the analysis utilized rabbit antibodies against the major allergens of *A. alternata*, *C. herbarum*, and *A. fumigatus* (87).

Standardization of mold allergen vaccines remains rather difficult, but a deeper understanding of the physiology of the organisms hopefully will help to identify relevant growth conditions and marker allergens.

F. Latex

Natural rubber (i.e., latex, *Hevea brasiliensis*) allergy is predominantly found among health care workers and patients, such as children with spina bifida who undergo repeated surgery and other invasive procedures (88) (Table 8). Field latex contains up to 2% protein. One third of the protein content is bound to insoluble rubber particles, including the major allergens, Hev b 1 (rubber elongation factor) and Hev b 3, which is homologous to Hev b 1. The soluble fraction contains 60 IgE-binding proteins, including the two-domain 20 kDa major allergen, prohevein (Hev b 6.01), which is processed into a 5 kDa hevein (Hev b 6.02), and a C-terminal 14 kDa fragment (Hev b 6.03). Clinical cross-reactivity

Table 8 Latex Allergens

Rubber Latex, *Hevea brasiliensis*			
Hev b 1	rubber elongation factor	58	GB:X56535
Hev b 2	beta 1,3-glucanase	34/36	GB:U22147
Hev b 3		24	EMBL:AJ223388
Hev b 4	component of microhelix protein complex	100–115	
Hev b 5		16	GB:U42640
Hev b 6.01	hevein precursor	20	SW:P02877
Hev b 6.02	hevein	5	SW:P02877
Hev b 6.03	C-terminal fragment	14	SW:P02877
Hev b 7	patatin homologue	46	GB:U80598
Hev b 8	profilin	14	EMBL:Y15042
	Mn-superoxide dismutase		GB:L11707

Allergen names are listed according to the official allergen nomenclature (5). Old names may be given in parentheses. Biological function of the allergen is indicated where applicable. The third column lists the molecular weight in kDa as determined by SDS-PAGE. References can be found through the accession numbers provided. The electronic sequence databases are available through the Internet. Abbreviations: GB: GeneBank, http://www.ncbi.nlm.nih.gov/; EMBL: European Molecular Biology Laboratory, http://www.embl-heidelberg.de/; SW: Swis-Prot, http://expasy.hcuge.ch/; PIR: The Protein Information Resource, http://nbrfa.georgetown.edu/pir/.

has been reported between latex and pollen allergens or plant foods. Several latex allergens share sequence homology with other plant proteins, including Hev b 5, which has high homology to a protein present in kiwi fruit; Hev b 7, a 46 kDa allergen homologous to patatins, which are storage proteins described in Solanaceae species such as potato and tomato; and finally Hev b 8, a profilin.

G. Foods

Food allergy defined as an IgE-mediated reaction is far less common than generally suspected (89–91) (Table 9). Many specific problems pertain to the production of food vaccines, however, and these are described in some detail below.

Identification, purification, and characterization of food allergens generally have been somewhat limited in comparison with other allergens. These limitations have been due partly to the problems of establishing the pathogenesis of some untoward reactions to foods. In recent years, however, an increasing number of reports have been published on the identification, purification, and characterization of food allergens.

There are great geographical and cultural variations in food consumption. The most common sources of food allergy are cow's milk, eggs, legumes (especially peanuts and soybeans), nuts, seeds, fish and various seafood, but allergic reactions have been reported for a number of other foods, such as fruits and vegetables.

As for other allergen sources, multiple allergenic components are often found among an even larger number of antigenic components in the source materials. A special feature of the food allergens compared to other allergens is the immense amount (often gram quantities) of allergenic material present in the daily intake. A number of these allergens (e.g., cow's milk proteins) have been purified and characterized for purposes other than allergy research (e.g., nutritional studies). Most of the major food allergens are glycoproteins in the molecular-weight range of 10–40 kD. In general, food allergens share the following characteristics: heat and acid stable, resistant to proteolytic digestion, and potent IgE binding even when denatured. Exceptions to these general characteristics are the fruit allergens, which are often susceptible to heat, acid, and proteolysis.

The production of food vaccines raises some special questions concerning the food processing. Raw peanuts, for example, contain relatively more allergen than roasted peanuts, but consumption of raw peanuts is very limited compared to roasted peanuts. Another special aspect is the digestion of the allergens, which might possibly generate additional allergenic components. This has been demonstrated for milk allergens in both animals and humans (92).

Food allergen vaccines are particularly difficult to produce and characterize, highlighting special demands for standardization to assure the proper quality for diagnostic use.

Table 9 Food Allergens

Cow's milk, *Bos domesticus* (see also cow's dander)			
Bos d 4	alpha-lactalbumin	14.2	GB:M18780
Bos d 5	beta-lactoglobulin	18.3	GB:X14712
Bos d 6	serum albumin	67	GB:M73993
	immunoglobulin	160	
	caseins	20–30	
Chicken's egg, *Gallus domesticus*			
Gal d 1	ovomucoid	28	GB:J00902
Gal d 2	ovalbumin	44	GB:J00895
Gal d 3	ovotransferrin	78	SW:P02789
Gal d 4	lysozyme	14	SW:P00698
Peanut, *Arachis hypogaea*			
Ara h 1	vicilin	63.5	GB:L34402
Ara h 2	conglutin	17	GB:L77197
Soybean, *Glycine max*			
	Kunitz protease inhibitor	20	
Gly m 1	hydrophobic seed protein	7.5	GB:999355
Gly m 2		8	PIR:A57106
Gly m 3	profilin	14	EMBL:AJ223982
Cod, *Gadus callarias*			
Gad c 1	(allergen M) parvalbumin beta	12	SW:P02622
Atlantic salmon, *Salmo salar*			
Sal s 1	parvalbumin	12	EMBL:X97824
Shrimp, *Metapenaeus ensis*			
Met e 1	tropomyosin	34	GB:U08008
Shrimp, *Penaeus aztecus*			
Pen a 1	tropomyosin	36	GB:632782
Shrimp, *Penaeus indicus*			
Pen i 1	tropomyosin	34	
Lobster, *Panulirus stimpsoni*			
Pan s 1	tropomyosin		EMBL:AF030063
Abalone, *Haliotis midae*			
Hal m 1		49	
Wheat, *Triticum aestivum*			
	27 kDa allergen	27	
	alpha-amylase inhibitor, CM16	13	SW:P16159
	alpha-amylase inhibitor, WMAI-1	13	SW:P01083
	agglutinin	17	PIR:S09623
	profilin		EMBL:X89825
Barley, *Hordeum vulgare*			
	alpha-amylase inhibitor, BMAI-1	14	SW:P16968
	alpha-amylase inhibitor, BDAI-1	13	SW:P13691

Table 9 Continued

Hor v 5		30	GB:U06640
	alpha-amylase	64	EMBL:Y11276
	beta-amylase	60	SW:P16098
Rice, *Oryza sativa*			
Ory s 1			GB:U31771
Apple, *Malus domestica*			
Mal d 1	Bet v 1 homologue		PIR:JC4276
Mal d 3	lipid transfer protein	9	
Pear, *Pyrus communis*			
Pyr c 1	Bet v 1 homologue		EMBL:AF057030
Apricot, *Prunus armeniaca*			
Pru ar 1	Bet v 1 homologue		GB:U93165
Sweet cherry, *Prunus avium*			
Pru av 1	Bet v 1 homologue		GB:U66076
Peach, *Prunus persica*			
Pru p 1	lipid transfer protein	10	SW:P81402
Kiwifruit, *Actinidia chinensis*			
Act c 1	cysteine protease	30	SW:P00785
Celery, *Apium graveolens*			
Api g 1	Bet v 1 homologue		GB:Z48967
Api g 2			EMBL:Z75662
Yellow mustard, *Sinapis alba*			
Sin a 1	2S albumin	14	
Sin a 1,	large chain		PIR:S01792
Sin a 1,	small chain		PIR:S01791
Oriental mustard, *Brassica juncea*			
Bra j 1	2S albumin	14	
Bra j 1,	large chain		EMBL:P80207
Bra j 1,	small chain		EMBL:P80215
Rape, *Brassica napus*			
Bra n 1	calcium-binding protein		PIR:S65149
Bra n 2	calcium-binding protein		PIR:S65150
Turnip, *Brassica rapa*			
Bra r 1	calcium-binding protein		PIR:S65151
Bra r 2	calcium-binding protein		PIR:S65152
Castor bean, *Ricinus communis*			
Ric c 1	2S albumin		SW:P01089
Potato, *Solanum tuberosum*			
Sol t 1	patatin	43	SW:P15476

Allergen names are listed according to the official allergen nomenclature (5). Old names may be given in parentheses. Biological function of the allergen is indicated where applicable. The third column lists the molecular weight in kDa as determined by SDS-PAGE. References can be found through the accession numbers provided. The electronic sequence databases are available through the Internet. Abbreviations: GB: GeneBank, http://www.ncbi.nlm.nih.gov/; EMBL: European Molecular Biology Laboratory, http://www.embl-heidelberg.de/; SW: Swis-Prot, http://expasy.hcuge.ch/; PIR: The Protein Information Resource, http://nbrfa.georgetown.edu/pir/.

1. Cow's Milk

Cow's milk contains 3.6% protein. Milk protein allergens are divided into caseins (80%) and whey proteins (20%). In cow's milk, the whey alone has been shown to contain at least 36 antigenic components, of which alpha-lactalbumin, beta-lactoglobulin, bovine serum albumin, and immunoglobulin are the most important allergens (93). Caseins are also important allergens. The caseins complex with calcium phosphate to form hydrated spherical micelles that give milk its turbid appearance. Immunoglobulin E antibodies cross-reacting between cow's milk and cow's dander allergens have been reported (94).

No differences in allergenicity between raw, pasteurized or homogenized and pasteurized cow's milk were noted in skin prick test and oral challenge (95). However, beta-lactoglobulin and alpha-lactalbumin are somewhat degraded in sterilized milk products.

2. Hen's Egg

Eggs from chicken (*Gallus domesticus*) contain 60% egg white and 30% egg yolk. Egg white is generally more allergenic than egg yolk, but IgE against egg yolk proteins also occurs (96). Major allergens in hen's egg white include ovalbumin, ovomucoid, and conalbumin, but lysozyme also strongly binds IgE from human sera of egg-allergic individuals. Heating egg white decreases allergic reactions in 50% of egg-allergic patients, but the other 50% still react after eating eggs. This may be explained by the fact that ovomucoid is very heat stable.

3. Peanut

Peanut allergy is characterized by acute and dramatic reactions (97). Different varieties of peanut (*Arachis hypogaea*) are grown commercially. In the United States, the predominant varieties are Virginia, Spanish, and Runner. The peanut kernel contains 27% protein. The skin contains tannins and pigments that will color the vaccine if not removed prior to extraction. Peanut proteins were originally divided into albumin (water-soluble) and globulin (salt-soluble) fractions. The globulin fraction was further subdivided into arachin (legumin) and conarachin (vicilin) fractions, based on precipitation with ammonium sulfate. Peanut allergens are found in various parts of the plant and are relatively heat stable. Thus, the allergens are present both in raw and roasted peanuts, but the raw peanuts contain more protein and hence more allergens. Peanut has two major allergens: vicilin (Ara h 1, 63.5 kDa) and conglutin (Ara h 2, 17 kDa).

4. Soybean

The oil from soybeans (*Glycine max*) is mostly used for human consumption, whereas the protein-containing part is fed to animals. Soybean flour is also used in breast milk substitutes, and allergy to soybeans is predominantly found in infants fed such formulas. However, inhalant allergy to soybean flour and dust has also been reported. Soybeans contain approximately 35% protein, which can be separated into globulin (precipitates at pH 4.5) and whey fractions. In SDS-PAGE, up to 17 individual Coomassie staining bands can be detected (98). The ''Kunitz' soybean-trypsin inhibitor'' (20 kDa) is an allergen shown to cause anaphylactic reactions after soybean ingestion. Another major allergen is Gly m 1, a hydrophobic seed protein. Soybean profilin has also been characterized.

5. Hazelnut

Polyacrylamide gel electrophoresis with sodium dodecylsulfate of hazelnut (*Corylus avellana*) extracts has revealed several bands between 13 and 46 kDa (99). Of these bands, the 18 kDa Bet v 1 homologue is the predominant hazelnut allergen. Hazelnut profilin also has been found in both pollen and nut vaccines.

6. Fish

Codfish muscle contains 18% protein. The major cod allergen, Gad c 1, was first purified and characterized in 1971 (100). This allergen is a parvalbumin, which controls the flow of Ca^{2+} in and out of the muscle cells of fish and amphibians. Gad c 1 is a very stable protein, resistant to digestion, cooking, and proteolysis. Vaccines of several other fish species (including tuna, salmon, perch, carp, and eel) also contain heat-stable IgE-binding proteins (13 kDa) that cross-react with Gad c 1 (101). Sal s 1, the major allergen of the Atlantic salmon (*Salmo salar*), has been characterized in detail and is indeed a parvalbumin, which is 74% homologous to Gad c 1. Protein bands in the range of 40 to 90 kDa molecular weights as determined by SDS-PAGE appear to be more sensitive to heat denaturation. Reports of the loss of IgE binding in canned fish seem inconsistent with the stability of fish vaccines, but allergen accessibility to proteolytic decomposition and the activity of specific proteases may be very different in vaccines compared to intact tissue.

Individuals who experience allergic reactions after eating fish but have negative skin tests to fish proteins often may react to nematode parasites, such as *Anisakis simplex* or *Hysterothylacium aduncum*, which infest fish.

7. Shrimp

Shrimp contain two major allergens, a heat-labile allergen (21 kDa) and a heat-stable major allergen (38 kDa) (102). The heat-stable allergen, tropomyosin, has been characterized in several shrimp species including Indian prawn (*Penaeus indicus*; Pen i 1, 34 kDa), brown shrimp (*P. aztecus*; Pen a 1, 36 kDa), and

Metapenaeus ensis (Met e 1, 34 kDa). Cross-reactive homologues of Pen a 1 have been found in crab, lobster, and crawfish.

8. Cereal Grains

Species used for the production of cereal grains include wheat (*Triticum vulgaris*), oat (*Avena sativa*), rye (*Secale cereale*), barley (*Hordeum vulgare*), maize (*Zea mays*), and rice (*Oryza sativa*). These grains account for 72% of human protein consumption (103). Grain proteins can be divided into albumin (a water-soluble fraction), globulin (a salt-soluble fraction), prolamin (a fraction soluble in 70% ethanol), and glutelin (an acid- or alkali-soluble fraction).

Wheat grains contain a small proximal germ, and the major part of the grain consists of the endosperm, which stores 100% of the starch and 72% of the grain protein. The albumin and globulin fractions contain the majority of the IgE-binding proteins, but IgE antibodies to the prolamin (gliadin) and glutelin (glutenin) fractions have also been described. The latter two fractions together are also referred to as ''gluten,'' which is prepared by extensively washing and kneading the grain. Western blots using IgE of wheat vaccines show many bands (104), of which 15, 17, 27, and 47 kDa bands were the major IgE-binding proteins in sera obtained from asthmatic bakers (105). The 15-kDa band represents subunits of the alpha-amylase inhibitor, homologues of which are also present in other grains. The 17-kDa allergen is an agglutinin.

Large differences in allergenic composition between varieties of *T. aestivum* have been reported (105). The varieties Apollo, Avis, Bussard, and Fregatt contained the largest amounts of the 27 kDa major allergen, whereas the content of alpha-amylase inhibitor was very low. Unfortunately, wheat flour producers generally mix together different varieties of wheat flour to obtain a final product with a good baking characteristic, thus hampering the use of commercial flour for the production of standardized vaccines.

The major allergens of barley are alpha- and beta-amylases. Other allergens are alpha-amylase inhibitors, which are homologues of the wheat alpha-amylase inhibitors. They are also homologous to the 2S seed storage proteins shown to be allergenic in oriental mustard (*Brassica juncea*), yellow mustard (*Sinapis alba*), and castor bean (*Ricinus communis*).

Alpha-amylase inhibitors also serve as allergens in rice and rye. In addition, pollen proteins homologous to the grass group 1–6 have been described in rye (Sec c 5, a group 5 allergen), and a grass group 1 component has been described in maize.

9. Fruits

The apple contains less than 1% protein, making the extraction of apple allergens difficult. Furthermore, phenolic compounds and proteolytic enzymes easily degrade the proteins. It is therefore essential to reduce protein degradation by adding inhibitors or performing organic extraction to remove phenolic compounds before the aqueous extraction (106). The allergenic activity may vary with the ripeness of the apple. More than 30 individual apple antigens can be detected by SDS-PAGE. Several strains of apple are available, of which Granny Smith, Golden Delicious, Jonagold, Braeburn, Prime Rouge, Cox Orange, and Apollo contain the highest amounts of the 18 kDa Bet v 1 homologous major allergen. Important allergens have also been found at 8 and 10 kDa, including a lipid transfer protein homologous to lipid transfer proteins found in several other species.

As is the case for the apple, major allergens homologous to the Bet v 1 allergen of birch pollen have been identified in the pear, sweet cherry, and apricot. In the peach, however, most of the allergenic activity seems to be associated with an 8-kDa component and with the 10-kDa lipid transfer protein, Pru p 1. The fruits of the *Prunus* genus (peach, cherry, apricot, and plum) contain a major cross-reacting allergen (13 kDa), which is not associated with birch or grass pollinosis (107).

10. Other Food Allergens

Sensitization to celery (*Apium graveolens*) is common in individuals hypersensitive to birch, mugwort, or grass pollen and is caused by cross-reactivity of allergen-specific IgE antibodies. Profilin (15 kDa) has been identified as an important allergen for celery-allergic patients (108), as well as the 16 kDa, Bet v

Table 10 Other Allergens

Worm, *Ascaris suum*			
Asc s 1		10	GB:AF051702
Mosquito, *Aedes aegyptii*			
Aed a 1	apyrase	68	EMBL:L12389
Aed a 2		37	EMBL:M33156
Aed a 3			GB:AF001927

Allergen names are listed according to the official allergen nomenclature (5). Old names may be given in parentheses. Biological function of the allergen is indicated where applicable. The third column lists the molecular weight in kDa as determined by SDS-PAGE. References can be found through the accession numbers provided. The electronic sequence databases are available through the Internet. Abbreviations: GB: GeneBank, http://www.ncbi.nlm.nih.gov/; EMBL: European Molecular Biology Laboratory, http://www.embl-heidelberg.de/; SW: Swis-Prot, http://expasy.hcuge.ch/; PIR: The Protein Information Resource, http://nbrfa.georgetown.edu/pir/.

1 homologous protein also important in the ''oral allergy syndrome'' that is associated with pollen allergy (109). Bet v 1 homologues have also been found in parsley (*Petroselinum crispum*) and carrot (*Daucus carota*), which are also members of the Apiaceae.

In Oriental mustard (*B. juncea*) and yellow mustard (*S. alba*), important allergens are the 2S storage albumins, which are homologous to storage albumins in wheat, barley, and rice.

Finally, in rape (*Brassica napus*) and turnip (*B. rapa*), important allergens are calcium-binding proteins with EF-hand motifs that are also found in several other species.

H. Others

Other allergen sources include worms and mosquitoes (Table 10).

I. Homology and Cross-Reactivity

Most patients allergic to birch pollen also react to pollens from the related alder and hazel species. Theoretically this allergic reactivity could be explained either by consecutive sensitization to each of the species or by cross-reactivity, conditions in which IgE reacts to similar structures (i.e., epitopes) present in the pollens. Most allergens have homologous counterparts in closely related species. This is not surprising, because the biological function of the allergen is also required in the related species and phylogenetically related allergens are likely to be similar in structure. Cross-reactivity based on the occurrence of similar epitope structures among related species is therefore a prevalent phenomenon in allergy. Allergenic cross-reactivity is also well known among the domestic mites and for most grasses.

Cross-reactivity between more distantly related species has also been reported (110). An example is the association between allergy to birch pollen and the oral allergy syndrome characterized by sensitization to apple, pear, hazelnut, or celery. In this case, the cross-reactivity relies on the occurrence of Bet v 1 homologous molecules in several fruits and vegetables. The underlying mechanism can be illustrated by modeling of the major apple allergen, Mal d 1, on the three-dimensional Bet v 1 structure, which possesses conserved patches on the molecular surface large enough to accommodate IgE-binding epitopes (Fig. 3).

Most allergens today are investigated using molecular biology as a tool, and knowledge of the sequences enables examination for homology by performing similarity searches in the electronic databases. Such approaches facilitate the identification of homologous allergens responsible for the IgE cross-reactivity. However, not all homologies are clinically relevant, inasmuch as even minor variations in sequence may influence IgE-binding. Sequence-based homologies or cross-reactivity determined by in vitro experimental technology based on principles similar to direct RAST or even in vivo skin prick testing can therefore not be extrapolated to clinical relevance.

In vitro assessment of cross-reactivity has to rely on carefully controlled quantitative inhibition assays. Even in this case, identified cross-reactivity is not necessarily clinically relevant. Low-affinity IgE directed toward carbohydrate moieties of glycoproteins could serve as an example (111).

The remainder of this chapter will address homologies and cross-reactivities among allergens.

1. Bet v 1 Homologues

Isoallergens and variants within the Fagales major allergens Bet v 1, Aln g 1, Car b 1, and Cor a 1, share more than 70% homology. The intraspecies variation for Bet v 1 is quantitatively similar to the interspecies variation. Major allergens from apple (*Malus domestica*, Mal d 1), pear (*Pyrus communis*, Pyr c 1), apricot (*Prunus armeniaca*, Pru ar 1), and sweet cherry (*P. avium*, Pru av 1) are homologous to levels that have been shown to be clinically relevant. Furthermore, Bet v 1 shares lesser homologies with disease-response proteins from alfalfa, pea, bean, lupine, soybean, potato, parsley, tomato, ginseng, celery, and others. The clinical relevance of these similarities has not been described in detail.

2. Profilin

Profilins bind to actin and affect the structure of the cytoskeleton. Profilins sharing homologies greater than 85%, and identities greater than 75% have been described from the following species: birch (*Betula verrucosa*: Bet v 2), sunflower (*Helianthus annuus*: Hel a 2), annual mercury (*Mercurialis annua*: Mer a 1), olive (*Olea europea*: Ole e 2), grass group 12 (*Cynodon dactylon* and *Phleum pratense*), latex (*H. brasiliensis*: Hev b 8), soybean (*G. max*: Gly m 3), and wheat (*T. aestivum*). Homologous profilins have also been described in barley, tomato, maize, and French bean, but these profilins have not been characterized with respect to IgE-binding.

3. Proteases

Serine proteases belonging to the trypsin family have been described primarily as allergens in domestic mites. *Dermatophagoides* group 3 allergens are trypsins, group 6 allergens are chymotrypsins, and group 9 allergens are collagenolytic serine proteases. Hymenoptera venoms also contain allergenic serine proteases, the group 4 allergens described in bumblebee (*Bombus pennsylvanicus*: Bom p 4) and Mediterranean paper wasp (*Polistes dominulus*: Pol d 4). Furthermore, Asp o 13 is an allergenic serine protease in the subtilase family which has been described in *Asper. oryzae*.

Aspartic proteases have been described in German cockroach (*B. germanica*: Bla g 2) and in *Asp. fumigatus* (Asp f 10, aspergillopepsin). Immunochemical cross-reactivity has not been reported.

Cysteine (thiol) proteases of the papain family are among the most important allergens from the domestic mite, *Dermatophagoides* group 1. Homologous and cross-reactive allergens are found in storage mites, such as *Euroglyphus maynei*: Eur m 1. Actinidin from kiwi fruit (*Actinidia chinensis*: Act c 1) has also been shown to be allergenic, although no studies on cross-reactivity have been reported.

4. Albumin

Albumins are present in most animal dander vaccines, and they are used as marker proteins for the quantification of serum proteins. Although they are not major allergens, albumins often cross-react between different mammalian species. The clinical significance of this IgE cross-reactivity, however, has not been studied in detail.

5. EF-Hand Calcium-Binding Proteins

EF-hand calcium-binding domains have been found in the 8 kDa allergen Bet v 4. Homologous motifs have also been found in alder (*Alnus glutinosa*: Aln g 2), olive (*O. europea*: Ole e 3), rape (*B. napus*: Bra n 1 and 2), turnip (*B. rapa*: Bra r 1 and Bra r 2), prickly juniper (*Juniperus oxycedrus*: Jun o 2), and grass group 7 (Cynodon dactylon and *P. pratense*), as well as in cow's dander (*Bos domesticus*).

6. Lipid Transport Proteins

Two lines of homologous lipid transport proteins have been described as allergens. One line includes Mal d 3 from apple (*Malus domestica*), an unnamed allergen from almond (*Prunus dulcis*), Pru p 1 from peach (*P. persica*), and Hel a 1 from sunflower (*H. annuus*). Also included in this homology are proteins from cotton, spinach, tobacco, sorghum, tomato, rice, maize, and French bean, but they have not been characterized with respect to IgE binding.

The other line of homologous lipid transport proteins includes Amb a 6 from short ragweed (*Ambrosia artemisiifolia*) and Par j 1 from *Parietaria judaica*. Other members are proteins from tobacco, rice, barley, maize, and Castor bean, but these proteins likewise have not been characterized with respect to IgE binding.

7. Tropomyosin

Tropomyosin is a conserved protein involved in striated muscle contraction. Tropomyosin has been found in domestic mite group 10 and in American cockroach (*Periplaneta americana*: Per a 7), as well as in various seafood, such as shrimp (*M. ensis*: Met e 1; *P. aztecus*: Pen a 1; *P. indicus*: Pen i 1), and lobster (*Panulirus stimpsoni*: Pan s 1). Immunoglobulin E from shrimp-allergic individuals has been shown to bind not only to shellfish vaccines but also to insect vaccines, such as cockroach (112).

8. Superoxide Dismutase

The biological function of superoxide dismutase is to remove chemical radicals, which are normally produced within living cells and are toxic to biological systems. Homologous allergenic mitochondrial manganese superoxide dismutases have been described in *A. fumigatus* (Asp f 6) and *H. brasiliensis*. An allergenic cytoplasmic copper-zinc superoxide dismutase from *O. europea* (Ole e 5), is not homologous to the other two.

9. Lipocalin

Lipocalins are secreted into saliva, tears, or milk. Lipocalins from dog (*C. familiaris*: Can f 1 and Can f 2) are homologous to lipocalins from horse (*Equus caballus*: Equ c 1) and about 40% homologous to bovine beta-lactoglobulin (Bos d 5). Bovine lipocalin (Bos d 2), the major allergen of cow's dander, is about 50% homologous to horse lipocalin. Members of this protein family are also the major allergens from the rat (*R. norvegicus*: Rat n 2). Other homologous sequences include calycin (Bla g 4) from the German cockroach, *B. germanica*.

10. Uteroglobin

The major allergen from the cat (*F. domesticus*: Fel d 1) is a heterotetramer composed of two noncovalently linked, disulfide-linked heterodimers of chain 1 and chain 2. Fel d 1 is secreted into the saliva and into the lachrymal fluid. A similar molecule (70% homology) recently has been described as an allergen in the mouse (*M. musculus*).

11. Prealbumin (Transthyretin)

The major urinary allergens from mouse (*M. musculus*: Mus m 1) and rat (*R. norvegicus*: Rat n 1) are thyroid hormone-binding proteins (transthyretins). These proteins exist as homotetramers.

12. 2S Albumin

2S albumins are seed storage proteins composed of heterodimers linked by disulfide bonds. Homologous allergens have been described in Oriental mustard (*B. juncea*: Bra j 1), yellow mustard (*S. alba*: Sin a 1), and Castor bean (*Ricinus communis*: Ric c 1).

13. Amylases

Amylases are enzymes that cleave polysaccharides, such as starch. Alpha- and beta-amylases, which are chemically and immunochemically distinct, have been described as allergens in barley (*H. vulgare*) and wheat (*T. aestivum*). Asp o 2, an allergen from *A. oryzae*, is also an important allergen in the baking industry. Furthermore, amylase has been described as an allergen in *Dermatophagoides pteronyssinus* (Der p 4), but there is no homology to the plant or fungal amylases.

14. Amylase Inhibitors

Protein inhibitors of amylase have been described as allergens in barley (*H. vulgare*), wheat (*T. aestivum*), and rye (*S. cereale*).

15. Pectinases

Sequence homology to pectate lyases indicates the biological function of Amb a 1 and Amb a 2, the major allergens from short ragweed (*Ambrosia artemisiifolia*), and Cry j 1, the major allergen from Japanese cedar (*Cryptomeria japonica*).

IV. SALIENT POINTS

1. All allergens are proteins and all soluble proteins are potential allergens.
2. Allergen vaccines are complex biological mixtures, and standardization is essential to ensure specificity and sensitivity of diagnosis.
3. Statistically, patients' IgE binds to some antigens more frequently than to others, thereby defining major allergens.
4. Source materials should be selected with special attention to specificity and to inclusion of all relevant biological material.
5. The process of extraction is highly dependent on physicochemical conditions. Extreme conditions are likely to destroy allergen epitopes and affect biological activity.
6. The existence and use of internal and external standards are essential for standardization and control of allergen vaccines.
7. The quality of an allergen vaccine is a result both of its qualitative and its quantitative composition.
8. The standardization procedure should include the assessment of vaccine composition, the concentration(s) of one or more major allergens or marker proteins, and the total IgE-binding potency.

REFERENCES

1. Løwenstein H. Selection of reference preparation. IUIS reference preparation criteria. Arb Paul Ehrlich Inst 1987;80:75–78.
2. Wahn U, Schweter C, Lind P, Løwenstein H. Prospective study on immunologic changes induced by two different *Dermatophagoides pteronyssinus* extracts prepared from whole mite culture and mite bodies. J Allergy Clin Immunol 1988;82: 360–370.
3. Lemanske RF, Taylor SL. Standardized extracts, foods. Clin Rev Allergy 1987;5: 23–36.
4. Løwenstein H, Marsh DG. Antigens of *Ambrosia elatior* (short ragweed) pollen. I. Crossed immunoelectrophoretic analyses. J Immunol 1981;126:943–948.
5. King TP, Hoffman D, Løwenstein H, Marsh DG, Platts-Mills TAE, Thomas W. Allergen nomenclature. J Allergy Clin Immunol 1995;96:5–14.
6. Dreborg S, Einarsson R. The major allergen content of allergenic preparations reflects their biological activity. Allergy 1992;47:418–423.
7. Helm RM, Gauerke MB, Baer H, Løwenstein H, Ford A, Levy DA, Norman PS, Yunginger JW. Production and testing of an international reference standard of short ragweed pollen extract. J Allergy Clin Immunol 1984;73:790–800.
8. Gjesing B, Jäger L, Marsh DG, Løwenstein H. The international collaborative study establishing the first international standard for timothy (*Phleum pratense*) grass pollen allergenic extract. J Allergy Clin Immunol 1985;75:258–267.
9. Ford A, Seagroatt V, Platts-Mills TAE, Løwenstein H. A collaborative study on the first international standard of *Dermatophagoides pteronyssinus* (house dust mite) extract. J Allergy Clin Immunol 1985;75:676–686.
10. Arntzen FC, Wilhelmsen TW, Løwenstein H, Gjesing B, Maasch HJ, Stromberg R, Einarsson R, Backman A, Makinen-Kiljunen S, Ford A. The international collaborative study on the first international standard of birch (*Betula verrucosa*) pollen extract. J Allergy Clin Immunol 1989;83:66–82.
11. Larsen JN, Ford A, Gjesing B, Levy D, Petrunov B, Silvestri L, Løwenstein H. The collaborative study of the international standard of dog, *Canis domesticus*, hair/dander extract. J Allergy Clin Immunol 1988;82:318–330.
12. Helm RM, Squillace DL, Yunginger JW, members of the international collaborative trial. Production of a proposed international reference standard *Alternaria* extract II. Results of a collaborative trial. J Allergy Clin Immunol 1988;81:651–663.
13. Baer H, Anderson MC, Helm RM, Yunginger JW, Løwenstein H, Gjesing B, White W, Douglass G, Phillips PR, Schumacher M, Hewitt B, Guerin BG, Charpin J, Carreira J, Lombardero M, Ekramoddoullah AKM, Kisil F, Einarsson R. The preparation and testing of the proposed international reference (IRP) Bermuda grass (*Cynodon dactylon*)-pollen extract. J Allergy Clin Immunol 1986;78:624–631.
14. Stewart GA, Turner KJ, Baldo BA, Cripps AW, Ford A, Seagroatt V, Løwenstein H, Ekramoddoullah AKM. Standardization of rye-grass pollen (*Lolium perenne*) extract. An immunochemical and physicochemical assessment of six candidate international reference preparations. Int Arch Allergy Appl Immunol 1988;86:9–18.
15. Løwenstein H. Physico-chemical and immunochemical methods for the control of potency and quality of allergenic extracts. Arb Paul Ehrlich Inst 1980;75:122–132.

16. Laemmli UK. Cleavage of structural proteins during the assembly of the head of bacteriophage T4. Nature 1970;227:680–685.
17. Kyhse-Andersen J. Electroblotting of multiple gels: a simple apparatus without buffer tank for rapid transfer of proteins from polyacrylamide to nitrocellulose. J Biochem Biophys Methods 1984;10:203–209.
18. Ipsen H, Larsen JN. Detection of antigen-specific IgE antibodies in sera from allergic patients by SDS-PAGE immunoblotting and crossed radioimmunoelectrophoresis. In: Bjerrum O, Heegaard NHH, eds. Handbook of Immunoblotting of Proteins. Vol II. Boca Raton, FL: Chemical Rubber Company 1988:159–166.
19. Brighton WD. Profiles of allergen extract components by isoelectric focussing and radioimmunoassay. Dev Biol Stand 1975;29:362–369.
20. Løwenstein H. Quantitative immunoelectrophoretic methods as a tool for the analysis and isolation of allergens. Prog Allergy 1978;25:1.
21. Weeke B, Søndergaard I, Lind P, Aukrust L, Løwenstein H. Crossed radioimmunoelectrophoresis (CRIE) for the identification of allergens and determination of the antigenic specificities of patients' IgE. In: Axelsen NH, ed. Handbook of Immunoprecipitation-In-Gel Techniques. Scand J Immunol 1983;17(suppl 10):265–272.
22. Engvall E, Perlmann P. Enzyme-linked immunosorbent assay, ELISA. III. Quantitation of specific antibodies by enzyme-labelled anti-immunoglobulin in antigen-coated tubes. J Immunol 1972;109:129–135.
23. Ceska M, Eriksson R, Varga JM. Radioimmunosorbent assay of allergens. J Allergy Clin Immunol 1972;49:1–9.
24. Siraganian RP. Automated histamine analysis for in vitro allergy testing. II. Correlation of skin test results with in vitro whole blood histamine release in 82 patients. J Allergy Clin Immunol 1977;59:214–222.
25. Platts-Mills TAE, Chapman MD. Allergen standardization. J Allergy Clin Immunol 1991;87:621–625.
26. D'Amato G, Spieksma FT. Liccardi G, Jager S, Russo M, Kontou-Fili K, Nikkels H, Wuthrich B, Bonini S. Pollen-related allergy in Europe. Allergy 1998;53:567–578.
27. Ipsen H, Løwenstein H. Isolation and immunochemical characterization of the major allergen of birch pollen (*Betula verrucosa*). J Allergy Clin Immunol 1983;72: 150–159.
28. Ipsen H, Hansen OC. The NH2-terminal amino acid sequence of the immunochemically partial identical major allergens of alder (*Alnus glutinosa*) Aln g 1, birch (*Betula verrucosa*) Bet v 1, hornbeam (*Carpinus betulus*) Car b 1, and oak (*Quercus alba*) Que a 1 pollens. Mol Immunol 1991;28:1279–1288.
29. Ipsen H, Wihl JA, Petersen BN, Løwenstein H. Specificity mapping of patients IgE response towards the tree pollen major allergens Aln g I, Bet v I and Cor a I. Clin Exp Allergy 1992;22:391–399.
30. Gajhede M, Osmark P, Poulsen FM, Ipsen H, Larsen JN, Joost van Neerven RJ, Schou C, Løwenstein H, Spangfort MD. X-ray and NMR structure of Bet v 1, the origin of birch pollen allergy. Nat Struct Biol 1996;3:1040–1045.
31. Valenta R, Duchene M, Pettenburger K, Sillaber C, Valent P, Bettelheim P, Breitenbach M, Rumpold H, Kraft D, Scheiner O. Identification of profilin as a novel pollen allergen; IgE autoreactivity in sensitized individuals. Science 1991;253:557–560.

32. Hashimoto M, Nigi H, Sakaguchi M, Inouye S, Imaoka K, Miyazawa H, Taniguchi Y, Kurimoto M, Yasueda H, Ogawa T. Sensitivity to two major allergens (Cry j I and Cry j II) in patients with Japanese cedar (*Cryptomeria japonica*) pollinosis. Clin Exp Allergy 1995;25:848–852.
33. Lauzurica P, Marubi N, Galocha B, Gonzalez J, Diaz R, Palomiro P, Hernandez D, Garcia R, Lahoz C. Olive (*Olea europea*) pollen allergens. II. Isolation and characterization of two major antigens. Mol Immunol 1988;25:337–344.
34. Obispo TM, Melero JA, Carpizo JA, Carreira J, Lombardero M. The main allergen of *Olea europaea* (Ole e I) is also present in other species of the Oleaceae family. Clin Exp Allergy 1993;23:311–316.
35. Løwenstein H, Marsh DG. Antigens of *Ambrosia elatior* (short ragweed) pollen. III. Crossed radioimmunoelectrophoresis of ragweed-allergic patients' sera with special attention to quantification of IgE responses. J Immunol 1983;130:727–731.
36. Rafnar T, Griffith IJ, Kuo MC, Bond JF, Rogers BL, Klapper DG. Cloning of Amb a I (antigen E), the major allergen family of short ragweed pollen. J Biol Chem 1991;266:1229–1236.
37. Metzler WJ, Valentine K, Roebber M, Friedrichs MS, Marsh DG, Mueller I. Determination of the three-dimensional solution structure of ragweed allergen Amb t V by nuclear magnetic resonance spectroscopy. Biochemistry 1992;31: 5117–5127.
38. Nilsen BM, Grimsoen A, Paulsen BS. Identification and characterization of important allergens from mugwort pollen by IEF, SDS-PAGE and immunoblotting. Mol Immunol 1991;28:733–742.
39. D'Amato G, Ruffilli A, Sacerdoti G, Bonini S. Parietaria pollinosis: a review. Allergy 1992;47:443–449.
40. Matthiesen F, Løwenstein H. Group V allergens in grass pollens. II. Investigation of group V allergens in pollens from 10 grasses. Clin Exp Allergy 1991;21:309–320.
41. Ipsen H, Løwenstein H. Basic features of crossreactivity in tree and grass pollen allergy. Clin Rev Allergy Immunol 1997;15:389–396.
42. Schumacher MJ, Grabowski J, Wagner CM. Anti-Bermuda grass RAST binding is minimally inhibited by pollen extracts from ten other grasses. Ann Allergy 1985; 55:584–587.
43. Bufe A, Schramm G, Keown MB, Schlaak M, Becker WM. Major allergen Phl p Vb in timothy grass is a novel pollen Rnase. FEBS Lett 1995;363:6–12.
44. Dust mite allergens and asthma—a worldwide problem. J Allergy Clin Immunol 1989;83:416–427.
45. Lind P, Weeke B, Løwenstein H. A reference allergen preparation of the house dust mite *D. pteronyssinus*, produced from whole mite culture—a part of the DAS 76 study. Comparison with allergen preparations from other raw materials. Allergy 1984;39:259–274.
46. Heymann PW, Chapman MD, Platts-Mills TA. Antigen Der f I from the dust mite *Dermatophagoides farinae*: structural comparison with Der p I from *Dermatophagoides pteronyssinus* and epitope specificity of murine IgG and human IgE antibodies. J Immunol 1986;137:2841–2847.
47. Heymann PW, Chapman MD, Aalberse RC, Fox JW, Platts-Mills TA. Antigenic

and structural analysis of group II allergens (Der f II and Der p II) from house dust mites (*Dermatophagoides* spp). J Allergy Clin Immunol 1989;83:1055–1067.
48. Ichikawa S, Hatanaka H, Yuuki T, Iwamoto N, Kojima S, Nishiyama C, Ogura, K, Okumura Y, Inagaki F. Solution structure of Der f 2, the major mite allergen for atopic diseases. J Biol Chem 1998;273:356–360.
49. Cuthbert OD. Storage mite allergy, Clin Rev Allergy 1990;8:69–86.
50. Wraith DG, Cunnington AM, Seymour WM. The role and allergenic importance of storage mites in house dust and other environments. Clin Allergy 1979;9:545–561.
51. Fernandez-Caldas E. Allergenicity of *Blomia tropicalis*. J Invest Allergol Clin Immunol 1997;7:402–404.
52. Løwenstein H, Lind P, Weeke B. Indentification and clinical significance of allergenic molecules of cat origin. Part of the DAS 76 study. Allergy 1985;40:430–441.
53. Duffort OA, Carreira J, Nitti G, Polo F, Lombardero M. Studies on the biochemical structure of the major cat allergen *Felis domesticus* I. Mol Immunol 1991;28:301–309.
54. Chapman MD, Aalberse RC, Brown MJ, Platts-Mills TA. Monoclonal antibodies to the major feline allergen Fel d I. II. Single step affinity purification of Fel d I, N-terminal sequence analysis, and development of a sensitive two-site immunoassay to assess Fel d I exposure. J Immunol 1988;140:812–818.
55. van Neerven RJJ, van de Pol MM, van Milligen FJ, Jansen HM, Aalberse RC, Kapsenberg ML. Characterization of cat dander-specific T lymphocytes from atopic patients. J Immunol 1994;152:4203–4210.
56. Blands J, Løwenstein H, Weeke B. Characterization of extract of dog hair and dandruff from six different dog breeds by quantitative immunoelectrophoresis. Identification of allergens by crossed radioimmunoelectrophoresis (CRIE). Acta Allergol 1977;32:147–169.
57. de Groot H, Goei KG, van Swieten P, Aalberse RC. Affinity purification of a major and a minor allergen from dog extract: serologic activity of affinity-purified Can f I and of Can f I-depleted extract. J Allergy Clin Immunol 1991;87:1056–1065.
58. Schou C, Hansen GN, Lintner T, Løwenstein H. Assay for the major dog allergen, Can f I: investigation of house dust samples and commercial dog extracts. J Allergy Clin Immunol 1991;88:847–853.
59. Prahl P, Bucher D, Plesner T, Weeke B, Løwenstein H. Isolation and partial characterisation of three major allergens in an extract from cow hair and dander. Int Arch Allergy Appl Immunol 1982;67:293–301.
60. Løwenstein H, Markussen B, Weeke B. Isolation and partial characterization of three major allergens of horse hair and dandruff. Int Arch Allergy Appl Immunol 1976;51:48–67.
61. Venables KM, Tee RD, Hawkins ER, Gordon DJ, Wale CJ, Farrer NM, Lam TH, Baxter PJ, Newman Taylor AJ. Laboratory animal allergy in a pharmaceutical company. Br J Ind Med 1988;45:660–666.
62. Price JA, Longbottom JL. Allergy to mice. II. Further characterization of two major mouse allergens (AG 1 and AG 3) and immunohistochemical investigations of their sources. Clin Exp Allergy 1990;20:71–77.

63. GeneBank accession AF008595.
64. Platts-Mills TA, Longbottom J, Edwards J, Heymann PW. Asthma and rhinitis related to laboratory rats: use of a purified rat urinary allergen to study exposure in laboratories and the human immune response. N Engl Reg Allergy Proc 1987; 8:245–251.
65. Wojtczak A. Crystal structure of rat transthyretin at 2.5 A resolution: first report on a unique tetrameric structure. Acta Biochim Pol 1997;44:505–517.
66. Lutsky I, Fink JN, Kidd J, Dahlberg MJ, Yunginger JW. Allergenic properties of rat urine and pelt extracts. J Allergy Clin Immunol 1985;75:279–284.
67. Walls AF, Newman Taylor AJ, Longbottom JL. Allergy to guinea pigs: I. Allergenic activities of extracts derived from the pelt, saliva, urine and other sources. Clin Allergy 1985;15:241–251.
68. Price JA, Longbottom JL. Allergy to rabbits. II. Identification and characterization of a major rabbit allergen. Allergy 1988;43:39–48.
69. Hoffman DR. Hymenoptera venom proteins. Adv Exp Med Biol 1996;391:169–186.
70. Paull BR, Yunginger JW, Gleich GJ. Melittin: an allergen of honeybee venom. J Allergy Clin Immunol 1977;59:334–338.
71. Scott DL, Otwinowski Z, Gelb MH, Sigler PB. Crystal structure of bee-venom phospholipase A2 in a complex with a transition-state analogue. Science 1990;250: 1563–1566.
72. Scott DL, Otwinowski Z, Gelb MH, Sigler PB. Crystal structure of bee-venom phospholipase A2: correction. Science 1991;252:764.
73. Hoffman DR. Fire ant venom allergy. Allergy 1995;50:535–544.
74. Baldo BA, Panzani RC. Detection of IgE antibodies to a wide range of insect species in subjects with suspected inhalant allergies to insects. Int Arch Allergy Appl Immunol 1988;85:278–287.
75. Weber E, Steigemann W, Jones TA, Huber R. The structure of oxy-erythrocruorin at 1.4 A resolution. J Mol Biol 1978;120:327–336.
76. Stankus RP, O'Neil CE. Antigenic/allergenic characterization of American and German cockroach extracts. J Allergy Clin Immunol 1988;81:563–570.
77. Pollart SM, Mullins DE, Vailes LD, Hayden ML, Platts-Mills TA, Sutherland WM, Chapman MD. Identification, quantitation, and purification of cockroach allergens using monoclonal antibodies. J Allergy Clin Immunol 1991;87:511–521.
78. Schou C, Lind P, Fernandez-Caldas E, Lockey RF, Løwenstein H. Identification and purification of an important cross-reactive allergen from American (*Periplaneta americana*) and German (*Blattella germanica*) cockroach. J Allergy Clin Immunol 1990;86:935–946.
79. Lehrer SB, Horner WE, Menon P, Stankus RP. Comparison of cockroach allergenic activity in whole body and fecal extracts. J Allergy Clin Immunol 1991;87:574–580.
80. Marshall NA, Chapman MD, Saxon A. Species-specific allergens from the salivary glands of *Triatominae* (Heteroptera: Reduviidae). J Allergy Clin Immunol 1986; 78:430–435.
81. Chapman MD, Marshall NA, Saxon A. Identification and partial purification of species-specific allergens from *Triatoma protracta* (Heteroptera: Reduviidae). J Allergy Clin Immunol 1986;78:436–442.

82. Trudeau WL, Fernandez-Caldas E, Fox RW, Brenner R, Bucholtz GA, Lockey RF. Allergenicity of the cat flea. Clin Exp Allergy 1993;23:377–383.
83. D'Amato G, Spieksma FT. Aerobiologic and clinical aspects of mould allergy in Europe. Allergy 1995;50:870–877.
84. Bush RK, Yunginger JW. Standardization of fungal allergens. Clin Rev Allergy 1987;5:3–21.
85. Burge HA. Classification of the fungi. Clin Rev Allergy 1992;10:153–163.
86. Aukrust L. Crossed radioimmunoelectrophoretic studies of distinct allergens in two extracts of Cladosporium herbarum. Int Arch Allergy Appl Immunol 1979;58:375–390.
87. Matthiesen F, Larsen LS, Løwenstein H. Purification and characterization of two important mold allergens, Alt a 1 and Cla h 1 (abstr). Allergologie 1989; 12:21.
88. Posch A, Chen Z, Raulf-Heimsoth M, Baur X. Latex allergens. Clin Exp Allergy 1998;28:134–140.
89. Bindslev-Jensen C. Food allergy. Br Med J 1998;316:1299–1302.
90. Sampson HA. Food allergy. JAMA 1997;278:1888–1894.
91. Bruinjzeel-Koomen CAFM, Ortolani C, Aas K, Bindslev-Jensen C, Bjorksten B, Moneret-Vautrin DA, Wüthrich B. Adverse reactions to food. Academy of Allergology and Clinical Immunology Subcommittee. Allergy 1995;50:623–635.
92. Haddad ZH, Kalra V, Verma S. IgE antibodies to peptic and peptic-tryptic digests of beta-lactoglobulin: significance in food hypersensitivity. Ann Allergy 1979;42: 368–371.
93. Gjesing B, Østerballe O, Schwartz B, Wahn U, Løwenstein H. Allergen-specific IgE antibodies against antigenic components in cow milk and milk substitutes. Allergy 1986;41:51–56.
94. Szepfalusi Z, Ebner C, Urbanek R, Ebner H, Scheiner O, Boltz-Nitulescu G, Kraft D. Detection of IgE antibodies specific for allergens in cow milk and cow dander. Int Arch Allergy Immunol 1993;102:288–294.
95. Høst A, Samuelsson EG. Allergic reactions to raw, pasteurized, and homogenized/pasteurized cow milk: a comparison. A double-blind placebo-controlled study in milk allergic children. Allergy 1988;43:113–118.
96. Anet J, Back JF, Baker RS, Barnett D, Burley RW, Howden ME. Allergens in the white and yolk of hen's egg. A study of IgE binding by egg proteins. Int Arch Allergy Appl Immunol 1985;77:364–371.
97. Loza C, Brostoff J. Peanut allergy. Clin Exp Allergy 1995;25:493–502.
98. Gonzalez R, Polo F, Zapatero L, Caravaca F, Carreira J. Purification and characterization of major inhalant allergens from soybean hulls. Clin Exp Allergy 1992;22: 748–755.
99. Hirschwehr R, Valenta R, Ebner C, Ferreira F, Sperr WR, Valent P, Rohac M, Rumpold H, Scheiner O, Kraft D. Identification of common allergenic structures in hazel pollen and hazelnuts: a possible explanation for sensitivity to hazelnuts in patients allergic to tree pollen. J Allergy Clin Immunol 1992;90:927–936.
100. Elsayed S, Aas K. Isolation of purified allergens (cod) by isoelectric focusing. Int Arch Allergy Appl Immunol 1971;40:428–438.
101. Bernhisel-Broadbent J, Scanlon SM, Sampson HA. Fish hypersensitivity. I. In vitro

and oral challenge results in fish-allergic patients. J Allergy Clin Immunol 1992; 89:730–737.
102. Hoffman DR, Day ED Jr, Miller JS. The major heat stable allergen of shrimp. Ann Allergy 1981;47:17–22.
103. Payne PI. Breeding for protein quantity and protein quality in seed crops. In: Daussant J, Mosse J, Vaughan J, eds. Seed Proteins. London: Academic Press, 1983: 223–253.
104. Varjonen E, Savolainen J, Mattila L, Kalimo K. IgE-binding components of wheat, rye, barley and oats recognized by immunoblotting analysis with sera from adult atopic dermatitis patients. Clin Exp Allergy 1994;24:481–489.
105. Weiss W, Vogelmeier C, Gorg A. Electrophoretic characterization of wheat grain allergens from different cultivars involved in bakers' asthma. Electrophoresis 1993; 14:805–816.
106. Björksten F, Halmepuro L, Hannuksela M, Lahti A. Extraction and properties of apple allergens. Allergy 1980;35:671–677.
107. Pastorello EA, Ortolani C, Farioli L, Pravettoni V, Ispano M, Borga A, Bengtsson A, Incorvaia C, Berti C, Zanussi C. Allergenic cross-reactivity among peach, apricot, plum, and cherry in patients with oral allergy syndrome: an in vivo and in vitro study. J Allergy Clin Immunol 1994;94:699–707.
108. Vallier P, DeChamp C, Valenta R, Vial O, Deviller P. Purification and characterization of an allergen from celery immunochemically related to an allergen present in several other plant species. Identification as a profilin. Clin Exp Allergy 1992; 22:774–782.
109. Vieths S, Jankiewicz A, Wuthrich B, Baltes W. Immunoblot study of IgE binding allergens in celery roots. Ann Allergy Asthma Immunol 1995;75:48–55.
110. Caballero T, Martin-Esteban M. Association between pollen hypersensitivity and edible vegetable allergy: a review. J Investig Allergol Clin Immunol 1998;8:6–16.
111. van der Veen MJ, van Ree R, Aalberse RC, Akkerdaas J, Koppelman SJ, Jansen HM, van der Zee JS. Poor biologic activity of cross-reactive IgE directed to carbohydrate determinants of glycoproteins. J Allergy Clin Immunol 1997;100:327–334.
112. Leung PS, Chow WK, Duffey S, Kwan HS, Gershwin ME, Chu KH. IgE reactivity against a cross-reactive allergen in crustacea and mollusca: evidence for tropomyosin as the common allergen. J Allergy Clin Immunol 1996;98:954–961.

2

Percutaneous and Intracutaneous Diagnostic Tests of IgE-Mediated Diseases (Immediate Hypersensitivity)*

Paul C. Turkeltaub
Center for Biologics Evaluation and Research, Food and Drug Administration, Rockville, Maryland

* The views expressed in this article are the personal opinion of the author and not the official opinion of the U.S. Food and Drug Administration.

I. CLINICAL APPLICATION

The fundamental application of skin testing is to detect mast cell-bound immunoglobulin (IgE) specific for the allergen introduced in the skin (i.e., detection of sensitization). The allergy skin test in this context can be viewed as a human bioassay to detect cell-bound allergen-specific IgE analogous to in vitro tests that detect circulating allergen-specific IgE. In contrast to in vitro tests, cutaneous allergen-induced inflammation also reflects allergic disease in miniature. The immediate cutaneous inflammatory response occurs due to the release of mast cell inflammatory mediators triggered by binding of the allergen to mast cell-bound allergen-specific IgE, thus mimicking the natural disease. Skin testing also can help to determine the clinical relevance of an allergen. It can indicate the likelihood that other organs, or the organism as a whole, will exhibit an allergic inflammatory response to the same or a cross-reacting allergen after a systemic, local, natural, or iatrogenic exposure.

Sensitivity refers to the dose of allergen required to elicit a defined cutaneous response. *Reactivity* refers to the cutaneous response to a defined dose, usually the full-strength allergen. Both sensitivity and reactivity are surrogate measures of the quantity of cell-bound allergen-specific IgE.

The skin test is clinically relevant because it reflects the immunopathogenesis of the allergic disease of interest. Because it is based on the response of the intact organism, skin testing also provides clinical information pertinent to the allergen of interest unavailable by in vitro assay. Allergy skin test procedures and test vaccines have not been completely standardized, and their optimal use remains to be determined by adequate and well-controlled studies of diagnostic efficacy.

Diagnostic efficacy is defined operationally by demonstrating that skin tests enable accurate and reproducible clinical decisions. Such decisions might include: distinguishing allergic from nonallergic patients; identifying patients likely to respond to allergen avoidance/control measures intended to prevent elicitation of symptoms or tissue priming; distinguishing patients who likely would respond favorably to allergen immunotherapy from those who would not; identifying patients who might be at high risk of allergic reactions from allergen immunotherapy; and estimating a safe initial dose for immunotherapy.

Research skin test applications include: comparing allergen sensitivity among patients to assess risk of developing allergic disease; comparing allergen sensitivity within patients over time to determine the effectiveness of immunotherapy and antiallergic agents or the influence of environmental exposures; comparing the relative potency of one allergen with another to standardize allergens biologically; evaluating the accuracy, precision, and sensitivity of skin test devices and methods; and evaluating the proficiency of individuals who perform skin test procedures.

The variety of skin test methodologies used for the clinical applications cited above have been the subject of review articles and practice guidelines (1–6). The history of allergen skin testing has been reviewed (5–7). Blackley (1873) first described the application of pollen to the abraded skin of a pollen allergic individual. Smith (1909) used the Von Pirquet scarification technique to administer a food allergen. Noon and Freeman (1911) used the scratch test, whereas Cooke (1911) used intracutaneous tests to administer allergen. Lewis and Grant (1924) described the prick test, which was quantitatively analyzed by Squire (1950) to estimate the volume administered (3×10^{-6} mL). Pepys modified the prick test (1970), thus encouraging its widespread use.

II. ROUTES OF ADMINISTRATION

There are three skin test routes:

1. Epicutaneous: The prefix ''epi'' means ''on.'' *Epicutaneous* refers to application of the allergen on the skin surface (for example, open or closed patch testing for eliciting delayed contact hypersensitivity). Because allergen usually does not gain access to mast cells through intact skin unless it has been traumatized (8) percutaneously or intracutaneously, this method is not routinely used for detecting immediate hypersensitivity. In the natural history of contact urticaria (an epicutaneous route of exposure), the skin barrier is commonly impaired by concomitant chemical/solvent-induced irritant/contact dermatitis (9,10).
2. Percutaneous: The prefix ''per'' means ''through.'' *Percutaneous* refers to application of allergen through the skin surface (for example, scratching, pricking, or puncturing the skin).
3. Intracutaneous: The prefix ''intra'' means ''within.'' *Intracutaneous* refers to application of allergen within the topmost layers of the skin.

A. Percutaneous Test Methods/Devices

Scarification and scratch methods were used initially to traumatize the skin to permit entry of allergen. Scratch tests may result in nonspecific reactions due to trauma (11), and they are somewhat more variable (12) and less sensitive than prick tests (13).

In a puncture test, the dose of the skin-reactive substance is applied topically and a device—needles (solid or hollow), lancets, or tines—is inserted through the drop into the topmost layers of the skin (Fig. 1). When the device pierces the skin and the tip is lifted so that a tiny needle track in which the skin reactive substance can flow is formed, this is called a prick/puncture test when the device is lifted to form a tiny needle track through which the skin-reactive substance can traverse (5).

A large number of percutaneous devices are commercially available and have been evaluated for variability in reactivity (5,14–20). These devices vary in size, number of puncture needles/tines, shapes (e.g., lancets, hollow, or solid needles), depth of insertion, and force and angle with which the skin is pierced. Different techniques such as rotation, puncture, or prick/puncture methods may even be used for the same device, with differing effects on the size of positive and negative controls, reproducibility of results, and degree of patient discomfort (15,18). The proper technique for use within or between devices differs. Experienced technicians obtain differing reaction sizes with each device for both positive and negative controls. Therefore, each physician should establish criteria with each device for positive and negative skin prick tests for each technician (14). The differences in the number and dimensions of the percutaneous needles used and in the technique of administration influence both the level of discomfort experienced with each device and the size of the cutaneous response to both positive and negative controls (15). Device-related differences in cutaneous reactivity have been explained based on the degree of trauma induced (15) and as a result of the device's physical characteristics and the method and force of test application. Devices inducing the greatest trauma produce the largest responses

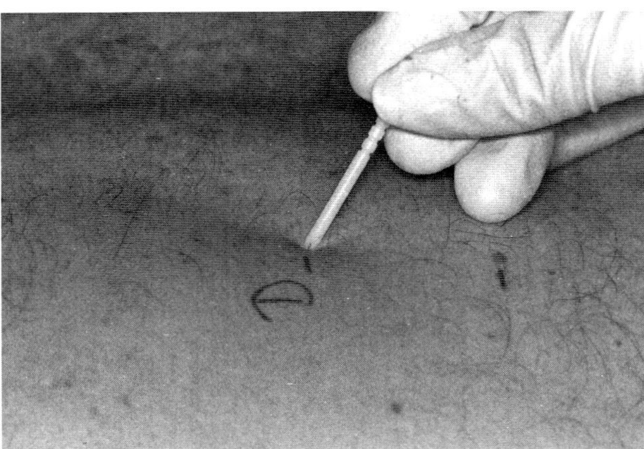

Figure 1 Percutaneous test using disposable device. Black lines applied to subject's back identify separate tests.

to histamine or allergen and are less likely to elicit a negative response on testing. They are also more likely to induce responses to the negative control and to cause discomfort.

The relative accuracy of percutaneous devices for detecting differences in known concentrations of skin reactive substances (20) has not been studied systematically. The relative sensitivity for many percutaneous devices based on analysis of dose-response lines (16,17) also has not been studied systematically. Although studies of the percutaneous reactivity to a single dose of histamine or glycerinated saline have been conducted, the dose of histamine used in many studies is not commercially available for physicians to replicate the results (14,15,19). Because data comparing the cutaneous response at two different histamine doses are limited, it is unclear whether the two dose responses can be differentiated (4). Moreover, there is a discrepancy in the histamine dose (histamine base 10 mg/mL) used for evaluating devices (14,15) and the histamine dose (histamine dihydrochloride 10 mg/mL) recommended for biological standardization in the Nordic countries (4,21,22). Assessment of adequate percutaneous device performance based on two different commercially available doses of histamine base (0.1 and 1.8 mg/mL) falling within specified but differing ranges of reactivity responses has been proposed (23).

Because data with percutaneous devices are operator dependent, these devices should be combined with a proficiency program to ensure that they can be used without excess negative responses with the positive control (analytic false negatives) and excess positive responses with the negative control (analytic false positives), respectively. Because the force with which the device is applied can be adjusted, the same device can give very different dose responses depending on the operator (16). Device instructions do not provide information to guide the physician on the expected cutaneous reaction sizes with doses of histamine. It will not be possible to evaluate the relative analytical performance of each device or to assess the proficiency of an operator until proficiency limits are specified for accuracy, precision, and sensitivity. Reactive substances may be applied using different techniques, even for the same device, thus influencing the response to the positive and negative controls as well as the subject's assessment of acceptability and comfort (15,18). The relative merits of different devices have yet to be determined in the absence of standards for assessing analytical performance with a common, validated method, skin test reagents which can be used to assess proficiency, and manufacturer-defined reactivity estimates provided to guide appropriate use. Because technique of application produces such marked test variability in devices, technician-specific response levels of significance must be established for each device and for both the positive and negative controls obtained with the specific device (14).

Although it is fraught with device, technique, and operator variability, percutaneous testing is generally accepted as the initial route for screening for cutaneous reactivity to allergen because of its convenience, deceptive simplicity, lesser degree of patient anxiety compared to that experienced with needle and syringe injections, and relative safety.

1. Percutaneous Controls

Because the size of the cutaneous response also depends on the degree of trauma induced by the test procedure, it is essential that appropriate positive and negative controls be administered. The positive control, usually histamine, verifies that the skin is capable of responding to an inflammatory mediator released through the allergic response. Verification that the positive control elicits a positive response avoids an analytic false negative skin test due to end organ unresponsiveness as may occur after the use of antihistamines, for example. In the United States, histamine doses approved for percutaneous testing are: histamine base 1.0 mg/mL (Center Labs, Port Washington, NY), histamine base 1.8 mg/mL (Allermed Labs, San Diego, CA), and histamine base 6 mg/mL (Hollister-Stier Labs LLC, Spokane, WA). The respective histamine package inserts discuss the cutaneous responses observed with specified percutaneous devices.

Opiates elicit secretion of mast cell inflammatory mediators and have been used as positive skin test controls. However, these agents have not been shown to have an advantage over histamine (4).

The vaccine diluent, commonly 50% glycerin, serves as the negative control, which verifies that the skin test device/technique/operator is not traumatically inducing an analytic false positive cutaneous response due to triple response (24), dermographism, or irritants contained in the diluent. Glycerin is viscous and forms coherent drops that are less likely to run than drops applied from aqueous vaccines.

B. Intracutaneous Test Method

The method of intracutaneous injection is straightforward (Fig. 2). The preferred syringe is a 0.5 mL allergy syringe that improves accuracy of delivery in the 10–50 μL range and has a unitized narrow gauge needle (e.g., 27 gauge) and an intradermal bevel to minimize trauma. The unitized design eliminates leakage at the syringe-needle interface. The larger intracutaneous injection volume (0.05 mL) is intended to increase reproducibility (5) by reducing the effect of any leakage on the amount delivered. Leakage will be a function of technique (i.e., whether the bevel is inserted sufficiently). An intradermal bevel decreases the length of needle tip insertion. Bevel down injection reduces leakage, increases comfort, and reduces trauma at the injection site (25) while avoiding eye splash

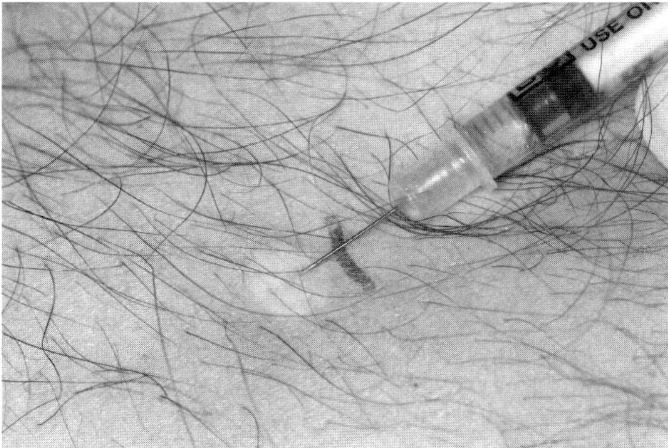

Figure 2 Intracutaneous test. Needle (bevel-down) produces wheal in subject's upper arm.

for the technician. A defined volume for intracutaneous injection is more reproducible than an undefined volume that creates a specified bleb size, because the depth of injection and the tissue characteristics may influence bleb size independent of the volume injected (26).

1. Intracutaneous Controls

The positive controls available for intracutaneous testing are histamine bases 0.1 mg/mL (5) (Center Labs, Port Washington, NY) and 0.0006 mg/mL (Hollister-Stier Laboratories LLC, Spokane, WA). The recommended intracutaneous dose is 0.1 μg of histamine base (27). The observed intracutaneous responses at the histamine doses tested (1 μg and 0.1 μg [Center Labs] and 0.12 μg [Hollister-Stier Laboratories LLC]) are provided in the respective package inserts.

The negative control for intracutaneous testing is the diluent used to prepare dilutions containing 0.03% human serum albumin (HSA) for stability enhancement (28,29). Dilutions prepared from 50% glycerin-containing vaccines should use a negative control diluent containing the same concentration of glycerin (e.g., 0.5–5.0%) as found in the intracutaneous vaccine dilution. This enables detection of nonspecific wheal and erythema responses to the residual glycerin. Although 0.6% glycerin diluent in one study did not elicit intracutaneous wheals and 6.0% glycerin did, erythema responses were not quantitated (30).

C. Percutaneous Versus Intracutaneous (Erythema Versus Wheal)

1. Relative Sensitivity

Because percutaneous testing delivers a very small amount (~3 ηL in one estimate) of skin-reactive substance (31), it is analytically insensitive compared to intracutaneous administration, where 10–50 μL are administered. Because the amount of material administered will vary by percutaneous device/method/technician, the relative analytic sensitivity will be device/technician dependent. A comparison of skin test sensitivity to short ragweed vaccine in a given subject based on erythema dose-response lines indicated that intracutaneous testing required about a 30,000-fold lower dose of allergen to elicit the identical erythema response as percutaneous testing with the bifurcated needle (Allergy Labs of Ohio) (32). However, the relative sensitivity of percutaneous versus intracutaneous routes is dependent on the skin reactive substance inasmuch as histamine requires only a 1000-fold lower intracutaneous dose to elicit the same percutaneous erythema response (32). Use of wheal dose-response lines is problematic because of the relatively large initial bleb induced by intracutaneous testing. Estimates of the relative sensitivity of intracutaneous versus percutaneous testing in which the wheal response is included and a variety of percutaneous devices are used indicate that intracutaneous tests require 100,000–400,000-fold lower doses (1).

2. Reproducibility

Intracutaneous wheals and erythema have significantly higher reproducibility than percutaneous wheals and erythema (21,33). Reproducibility of intracutaneous wheal and erythema responses is similar (32,33), whereas percutaneous erythema is more reproducible than percutaneous wheal (12). Percutaneous administration is the most variable injection method because it depends on individual differences in the device/technique/technician.

3. Slope

The slopes of intracutaneous erythema response lines are significantly steeper (~ 5–7-fold) than the slopes of intracutaneous wheal response lines (32,33), especially when the erythema response is quantitated near the endpoint (32). Similarly, the slopes of intracutaneous erythema response lines measured near the endpoint (32) are significantly steeper than the slopes of percutaneous wheal response lines (21). Steeper slopes yield more accurate and precise estimates (32) when discriminating between different doses of allergen and, by extension, between different quantities of cell-bound, allergen-specific IgE.

4. *Test Sequence*

A practical approach based on the relative sensitivity and safety (see Sec. XI) of the two routes of skin testing uses percutaneous testing for screening and intracutaneous testing for confirming equivocal or negative percutaneous test results (5).

D. Allergen Doses

1. Percutaneous

Relatively high doses are used to determine cutaneous responses because percutaneous testing is analytically insensitive. Indicated percutaneous doses for standardized vaccines in the United States are: 10,000 AU/mL for *Dermatophagoides farinae* or *D. pteronyssinus* mite; 10,000 BAU/mL for standardized cat or cat pelt; and 10,000 BAU/mL for the eight standardized grass vaccines (Bermuda, Kentucky bluegrass, meadow fescue, orchard, perennial ryegrass, Redtop, sweet vernal, and timothy) (34). Although 100,000 BAU/mL grass vaccines are available, they are unsuitable for initial testing because they may elicit huge wheal and erythema reactions in highly reactive subjects (34), and systemic adverse reactions have been reported when several grass vaccines are percutaneously administered at the same time (35). For short ragweed, Amb a 1 doses exceeding 130 U/mL are available for percutaneous testing. For unstandardized vaccines, 1:10 or 1:20 w/v vaccines are commonly used for percutaneous testing, and lower concentrations of 1:50 w/v to 1:100 w/v or 10,000 PNU/mL are used less commonly. Standardized vaccines are formulated with 50% glycerinated diluent, a very good preservative and stabilizer of allergenic potency (28).

2. Intracutaneous

The dosage for intracutaneous testing is 100 BAU/mL for standardized cat/cat pelt and grass pollen vaccines and 100 AU/mL for dust mite when the 10,000 BAU/mL or AU/mL dose, respectively, is negative by percutaneous testing. This is based on the observation that a 100-fold lower allergen dose is required to elicit a positive intracutaneous response in an allergic subject if the percutaneous test is negative (36). This dilution factor results in a 1:1000 w/v or 1:2000 w/v intracutaneous dose when 1:10 w/v and 1:20 w/v concentrations, respectively, are negative by percutaneous testing (5). Preparation of fresh dilutions at 3-month intervals has been recommended due to loss of in vitro potency at dilutions recommended for intracutaneous testing (29). However, intracutaneous skin testing cannot detect a three- to fourfold variability in potency (95% confidence interval) between identical vaccines (32). Therefore, the clinical relevance of in vitro potency differences, where the magnitude of the difference and the 95%

confidence interval are undefined (29), requires confirmation before this recommendation is accepted for clinical implementation.

Safe intracutaneous doses for highly puncture-reactive subjects are specified in the package inserts for the following 10,000 BAU/mL vaccines, the eight standardized grass pollen vaccines, standardized cat/cat pelt vaccines, and 10,000 AU/mL dust mite (*D. pteronyssinus* and *D. farinae*) vaccines. The range in mean reactivity observed in highly reactive subjects tested percutaneously with these doses using the bifurcated needle is: mean erythema diameter range 35.5–43.5 mm and mean wheal diameter range 7–8.5 mm (34). The mean intracutaneous dose for a 25 mm mean erythema diameter in these highly puncture-reactive subjects is ~ 0.02 BAU or AU/mL (34). Thus a similar safe intracutaneous dose in these highly reactive subjects was observed for each of the specified standardized vaccines regardless of allergen source.

III. ISSUES IN MEASUREMENT AND RECORDING THE CUTANEOUS RESPONSE

To assure consistency, a number of factors need to be specified in the measurement and recording of the response.

A. Time to Measure Response

The response should be measured at its peak, which is 12–15 min for wheal size (37), 8–9 min for histamine, and 12–17 min for allergen (38). To simplify, responses can be recorded at 15 min with reevaluation at a later time (e.g., 25–30 min) to capture slower reaction peaks (11).

B. Making a Permanent Record of the Response

At the specified time, the response can be captured for placement in the medical record. This can be achieved simply by using a pen to outline the response (both wheal and erythema), placing transparent tape over the outline, and lifting the tape with the transferred outline and attaching it to the medical record (1).

C. Measurement of the Response

The simplest standard method to measure the skin response is to average the sum of the longest and midpoint orthogonal diameters (1). Criteria for skin test positivity are generally based on these mean response diameters (in millimeters). Reference can also be found in the medical literature to area of skin response in terms of mm^2 (3). It should be noted that the precision estimates for acceptability of a percutaneous response differ depending on whether the estimate is mean diameter or area (3).

D. Erythema Versus Wheal

Because the erythema response is several times larger and has a steeper slope near the endpoint, it should be quantitated along with the wheal response (1). Comparison of percutaneous (39) and intracutaneous (33) wheal and erythema sizes over a wide range of wheal sizes has demonstrated that erythema is consistently larger by at least a factor of 10, and that erythema tends to increase more rapidly (it has a steeper slope) at smaller wheal sizes (39). The larger erythema response and steeper slope increase the ability of percutaneous responses to discriminate among persons based on the size of the skin test response. For example, a skin test survey of a population in the United States (n = 16,204) found that 80% of the percutaneous test reactors fell between 2–5 mm for wheal diameter compared to 5–30 mm for erythema diameter (40). The precision of estimating erythema reactions versus wheal is similar (1). Because erythema dose-response is steeper near the endpoint than wheal dose-response, histamine doses differing tenfold were able to be detected by differences in the erythema response, but not by differences in the wheal response (1). Similarly, accurate interpretations of positive and negative controls are enhanced when erythema is considered while assessing reactivity (14). Erythema size highly correlates with release of inflammatory mediators, such as histamine (41), and thermographic estimates of inflammation (33) during the early cutaneous response and with the release of leukotrienes during the late phase response (41). The U.S. Joint Task Force on Practice Parameters states that ''both erythema and wheal should be measured and recorded in mm and compared with positive . . . and negative controls'' (5).

E. Grading of Skin Responses

The simplest method for grading reactions is to report the mean diameter of erythema and wheal (5). Use of semiquantitative grades of 0–4+ suffers from imprecision and ambiguity. Imprecision exists because wheal/erythema size criteria differ in each system. Often grades are based on whether wheal or erythema response is present or absent (42), above or below some size (43) or size range (44), or simply relative to a positive (11) or negative control (43), regardless of the actual size (11,43). Different grading systems for percutaneous (11,42) and intracutaneous responses have been proposed (43,44). Therefore, the same grade may be assigned to skin reactions that differ in size and presence of wheal and erythema, or different grades may be assigned to the identical allergic response depending on the size of the positive or negative control. If the same physician uses different grading systems for percutaneous and intracutaneous testing results, then the same skin test grade will differ depending on the route of administration. Because most physicians do not delineate their grading system when reporting their skin tests, semiquantitative grades are based on the size of wheal and erythema complicates communication both clinically and scientifically, as (45).

Similarly, the concept of relating allergen-induced skin reactions to a fixed concentration of a well-defined reagent, such as histamine, is flawed (33). Variability in the response to histamine is marked, the correlation between skin reactivity (especially wheal) to histamine and allergen is poor, and the relationship between the response to histamine and the allergic inflammatory response estimated by thermography is virtually nonexistent (33).

Reporting the actual size of wheal and erythema is accurate, precise, unambiguous, and easily communicated. The need for accurate and precise data to enhance clinical decision-making and facilitate patient diagnosis and treatment are among the chief goals of proficiency testing.

IV. ISSUES IN INTERPRETING THE RESPONSE

A. Skin Test Proficiency

With enactment of the Clinical Laboratory Improvement Amendments of 1988 (CLIA), a congressional initiative to promote uniform quality and standards among all laboratories in the United States by means of proficiency testing, greater awareness has been given to the analytical performance of tests and the proficiency with which they are conducted (46). To apply the concept of proficiency to allergy skin testing (47) requires evaluation of the analytical performance of the test in estimating the analyte of interest, allergen-specific IgE.

B. Analytical Performance of Skin Test

Analytical test performance (48) refers to the accuracy, precision, and sensitivity of a test in measuring the analyte of interest (i.e., whether the test accurately discriminates between sensitization [detectable cell-bound allergen-specific IgE] and no sensitization [no detectable cell-bound allergen-specific IgE]). The analytical test performance needs to be distinguished from the clinical test performance (49,50). *Clinical test performance* is defined by the clinical accuracy of the test (i.e., whether the test accurately discriminates between allergic disease + sensitization and no allergic disease + sensitization).

The analyte of interest in the allergy skin test is the quantity of cell-bound allergen-specific IgE. The cutaneous inflammatory response is the detection signal for this analyte because the analyte cannot be directly measured, and the cutaneous response is due to mast cell degranulation and inflammatory mediator release that results from allergen binding to cell-surface allergen-specific IgE (see Sec. V). In any test system, the dose-response relationship is critical in determining the accuracy, precision, and sensitivity of the test results (51). For example, it can be hypothesized that two patients with identical skin test dose-responses (identical skin sensitivity) to the same allergen have the identical quantity of cell-bound allergen-specific IgE (52).

In this context, skin sensitivity refers to the dose of allergen eliciting a defined response. In order for the response to meaningfully reflect the quantity of analyte, it needs to be in the steep slope portion of the allergen dose-response where the magnitude of the allergic response (e.g., erythema response near the endpoint) is dramatically affected by small changes in dose (i.e., steep slope) (1,2,32). In a flat dose-response (e.g., wheal response), the magnitude of the allergic response is less affected by relatively large dose differences. That is, varying allergen doses produce similar responses (1,2). Flat dose responses will give inaccurate, imprecise estimates, whereas steep dose responses will give accurate, precise estimates of sensitivity (1,2,32). Therefore, the slope of the dose response is critical in defining the accuracy and precision of the skin test, and skin test variables resulting in steep dose-response lines will give more accurate estimates of the analyte. Because the dose response in biological systems is assumed to be sigmoidal, it is necessary to demonstrate that there is a consistent, defined relationship between allergen dose and skin response. The more cell-bound allergen-specific IgE, the larger the allergen skin response should be. However, the quantity of cell-bound IgE is constant in each patient. Therefore the skin test must be in a portion of the dose-response curve where the larger the allergen dose, the larger the skin response. Because the erythema response is steeper than the wheal response near the endpoint (32), the midpoint erythema response—or dilution for sum of erythema = 50 mm (the D_{50})—can be used to compare skin sensitivity as long as there is a defined linear response ($r \geq 0.93$) and a steep slope (≥ 13) (53). Skin test titration can establish this response. Endpoint titration provides an inadequate estimate of sensitivity because it does not define the linearity of the response, the slope, or the midpoint of the assay (1,2,6,54).

The analytical performance of the skin test is defined operationally if the difference between two known histamine doses can be estimated by skin test dose-response lines (accuracy), the estimates of the difference fall within defined statistical limits (precision), and the skin sensitivity (D_{50}) is specified for each histamine dose. Technicians whose accuracy, precision, and sensitivity fall within the specified limits demonstrate proficiency (47). A proficiency method has been proposed for intracutaneous testing (47), refined on the basis of increased clinical experience (55), implemented for regulatory purposes (23,56), and simplified for clinical application (57). This method is also applicable for evaluating the analytical performance of percutaneous tests (16) because the mean slope of the percutaneous dose-erythema response lines (~ 12) is very similar (32) to the acceptable lower slope limit ($\geq$ 13) for intracutaneous dose-erythema response lines (23).

In brief, the intracutaneous proficiency method for clinical practice entails the preparation of eight threefold dilutions from the respective histamine base concentrates of 1.8 mg/mL and 0.1 mg/mL. Each respective concentrate is labeled ''dilution #0.'' The threefold dilutions proceed from ''dilution #1'' to ''dilution #8.'' A new syringe and needle set is used to prepare each dilution. Because the expected relative potency is 18 (1.8/0.1), an accurate skin test procedure should detect an eighteenfold difference between these two histamine concentrations. For the titration, 0.05 mL is injected, beginning with ''dilution #8.'' Erythema and wheal are outlined and measured at 15 minutes. The purpose of the titration is to determine the endpoint (first dose with minimal erythema) and the next three serial doses where graded erythema brackets 50 mm (sum of erythema diameters). The dilution number producing a sum of erythema between 45–55 mm is the estimated D_{50} (ED_{50}). Interpolating between the two dilutions bracketing 50 mm can also derive the ED_{50}. The difference between the ED_{50} of each histamine concentrate is the $\log_3$ relative potency. The expected mean difference is 2.5 (2–3) threefold dilutions equivalent to a relative potency of $3^{2.5}$ (3^2 to 3^3) or 15.6 (9 to 27). Because the expected relative potency is 18, the acceptable accuracy of this skin test is 87% (15.6/18), with a range of 50–150% of the expected value when six subjects are tested. The standard deviation of the mean ED_{50} for acceptable precision should be below 0.6 when $n = 6$. For acceptable test sensitivity, the expected mean ED_{50} for histamine base 1.8 mg/mL and 0.1 mg/mL is 6.5 (5.5–7.5) and 4 (3–5), respectively.

Percutaneous proficiency testing using a model similar to the above would require a histamine concentration (16,20) that is commercially unavailable.

C. Reactivity Versus Sensitivity

For convenience, most allergy skin testing records the cutaneous response to a single dose of allergen rather than defining the allergen dose response. The skin test response at a single dose can be defined as *skin test reactivity*. Because the portion of the dose-response line in which skin test reactivity is elicited is not determined, the analytical accuracy and sensitivity of this response cannot be ascertained. Skin testing is designed to detect any cell-bound allergen-specific IgE. Thus the most concentrated allergen doses are conventionally used to determine reactivity. Inasmuch as skin test reactivity does not define the dose response, the response may occur in the flat portion of the curve, and different doses may give the same response. Differences of 100-fold in vaccine potency may yield identical percutaneous wheal responses (6), and patients with the same reactivity may have very different sensitivities. For example, percutaneous erythema reactivity has been correlated with intracutaneous sensitivity defined as the dose eliciting a 50 mm sum of erythema diameter response (47). Although reactivity was correlated with sensitivity, the same percutaneous erythema reactivity could be associated with intracutaneous erythema sensitivity estimates differing more than 100-fold. Similarly, percutaneous wheal reactivity is also associated with intracutaneous wheal sensitivity, but the same wheal reaction may also yield sensitivity estimates varying 100- to 1000-fold (58) or wheal reactivity varying ±1 mm could differ over 10,000-fold in sensitivity (59). This will result in situations where skin test reactivity does not accurately predict skin test sensitivity and the clinical significance of skin test reactivity may be in question if it is used as a measure of sensitivity (60). Although patients with greater percutaneous reactivity are generally more sensitive, reactivity estimates may yield inaccurate and imprecise skin sensitivity estimates because of variability imposed by technique/technician/device factors as well as by not defining in which part of the dose-response curve reactivity is obtained.

Because reactivity estimates do not specify the portion of the dose-response relationship, proficiency methods cannot address accuracy and analytic sensitivity. However, they can specify the reproducibility of the response when replicates are conducted (3). One approach defines acceptable percutaneous erythema reactivity ranges as mean sums of erythema diameter of 10–30 mm (histamine base 0.1 mg/mL) and 35–65 mm (histamine base 1.8 mg/mL) when six subjects are tested with the bifurcated needle (Allergy Laboratories of Ohio, Columbus, OH) (23).

D. Criteria for a Positive Response

1. Percutaneous Test

The wheal cutoff for a positive percutaneous test relative to the negative control has varied from 1–5 mm (61) with recent recommendations from European and American allergy organizations as follows: wheal diameter ≥3 mm or more (11); wheal diameter >3 mm (3); and wheal response >3 mm (with equivalent erythema) (5). Smaller wheals (1–2 mm) with erythema and itching have also been considered as likely indicators of cell-bound allergen-specific IgE when the control sites are completely negative (6,61). Larger wheal cutoffs appropriate for each device/technique/technician need to be specified because of the larger negative control wheals many of these induce (Sec. II.A). Subtracting a negative control response from the allergen response is inadequate to correct for the variability in eliciting traumatic responses at negative control sites (15).

The erythema cutoff for a positive percutaneous test has been defined as 10–10.5 mm (40,62–65). This erythema cutoff has been favorably compared to varying wheal sizes (3–20 mm) in discriminating between symptomatic and asymptomatic patients (66), has been confirmed as a conservative, reliable estimate of immediate hypersensitivity (67), and is cited as an acceptable cutoff in recent reviews of skin testing (5,6).

Elicited erythema may be considered as a positive test, despite little or no wheal formation (40,62–65). For example, the quantity of histamine required to elicit erythema is tenfold less than that required to elicit a wheal (68). Efforts to reduce the frequency of analytic false negative percutaneous reactions elicited by the positive control take advantage of the increased analytic sensitivity of the lower threshold for a positive erythema response. These consider as a positive skin test either the wheal or erythema response that exceeds the respective threshold (14). Defining a positive test by either wheal or erythema criteria for a positive percutaneous skin test to histamine rather than requiring satisfaction of both criteria reduced the rate of analytic false negative responses to the positive control ten- to twentyfold (14). However, cutoffs based on the larger erythema responses will give more conservative estimates of skin positivity (40,67) because small skin responses ($\leq$ 5 mm diameter) are associated with increased variability in measurement (1). Similarly, small wheals without accompanying erythema exceeding the erythema threshold should be considered doubtful because the wheal dose-response is flatter near the endpoint than the erythema dose response. However, erythema responses exceeding the threshold have been considered positive even in the absence of a wheal response (42).

2. Intracutaneous Test

The semiquantitative grading method of Norman and others (44) specifies a minimal cutoff for a positive intracutaneous test when the wheal diameter is within 5–10 mm and the surrounding erythema diameter is either 11–20 mm or 21–30 mm (69). The 11–20 mm erythema diameter is associated with a 3–5.9 mm wheal, whereas the 21–30 mm-diameter erythema corresponds to a 6–9 mm wheal diameter (59). Either cutoff is acceptable because both the smaller (69) and larger (59) intracutaneous wheal and erythema diameter ranges are associated at high dilutions with allergen-specific IgE. However, a minimal cutoff of 6 mm wheal diameter and 21 mm erythema diameter is the more conservative intracutaneous cutoff based on the preceding observations and is more consistent with the 5–10 mm wheal diameter range associated with erythema that Norman and others specified for a positive intracutaneous response (69). In this regard, an intracutaneous endpoint cutoff of 20 mm erythema diameter was used to diagnose cat allergy and it detected significant decreases in skin sensitivity following cat immunotherapy (70). Although any intracutaneous response larger than the negative control may indicate the presence of specific IgE (5), concern has been raised regarding the clinical significance of small positive intracutaneous reactions (5) and the need for a more conservative intracutaneous cutoff (71).

V. IMMEDIATE AND LATE-PHASE REACTIONS

Binding of allergen to mast cell allergen-specific IgE results in the immediate release of preformed mediators (mast cell degranulation) and de novo synthesis of inflammatory mediators over a period of hours. The exposure of cutaneous receptors to the liberated neuroinflammatory mediators results in a cutaneous response characterized by local vasodilatation followed by plasma leakage from postcapillary venules (wheal) and stimulation of peptidergic nerves causing the axon reflex (erythema) (68) and itch.

The kinetics of the allergic response consists of the early (10–20 min) wheal and erythema response, which regresses after 1 h. A late response develops in a large percentage of subjects as the allergen dose is increased and progressive subcutaneous swelling with erythema reappears at 3–4 h, peaks at 9 h (5–22 h), and subsides 24–48 h later (41,72).

Both the early- and late-phase reactions are allergen-specific IgE-dependent (54,72), and the likelihood of eliciting a late-phase response at lower allergen doses is increased in the more sensitive allergic subjects (72). One dosing strategy is to conduct an intracutaneous titration to determine the dose eliciting an immediate wheal response of $\geq$10 mm (or wheal with pseudopods) and erythema $\geq$40–45 mm (41,73). The late-phase reaction dose is tenfold higher than this dose. This strategy induces late-phase reactions in 87% of subjects, but it is associated with a high risk of adverse reactions (41). The erythema size correlates very closely with the peak of histamine during the immediate allergic response and with leukotrienes 6 to 7 h after challenge (41).

Several cellular changes are associated with these allergic reactions (72,74). There is an early eosinophil influx at 5 min to 1 h. In the late phase, there is progressive neutrophil leukocytosis with eosinophils and basophils. During the latter portion of the late phase, there is a shift to mononuclear cells. Inflammatory mediators in the early phase consist of histamine, tryptase, prostaglandin D_2 (PGD_2), and leukotriene C_4 (LTC_4), with a subsequent late rise in histamine without tryptase. PGD_2 and LTC_4 remain elevated. Interleukin (IL)-1β, IL-6, E-selectin endothelial-leukocyte adhesion molecule-1 (ELAM-1), IL-4, and IL-5 RNA appear as early as 1–1.5 h after reaction onset with subsequent detection of granulocyte-macrophase colony-stimulating factor (GM-CSF), tumor necrosis factor (TNF)α, regulated on activation, normal T-cell-expressed, and secreted (RANTES), monocyte chemotactic peptides (MCP-3), and platelet activating factor (PAF), followed by IL-2 and interferon (IFN)γ signals detected at 48 h. Corticosteroids do not influence the early response significantly but diminish the late response and its associated eosinophilic and basophilic infiltration. H1 antagonists (antihistamines) inhibit the early response without affecting the late response. The early immediate allergic cutaneous response is mainly mediated by mast cells, whereas basophils, eosinophils, neutrophils, and lymphocytes are responsible for the late phase.

Neurogenic inflammation is likely to contribute to the cutaneous allergic response in addition to the cells and inflammatory mediators identified (74–76). The identity of the neurotransmitters responsible for the human allergen-induced cutaneous axon reflex response (erythema and pruritus) remains unknown (75).

VI. CLINICAL PERFORMANCE: PERCUTANEOUS/INTRACUTANEOUS TESTS

A. Diagnostic Accuracy: Sensitivity/Specificity

The *clinical performance* of a test relates to its ability to discriminate between clinical states, whereas *analytic performance* pertains to a test's ability to discriminate between differences in the quantity of an analyte, such as mast cell-bound allergen-specific IgE (Sec. IV.B).

Because skin testing, except for intracutaneous testing (23), has not been adequately standardized on the basis of analytic performance, published studies describing clinical performance of skin testing may not be applicable to the vaccines, skin test methods, and devices used in clinical practice.

The terms ''sensitivity'' and ''specificity'' are commonly used in discussions of clinical test performance (49,50). Clinical *sensitivity* is defined as the test-positive fraction that has the clinical condition of interest (i.e., the true positive fraction). *Specificity* is defined as the test-negative fraction that does not have the clinical condition of interest (i.e., the true negative fraction). The equation (1 − specificity) defines the false positive fraction.

Optimal clinical performance is defined on the basis of the test cutoff, which maximizes clinical sensitivity (the true positive rate) and minimizes the false positive rate (1 − specificity). Predicated on the use of the terms clinical sensitivity and specificity is the proviso that the test has defined analytic performance/proficiency and that the true clinical condition is diagnosed using a ''gold standard.'' Example of gold standards include defining insect sting allergy based on the response to an insect sting challenge; defining ragweed allergy based on the response to natural airborne exposure to ragweed pollen; and diagnosing food allergy based on a double-blind, placebo-controlled food challenge.

Gold standard studies are labor intensive, costly, and require special precautions to reduce and control the risk associated with exposure to the suspect allergen. Thus they are not frequently used. Surrogates such as patient history or end organ (e.g., nasal, bronchial) challenges have been used in lieu of a gold standard definition of the true clinical state. Because percutaneous test methodologies have not been standardized (5), their analytic test performance has not been determined, many test vaccines are not standardized, and gold standard studies are often not used to establish the true clinical state of the patient. Published studies of clinical skin test performance may not accurately reflect their true clinical performance, and it may not be possible to extrapolate them to skin test methodologies used in clinical practice. Therefore, the diagnostic efficacy of percutaneous testing remains to be established (6).

B. Clinical Utility

An approach to defining clinical performance/diagnostic efficacy is to demonstrate a test's clinical utility in discriminating among patients with differing clinical responses to the allergen of interest. For example, a standardized skin test method (47,53) with defined analytic performance, proficiency, and cutoff (intracutaneous D_{50}) enabled investigators to distinguish between subjects with regard to symptom severity to natural ragweed pollen exposure (60), risk of systemic reaction to ragweed immunotherapy (60), and degree of symptomatic benefit derived from ragweed immunotherapy (60).

Another study noted a similar relationship between intracutaneous ragweed sensitivity and symptom severity on natural exposure to ragweed (69). In both studies, the intracutaneous D_{50} associated with increased symptom severity after natural ragweed exposure was $\leq 10^{-5}$ µg/mL Amb a 1 for sum of erythema diameter ~50 mm. The predictive value of the specified positive intracutaneous ragweed test at this dose exceeds 90% in patients claiming to have hay fever symptoms associated with the fall ragweed pollen count (47).

C. Analytic True Positive Test: Sensitization (Circulating Allergen-Specific IgE as a Surrogate for Cell-Bound Allergen-Specific IgE)

Skin testing has been used to quantitate the degree of sensitization (quantity of cell-bound allergen-specific IgE) in addition to distinguishing different disease states, clinical conditions, and therapeutic and safety outcomes in response to interventions. This measurement is really an estimate of the analytic accuracy of the skin test, because cell-fixed allergen-specific IgE is the critical analyte assayed by the skin test. It can be present independent of the disease state (i.e., asymptomatic sensitization) (5,6). Direct measurement of basophil-bound allergen-specific IgE is problematic (77), let alone the ability to quantify mast cell-bound allergen-specific IgE that is chiefly responsible for the immediate cutaneous response to allergen (41,74). In this respect the cutoffs recommended as the lower limit for a positive skin test (Sec. IV.D) are considered indicative of mast cell sensitization (analytic true positive test), but not necessarily indicative of allergic disease (clinical false positive test). Assays of circulating allergen-specific IgE (which is in equilibrium with cell-bound allergen-specific IgE [78,79]) have been used as surrogates for cell-bound IgE. They show a significant association between intracutaneous skin test sensitivity for the dust mite, *D. pteronyssinus* (wheal = 8 mm) (59), and short ragweed (wheal diameter 5–10 mm, erythema diameter 22–60 mm range) (69) at ≤1 : 10,000 v/v skin test dilutions of the respective vaccine concentrates. At more concentrated intracutaneous dilutions that yield positive skin tests, the association is less significant or circulating specific IgE is not detectable (59,69). Similarly, a significant association between intracutaneous sensitivity (dose for erythema diameter = 10 mm) to five purified major allergens (Der p 1 and Der p 2 mite allergens, Fel d 1 cat allergen, and Lol p 1 and Lol p 2 grass allergens) and their respective circulating allergen-specific IgE levels was observed at doses ≤1 : 100 v/v dilution of the grass and cat allergens and at doses ≤1 : 10,000 v/v dilution of the mite allergens (80).

A significant association has been reported between circulating allergen-specific IgE and percutaneous wheal size using a lower limit wheal diameter cutoff of 1 mm or greater (81) and 3 mm or greater (82,83). However, the correlation observed when using skin sensitivity estimates is reportedly higher than the association based on skin reactivity estimates using a single full-strength vaccine dose (80).

Despite the correlation between skin test reactivity and circulating allergen-specific IgE, which is assay dependent (84), approximately 20% of patients with a positive intracutaneous test (85) and 30% (17% for pollens; 41% for dog, cat, house dust) of patients with a positive (≥ 3 mm) percutaneous test (83) have undetectable circulating allergen-specific IgE to the skin reactive allergen. A review (59) of studies comparing circulating allergen-specific IgE and percutaneous test positivity also reported that 10–25% of patients with a positive percutaneous test have no detectable circulating allergen-specific IgE to the skin reactive allergen, thus demonstrating the higher sensitivity of the skin test. If the circulating allergen-specific IgE was intended to be a surrogate for cell-bound allergen-specific IgE, then the negative in vitro tests were analytic false negative tests inasmuch as the skin test detected cell-bound allergen-specific IgE.

Many subjects with positive intracutaneous tests at less than 1 : 1000 v/v dilution of the concentrate but no circulating allergen-specific IgE were found to have cell-bound allergen-specific IgE using basophil histamine release measurements (85). In subjects who reacted at the highest intracutaneous dose (1 : 1000 v/v dilution of the concentrate), many of the basophils did not release histamine on allergen challenge, but these cells also did not respond to the positive control (anti-IgE). Thus, the basophils were desensitized (78), and it could not be concluded that allergen-specific cell-bound IgE was absent (85). Serologic assays are analytically less sensitive than skin tests for detecting cell-bound allergen-specific IgE (69,85). Biologically irrelevant IgE specific for cross-reactive carbohydrate determinants may account for positive intracutaneous test responses at very high test concentrations (1 : 10–1 : 100 v/v dilutions of the concentrate) in percutaneous negative, RAST-positive subjects (86).

D. Diagnostic Accuracy: Clinical History as "Non-Gold Standard"

Estimates of clinical sensitivity (true positive fraction) and specificity of skin testing using the patient history as the "non-gold standard" are not possible because the true clinical state is unknown. Inasmuch as published studies refer to these terms, however, they will be used for illustrative purposes. Clinical performance of a percutaneous test using timothy grass (1:20 w/v) and a minimal skin test cutoff of erythema with wheal as a positive response estimated the sensitivity as 0.75 and specificity as 0.89 (false positive fraction 0.11) (87). For cat (1:50 w/v), estimated sensitivity was 0.57 and specificity 0.84 (87). Using intracutaneous reactivity (100-fold dilution of concentrate) with a cutoff of 8–12 mm wheal with erythema, the sensitivity slightly increased for timothy (0.79), but the specificity decreased (0.84). Similarly, the intracutaneous positivity for cat increased sensitivity (0.81), but decreased specificity (0.67) (87). Another study (66) using standardized cat vaccine at a dose equivalent to 5000 BAU/mL and percutaneous reactivity defined as erythema of 10 mm or more (or wheal $\geq$ 3 mm) estimated clinical sensitivity as 0.91 (or 0.90) and specificity as 0.90 (0.90). These indicated that clinical performance was similar for both erythema and wheal cutoffs. Percutaneous testing using the wheal cutoff at 500 BAU/mL substantially reduced sensitivity to 0.57, but increased the specificity to 0.96. Thus the overall accuracy of the test was slightly improved at the tenfold lower dose (66). Another study aimed at optimizing clinical performance found optimal sensitivity and specificity when timothy and dust mite (*D. pteronyssinus*) vaccines were diluted tenfold for percutaneous testing and 1000-fold for intracutaneous testing (88). The approximate cutoffs of percutaneous wheal larger than 2 mm and intracutaneous wheal larger than 7 mm yielded sensitivity/specificity estimates of 0.85/0.79 and 0.75/0.70, respectively (89).

Reasonable estimates of sensitivity and specificity thus can be obtained by using either the percutaneous or intracutaneous route with commercially available vaccines at the recommended doses and cutoffs (5). It should be noted that increasing the skin test dose of allergen increases sensitivity but decreases specificity (i.e., increase the clinical false positive rate), whereas lower doses decrease sensitivity but increase specificity (i.e., lower the clinical false positive rate) (66,88). The converse is true at any dose tested for lowering (i.e., increased sensitivity/decreased specificity) or raising the cutoff value (i.e., decreased sensitivity/increased specificity) (88).

The use of patient history is inadequate as a gold standard (90). To detect the true clinical state of the patient, the gold standard must be based on an allergen challenge (preferably double blind) that simulates natural exposure. Examples include establishing insect sting allergy based on the response to an insect sting challenge or diagnosing food allergy on the basis of a double-blind, placebo-controlled food challenge.

1. Differentiating Sensitized Symptomatic Patients from Sensitized Asymptomatic Patients

Individuals with a family history but without a personal history of allergy may have a high prevalence (45%) of percutaneous reactivity, although it is lower than the prevalence (90%) in persons with a personal history of allergy (66). Even those with no personal or family history of allergy may have a prevalence of percutaneous reactivity as high as 30% (66) or 58% (71). Similarly, percutaneous reactivity to dust mite may be increased in nonallergic persons (66) and may result in an increased rate of false positives, even with a tenfold dilution of the concentrate, when patient history and levels of circulating dust mite-specific IgE are used as the non-gold standards (89). A mean percutaneous wheal diameter exceeding 6 mm has been recommended as a cutoff with 0.61 sensitivity and 0.60 specificity to differentiate between sensitized, symptomatic from sensitized, asymptomatic persons (91).

2. Gold Standard Studies: Percutaneous Versus Intracutaneous

The clinical performance of timothy grass skin testing was determined in relation to a gold standard defined in subjects with a history of grass rhinitis by the response to timothy pollen nasal challenge and by symptom diaries kept during the grass pollen season (92). Subjects with negative percutaneous but positive intracutaneous tests (wheal ≥ 6 mm with erythema) to timothy 1000 AU/mL were no more likely to have grass allergic rhinitis than a skin test negative group with a history of grass rhinitis (92). Of the individuals with a history of grass pollen allergy who had positive percutaneous tests (wheal ≥ 3 mm and erythema ≥ 5 mm) to timothy 100,000 AU/mL, 46% were diagnosed as true positives (92). Although different doses (100,000 AU/mL and 10,000 AU/mL) of timothy vaccine were used for percutaneous testing, with minimal differences in mean wheal and erythema size between the two doses (35,92), no estimates of sensitivity/specificity were obtained. The 10,000 AU/mL dose would be expected to have higher specificity and thus higher accuracy, because only one grass-allergic subject reportedly was missed at this dose (92). Moreover, different recommended, more conservative cutoffs (e.g., erythema ≥ 10 mm) that would increase specificity at both doses were not evaluated.

The percutaneous timothy skin test true positive rate of 46% in the diagnosis of rhinitis (92) based on timothy pollen nasal challenge and natural pollen exposure is similar to the true positive rates reported for gold standard challenges in insect sting, latex, and food allergy. The intracutaneous venom skin test true positive rate for diagnosing anaphylactic insect sting allergy is approximately 60% based on a gold standard insect sting challenge (93). The percutaneous latex skin test true positive rate is about 50% for diagnosing latex asthma based on gold standard natural latex glove inhalation challenge (94). The percutaneous (wheal $\geq$ 3 mm to 1:10–1:20 w/v glycerinated food extracts) true positive rate for food allergy is less than 50% based on a gold standard double-blind food challenge (95). These data suggest that further optimization in the allergen dose or cutoff is desirable to increase sensitivity and specificity. It should be noted that the negative predictive value of a percutaneous test (wheal $<$3 mm) to good quality food extracts is considered to be more than 95%. Thus, a negative percutaneous test excludes IgE-mediated food allergy (95).

Intracutaneous positive, percutaneous negative food tests are not associated with food allergy based on double-blind food challenges (i.e., they have very high clinical false positive rates) and the intracutaneous route is not recommended for routine food testing (95). Intracutaneous testing of venoms is recommended to determine clinically significant sensitization that would require the initiation of venom immunotherapy and, conversely, determine when sensitization has been lost and venom immunotherapy can be discontinued safely (93). Intracutaneous testing of drugs at appropriate doses is also recommended to determine clinically significant sensitization that requires drug avoidance (96) or possible desensitization that would permit certain drugs (e.g., penicillin) to be readministered safely ($\sim$ 95% negative predictive value; 50% positive predictive value) (96). (T.J. Sullivan, personal communication).

VII. VARIABLES INFLUENCING SKIN TEST RESULTS

A. Site of Injection

The back elicits significantly larger percutaneous allergen wheals (27%) and erythema (14%) responses than the arm (97). Based on parallel-line intracutaneous tests comparing the back to the arm using standardized Bermuda grass, the back was 37% more reactive than the arm ($p \sim 0.05$) based on the erythema response (P.C. Turkeltaub and J.J. Murray, unpublished data). The rate of percutaneous reactivity to eight allergens was increased 2.3% when tested on the back rather than the forearm (97). Percutaneous wheal and erythema are largest in the mid-back and smallest at the lower back (12). Differences in reactivity of the forearm have been reported, with minimal reactivity at the wrist and maximal reactivity at the antecubital fossa, volar more reactive than dorsal, and ulnar more reactive than radial (38).

B. Distance Between Injection Sites

To prevent interaction between skin test sites due to overlap of erythema or lymphatic spread of cellular mediators or vaccine, it is recommended that skin test sites should be at least 5.0 cm apart (38). Analytic false positive percutaneous reactions are noted more commonly in proximity to a positive allergen response than to a histamine control, probably due to the larger size of the allergen response (33). The rate of false positive responses is decreased from 1.5–2.0% to less than 1.0% at a distance of 7.5 cm between sites (97). This report did not analyze subjects with very large skin responses and ≥7.5 cm may be a reasonable intersite distance to use when large responses are anticipated (33). Because the analytic false positive rate is relatively low (1.5–2.0%) at shorter distances of 2.0 to 5.0 cm (97), it would be prudent to use the higher end of this range simply to reduce the likelihood of an overlap of adjacent erythema responses.

C. Time of Day/Season

Allergen (98) and histamine (99) reactivity has been reported to be larger in the morning, but without clinical significance. An increase (~ 5%) in the prevalence of percutaneous reactivity to ragweed was observed in the U.S. population just after the ragweed pollen season in high ragweed pollen regions (40). A boost in ragweed reactivity also has been observed at the end of ragweed pollination, but this was accompanied by an increase in histamine reactivity as well as reactivity to perennial allergens and tree pollens (100). Another study reported an increase in grass and tree pollen reactivity in the fall, no increase in histamine reactivity, and a decrease in reactivity to animal dander and house dust (82). These data suggest a seasonal effect, but they should not affect clinical interpretation (6).

D. Age

Percutaneous reactivity to allergens is age dependent. Reactivity peaks between ages 12–24 years with progressive decrease with advancing age and progressive increase from childhood (40,63). In the same age range, the rate of reactivity to histamine based on the erythema response remains relatively constant until age 55 when it decreases slightly (40). Percutaneous histamine wheal response reportedly increases gradually from infancy to a peak between 15–50 years, with decreased wheal size in later years (101) and before the age of 6 months (102).

E. Race

Rates of percutaneous allergen reactivity (erythema ≥ 10.5 mm) were observed to be higher in blacks compared to whites in the U.S. population, but the difference was not statistically significant (40,63). Similarly, the rate of histamine reactivity using either wheal or erythema response was slightly lower in both percent-positive and mean size in American blacks, but in neither case did the difference reach statistical significance (40).

F. Gender

In the U.S. population white males statistically have a higher prevalence of allergen reactivity than white females (63). Increased skin test reactivity of males has been observed in other studies (103,104).

G. Socioeconomic Status

The prevalence of allergen skin test reactivity in high income families is significantly increased compared to families living at or below the poverty level in the United States (63). There is also a positive association between years of education and prevalence of percutaneous reactivity, with nearly double the rate of reactivity at the extremes of educational attainment (63). Another report confirmed this association with educational level, which could not be explained by an inverse association of prevalence of percutaneous reactivity with family size (105).

H. Tobacco Smoke Exposure

No effect of smoking was observed in the U.S. population on the prevalence of allergen skin test reactivity or mean size of allergen erythema or wheal in perennial nonsmokers and former or active smokers (including those who smoked 1–10, 11–20, or 21+ cigarettes per day) (65).

I. Medication

The medications that most commonly suppress skin test reactivity to allergen and histamine are H1 antagonists (antihistamines). Skin test suppression may be variable and persist from 24 hours to 1 week depending on the antihistamine and its dose. Astemizole may suppress skin tests for up to 1–2 months (6). Tricyclic antidepressants also exert suppressive effects on skin tests, which may persist for 1 week or more (6). Retention of histamine reactivity in the positive skin test control should permit evaluation of allergen reactivity unless the agent interferes with mast cell degranulation.

VIII. NUMBER OF TESTS

The number of tests (5) is tailored to the patient's history and probability of allergen exposure. Consideration needs to be given to the different locales and environments to which the patient may be exposed, whether at home, work, school, daycare, vacation, or elsewhere. The taxonomic relationship, cross-reactivity, and airborne dispersal, if any, need to be considered to reduce the number and redundancy of vaccines tested.

Skin testing with mixtures of unrelated allergens may dilute clinically relevant allergens within the mixture so much that analytic false negative tests result.

An upper limit on the number of skin tests (e.g., 70 percutaneous tests and up to 40 intracutaneous tests) has been proposed, but such limitations may be a problem in selected patients.

IX. PATIENT SELECTION FACTORS

Any patient for whom a determination of allergen sensitization is considered clinically relevant is a candidate for skin testing. The skin surface used for testing should be normal (e.g., no urticaria or dermatographism). Cutaneous reactivity may be reduced in diabetes, chronic renal failure, spinal cord injuries, cancer, and eczema (6).

X. FREQUENCY OF SKIN TESTING

Indications for additional testing include a change in the pattern of symptoms (e.g., development of new symptoms) or a change in exposure (e.g., geographic relocation).

Repeat skin testing during immunotherapy is indicated if symptoms persist or new symptoms develop after adequate dosing. Repeat testing to determine whether venom hypersensitivity has waned is indicated after 3 years. Comparative skin testing of a current treatment formulation with respect to a replacement treatment formulation is also an indication for additional skin testing.

XI. SAFETY

Percutaneous allergy testing in a cross-section of the U.S. population (n = 16,204) was found to pose minimal risk with a rate of adverse reactions of 0.04% (none allergic), which is comparable to other minimal risk procedures, such as venipuncture (0.49%) and body measurements (0.006%) (106). Anaphylactic reactions are more likely to occur in patients suspected of allergy. In a safety survey of 18,311 patients suspected of allergy who were tested by the percutaneous route, the adverse reaction rate was 0.04%. However, all were systemic allergic reactions with an asthma component (107). In a 1-year survey of an allergy practice in which 1144 patients received percutaneous allergen skin tests followed by intracutaneous tests when indicated, systemic reactions occurred in 6% of tested patients (108). An allergic systemic reaction rate of 1.4% was observed in a survey ($n = 3236$) of the safety of venom skin testing in which the intracutaneous route was used (109). Fatalities after skin testing are extremely rare and occur more frequently after intracutaneous testing, especially when percutaneous testing is not used initially to screen for reactivity (110). Only one fatality due to skin testing has been reported in the United States this decade, and this occurred after intracutaneous testing in an asthmatic individual (111)

Although allergy skin testing is safe, patients and physicians should take precautions to reduce the risk of a serious adverse event. All patients should be tested under the supervision of an appropriately trained physician and qualified medical personnel who have ready access to emergency medical supplies (112). A patient's medical status should be evaluated 20 min after testing before he or she is permitted to leave the office (113). Concomitant use of beta-blockers or angiotensin-converting enzyme inhibitors may result in refractory anaphylaxis if the allergen elicits a systemic reaction (113).

XII. SALIENT POINTS

1. The allergen skin test is a human bioassay that detects mast cell-bound allergen-specific IgE.
2. The three cutaneous routes of allergen administration are (1) epicutaneous–patch test; (2) percutaneous–prick, puncture, or scratch test; and (3) intracutaneous (intradermal) test.
3. Percutaneous tests inherently produce more variable results than intracutaneous tests because of differences in devices, techniques of administration, and technicians.
4. Percutaneous testing is generally accepted as the initial route for screening for immediate hypersensitivity because of its convenience, deceptive simplicity, less patient anxiety than that experienced with syringes and needles, and relative safety.
5. Because the percutaneous route is relatively insensitive, negative or equivocal percutaneous results with allergen concentrates (e.g., 10,000 BAU/mL) can be confirmed as analytic true negative by the intracutaneous route with 100-fold test dilutions (e.g., 100 BAU/mL).
6. Both wheal and erythema should be measured and compared with positive and negative controls to detect a positive response. Proficiency is an important consideration in allergy skin testing.
7. Percutaneous cutoffs for a positive test are wheal of 3 mm or more and erythema of more than 10 mm. Semiquantitative grading systems (0–4+) should be discontinued because of their imprecision and ambiguity.

8. Conservative intracutaneous cutoffs for a positive test are wheal of 6 mm or larger and erythema of 21 mm or more.
9. The package inserts of standardized vaccines provide the intracutaneous dose for a 25-mm erythema response (~ 0.02 BAU/mL) in patients with large percutaneous responses (e.g., wheal 7 mm/erythema 40 mm) to the same allergen. This provides target intracutaneous test or initial immunotherapy allergen doses in patients with percutaneous responses similar to those specified in the insert.
10. Clinical history is inadequate to determine the true clinical state. In studies using this inadequate standard, sensitivity (a misnomer without knowledge of the true clinical state) ranged from 0.57–0.90 for percutaneous testing and 0.75–0.81 for intracutaneous testing. Specificity (also a misnomer) ranged from 0.84–0.96 for percutaneous testing and 0.67–0.84 for intracutaneous testing.
11. Standardized vaccines, standardized skin test methods, and proficiency programs are needed to distinguish patients with allergic disease due to specific allergen sensitization from those who are sensitized but have no symptoms related to the specific allergen.
12. The positive predictive value of skin testing based on a gold standard provocative challenge definition of the true clinical states for latex, Hymenoptera insect sting, food, penicillin, and timothy grass allergy is approximately 50%. The negative predictive value of food allergy or penicillin testing can exceed 95%.
13. The prevalence of percutaneous reactivity peaks in adolescents and young adults. Prevalence is higher in males and in individuals with higher socioeconomic status. Tobacco smoke inhalation does not influence allergen prevalence or reactivity.
14. Percutaneous allergy testing has a very low rate of adverse events: approximately 0.04%. The rate of intracutaneous test adverse events is somewhat higher: about 1%. Adverse events for both routes in up to 6% of patients have been reported when a wide array of allergens is tested. Fatalities due to skin testing are extremely rare and generally follow intracutaneous testing, especially when percutaneous testing is not used as an initial screen for reactivity.

ACKNOWLEDGMENT

Photographs of percutaneous and intracutaneous tests courteously provided by Stephen F. Kemp, M.D., University of Mississippi Medical Center, Jackson, Mississippi.

REFERENCES

1. Turkeltaub PC. In vivo methods of standardization. Clin Rev Allergy 1986;4:371–387.
2. Turkeltaub PC. Allergenic extracts. II. In-vivo standardization. In: Middleton E Jr, Reed CE, Ellis E, Adkinson NF, Jr, Yunginger JW, eds. Allergy Principles and Practice. 3rd ed. St. Louis: CV Mosby, 1988;388–401.
3. Dreborg S, Frew A, eds. Allergen standardization and skin tests. Position Papers. Allergy 1993;48 (suppl 14):48–82.
4. Nelson HS. Clinical application of immediate skin testing. In: Spector SL, ed. Provocation Testing in Clinical Practice. New York: Marcel Dekker, 1995;703–727.
5. Bernstein IL, Storms WW. Practice parameters for allergy diagnostic testing. Ann Allergy Asthma Immunol 1995;75 (no. 6, pt II): 543–625.
6. Demoly P, François-Bernard M, Bousquet J. In vivo methods for study of allergy skin tests, techniques, and interpretation. In: Middleton E Jr, Reed CE, Ellis E, Adkinson NF, Jr, Yunginger JW, Busse WW, eds. Allergy Principles and Practice. 5th ed. St. Louis: Mosby-Year Book, 1998;430–439.
7. Vaughn WT, Black JH. Practice of allergy. St. Louis: Mosby, 1954, p. 52.
8. Hamilton RG, Adkinson NF Jr. Validation of latex glove provocation procedure in latex-allergic subjects. Ann Allergy Asthma Immunol 1997;79:266–272.
9. Charous BL, Hamilton RG, Yunginger JW. Occupational latex exposure: characteristics of contact and systemic reactions in 47 workers. J Allergy Clin Immunol 1994;94:12–18.
10. Douglas R, Morton J, Czarny D, O'Hehir RE. Prevalence of IgE-mediated allergy to latex in hospital nursing staff. Aust NZ J Med 1997;27:165–169.
11. Skin tests used in type I allergy testing. Position paper. Dreborg S, editor. Allergy 1989;44 (suppl 10):1–59.
12. Galant SP, Maibach HI. Reproducibility of allergy epicutaneous test techniques. J Allergy Clin Immunol 1973;51:245–250.
13. Indrajana T, Spieksma FThM, Voorhorst R. Comparative study of the intracutaneous scratch and prick tests in allergy. Ann Allergy 1971;29:639–650.
14. Nelson HS, Lahr J, Buchmeier A, McCormick D. Evaluation of devices for skin prick testing. J Allergy Clin Immunol 1998;101:153–156.
15. Nelson HS, Rosloniec DM, McCall LI, Ikle D. Comparative performance of five commercial prick skin test devices. J Allergy Clin Immunol 1993;92:750–756.
16. Matthews J, Delasko J, Turkeltaub PC, Rastogi SC. The analytical performance of six puncture devices. J Allergy Clin Immunol 1993;91 (pt 2):280.
17. Engler DB, DeJarnatt AC, Sim TC, Le JL, Grant AJ. Comparison of the sensitivity and precision of four skin test devices. J Allergy Clin Immunol 1992;90:985–991.
18. Corder WT, Wilson NW. Comparison of three methods of using the DermaPIK with the standard prick method for epicutaneous skin testing. Ann Allergy Asthma Immunol 1995;70:434–438.
19. Adinoff A, Rosloniec DM, McCall LL, Nelson HS. A comparison of six epicutaneous devices in the performance of immediate hypersensitivity skin testing. J Allergy Clin Immunol 1989;84:168–174.

20. Turkeltaub PC, Zenger V, Rastogi SC. The accuracy and precision of percutaneous testing for estimating relative potency and patient sensitivity: a comparison of the bifurcated versus the 25 gauge needle. J Allergy Clin Immunol 1989;83 (pt 2): 257.
21. Malling HJ. Skin prick testing in biological standardization of allergenic products. Arb Paul Ehrlich Institut 1997;91:157–163.
22. Dreborg S, Basomba A, Belin L, Durham S, Einarsson R, Eriksson NE, Frostad AB, Grimmer O, Halvorsen R, Holgersson M, et al. Biological equilibration of allergen preparations: methodological aspects and reproducibility. Clin Allergy 1987;17:537–550.
23. Turkeltaub PC, Rastogi SC. Quantitative intradermal procedure to determine relative potency and compositional differences of allergenic extracts using parallel line bioassay: screening and proficiency method. Revised Nov 1994. In: Methods of the Allergenic Products Testing Laboratory, Congressional and Consumer Affairs, CBER, HFM 46, document 0148. Rockville, MD.
24. Lewis T. Vascular reactions of skin to injury; reaction to stroking; urticaria and factitia. Heart 1924;11:119–139.
25. Howard A, Mercer P, Nataraj HC, Kang BC. Bevel-down superior to bevel-up in intradermal skin testing. Ann Allergy Asthma Immunol 1997;78:594–596.
26. Rappaport BZ, Becker EL. Quantitative studies in skin testing. IV. The volume-response relationship. J Allergy 1949;20:358–363.
27. Report of the Committee on Standardization: I. A method of evaluating skin test response. Ann Allergy 1971;29:30–34.
28. Baer H, Anderson MC. Allergenic Extracts I. Sources, preparation and in vitro standardization. In: Middleton E Jr, Reed CE, Ellis E, Adkinson NF, Jr, Yunginger JW, eds. Allergy Principles and Practice. 3rd ed. St. Louis: CV Mosby, 1988:373–388.
29. Nelson H, Ikle D, Buchmeier A. Studies of allergen extract stability: the effects of dilution and mixing. J Allergy Clin Immunol 1996;98:382–388.
30. Lindblad JH, Farr RS. The incidence of positive intradermal reactions and the demonstration of skin sensitizing antibody to extracts of ragweed and dust in humans without history of rhinitis or asthma. J Allergy 1961;32:392–401.
31. Squire JR. The relationship between horse dandruff and horse serum antigens in asthma. Clin Sci 1950;9:127–150.
32. Turkeltaub PC, Rastogi SC, Baer H, Anderson MC, Norman PS. A standardized quantitative skin test assay of allergen stability: studies on the allergen dose-response curve and effect of wheal, erythema, and patient selection on assay results. J Allergy Clin Immunol 1982;70:343–352.
33. de Weck AL, Derer T. Critical evaluation of the use of skin tests and cellular tests in standardization of allergens. Arb Paul Ehrlich Institut 1994;87:89–117.
34. Turkeltaub PC. Biological Standardization. Arb Paul Ehrlich Institut 1997;91:145–156.
35. Redfern DC, Keane BB, Esch RE, Murray JJ. Optimal concentration of standardized grass extracts for epicutaneous testing. Ann Allergy 1993;70:92.
36. Stenius B. Skin and provocation tests with *Dermatophagoides pteronyssinus* in allergic rhinitis: comparison of prick and intracutaneous skin test methods and correlation with specific IgE. Acta Allergol 1973;28:81–100.

37. Hordle DA, Mehta V, Tomensen B, Wainscott G. Development of skin prick test for allergen assay. J Immunol Methods 1984;75:369–382.
38. Voorhorst R, van Krieken H. Atopic skin test reevaluated. Perfection of skin test technique. Ann Allergy 1973;31:137–142.
39. Lavins BJ, Dolen WK, Nelson HS, Weber RW. Use of standardized and conventional allergen extracts in skin prick testing. J Allergy Clin Immunol 1992;89:658–666.
40. Gergen PJ, Turkeltaub PC. Percutaneous immediate hypersensitivity to eight allergens, United States 1976–80. National Center for Health Statistics, Vital and Health Statistics. Series 11, No.235. DHHS Pub. No. (PHS) 86-1685. Public Health Service, Washington DC, US Government Printing Office, July 1986;1–73.
41. Reshef A, Kagey-Sobotka A, Adkinson NF Jr, Lichtenstein LM, Norman PS. The pattern and kinetics in human skin of erythema and mediators during the acute and late phase response. J Allergy Clin Immunol 1989;84:678–687.
42. Freedman SO. Asthma and allergic rhinitis. II. Clinical aspects. In: Freedman SO, Gold P, eds. Clinical Immunology. 2nd ed. Hagerstown: Harper & Row, 1976:131.
43. Terr AI. Allergic diseases. In: Fudenberg HH, Stites DP, Caldwell JL, Wells JV, eds. Basic and Clinical Immunology. 3rd ed. Los Altos: Lange Medical Publications, 1980:515.
44. Norman PS. In vivo methods of study of allergy: skin and mucosal test, techniques, and interpretation. In: Middleton E Jr, Reed CE, Ellis EF, eds. Allergy Principles and Practice. 2nd ed. St. Louis: CV Mosby, 1983:297.
45. Holbreich M, Nelson HS. Skin test recording techniques among allergists. J Allergy Clin Immunol 1998;101(no 1, pt 2):S249.
46. Stull TM, Hearn TL, Hancock JS, Handsfield JH, Collins CL. Variation in proficiency testing performance by testing site. JAMA 1998;279:463–467.
47. Turkeltaub PC. Biological standardization of allergenic extracts. Allergol Immunopathol (Madr.) 1989;17:53–65.
48. Doumas BT. The evaluation and limitations of accuracy and precision standards. Clin Chim Acta 1997;260:145–162.
49. Zweig MH, Ashwood ER, Collinsworth WL, Galen RS, Robinowitz M. Assessment of the clinical accuracy of laboratory tests using receiver operating characteristic (ROC) plots. Approved Guideline. NCCLS Document GP10-A, Vol. 13(no. 28), 1995. National Committee for Clinical Laboratory Standards, Wayne, PA.
50. Zweig M, Campbell G. Receiver-operating characteristic plots: a fundamental evaluation tool in clinical medicine. Clin Chem 1993;39:561–577.
51. Zweig MH, Kroll MH. Linear regression of minimal detectable concentration. Thyrotropin as an example. Arch Pathol Lab Med 1997;121:948–955.
52. Voorhorst F, Spieksma FThM, Varekamp H. House dust atopy and the house dust mite. Leiden: Stafleu's Scientific Publishing Co., 1969:18–31.
53. Turkeltaub P, Rastogi SC. Quantitative intradermal procedure for evaluation of subject sensitivity to standardized allergenic extracts using the $ID_{50}EAL$ (Intradermal Dilution for 50 mm sum of erythema determines the bioequivalent allergy unit) method. Revised Nov. 1994. In: Methods of the Allergenic Products Testing Laboratory, Congressional and Consumer Affairs, CBER, HFM 46, document #0148, Rockville, MD.

54. Van Metre TE Jr, Adkinson NF Jr, Kagey-Sobotka A, Marsh DG, Norman PS, Rosenberg GL. How should we use skin testing to quantify IgE sensitivity? J Allergy Clin Immunol 1990;86:583–586.
55. Turkeltaub PC, Mandel J, Zenger V. International collaborative evaluation of the accuracy and precision of relative potency estimated by parallel-line skin test. J Allergy Clin Immunol 1990;85(no 1, pt 2):292.
56. Methods of the Allergenic Products Testing Laboratory: Availability. (Docket No. 94N-0012) Federal Register 1994:59 (225);60362–60363.
57. Matthews J, Delasko J, Turkeltaub PC. An approach to evaluating proficiency of intradermal testing. J Allergy Clin Immunol 1992;89(no 1, pt 2):367.
58. Santilli J Jr, Potsus RL, Goodfriend L, Marsh DG. Skin reactivity to purified pollen allergens in highly ragweed sensitive individuals. J Allergy Clin Immunol 1980; 65:406–412.
59. Hamilton RG, Adkinson NF Jr. Assessment of human allergic diseases. In: Rich RR (editor-in-chief). Clinical Immunology: Principles and Practice. St. Louis: Mosby-Year Book, 1995:2169–2186.
60. Turkeltaub PC, Campbell G, Mosiman JE. Comparative safety and efficacy of short ragweed extracts differing in potency and composition in the treatment of fall hay fever. Allergy 1990;45:528–546.
61. Sears MR. Risk Factors: Immunoglobulin E and Atopy. In: Barnes PJ, Grunstein MM, Lieff AR, and Woolcock M, eds. Asthma. Philadelphia: Lippincott-Raven Publishers, 1997:71–82.
62. Ohman JL, Kendall S, Lowell, FC. IgE antibody to cat allergens in an allergic population. J Allergy Clin Immunol 1977;60:317–323.
63. Gergen P, Turkeltaub PC, Grace M. The prevalence of allergic skin test reactivity to eight common aeroallergens in the US population. Results from the Second National Health and Nutrition Examination Survey. J Allergy Clin Immunol 1987;80: 669–679.
64. Gergen PJ, Turkeltaub PC. The association of allergen skin test reactivity and respiratory disease among whites in the US population: data from the Second National Health and Nutrition Examination Survey 1976–80. Arch Intern Med 1991;151: 487–492.
65. Turkeltaub PC, Gergen PJ. Epidemiology of allergic disease and allergen skin test reactivity in the US population: data from the Second National Health and Nutrition Examination Survey (1976–80)-NHANES II. In: Kurth R, ed. Regulatory Control and Standardization of Allergenic Extracts. Sixth International Paul Ehrlich Seminar, Sept. 5–7, 1990. Stuttgart: Gustav Fischer Verlag, Arb. Paul Ehrlich Instit. 1992;85:59–82.
66. Adinoff AD, Rosloniec DM, McCall LL, Nelson HS. Immediate skin test reactivity to Food and Drug Administration approved standardized extracts. J Allergy Clin Immunol 1990;86:766–774.
67. Lucas SK, Buckley CE III. Quantitative studies of cutaneous hypersensitivity: the prevalence of epicutaneous flare reactions to allergenic pollen extracts. J Allergy Clin Immunol 1989;84:465–474.
68. Petersen LJ, Church MK, Skov PS. Histamine is released in the wheal but not the

flare following challenge of human skin in vivo: a microdialysis study. Clin Exp Allergy 1997;27:284–295.
69. Norman P, Lichtenstein LM, Ishizaka K. Diagnostic tests in ragweed hayfever. A comparison of direct skin tests, IgE antibody measurements, and basophil histamine release. J Allergy Clin Immnunol 1973;52:210–224.
70. Van Metre TE Jr, Marsh DG, Adkinson NF Jr, Kagey-Sobotka A, Khattignavong A, Norman PS, Rosenberg GL. Immunotherapy decreases skin sensitivity to cat extract. J Allergy Clin Immunol 1989;83:888–899.
71. Brown WG, Halonen MJ, Kaltenborn WT, Barbee RA. The relationship of respiratory allergy, skin test reactivity, and serum IgE in a community population sample. J Allergy Clin Immunol 1979;63:328–335.
72. Peters S, Zangrilli JG, Fish JE. Late phase allergic reactions. In: Middleton E Jr, Reed CE, Ellis E, Adkinson NF, Jr, Yunginger JW, Busse WW, eds. Allergy Principles and Practice. 5th ed. St. Louis: Mosby-Year Book, 1998:342–355.
73. Charlesworth EN, Hood AF, Soter NA, Kagey-Sobotka A, Norman PS, Lichtenstein CM. Cutaneous late phase response to allergen. Mediator release and inflammatory cell infiltration. J Allergy Clin Immunol 1989;83:1519–1526.
74. Charlesworth, EN. The role of basophils and mast cells in acute and late reactions in the skin. Allergy 1997;52(suppl 34):31–43.
75. Petersen LJ, Winge K, Brodin E, Skov PS. No release of histamine and substance P in capsaicin-induced neurogenic inflammation in intact human skin in vivo: a microdialysis study. Clin Exp Allergy 1997;27:957–965.
76. Wallingen I. The pathophysiology of itch. Clin Rep 1993;3:643–647.
77. Pruzansky JJ, Patterson R. Limiting concentrations of human basophil bound IgE antibody required for histamine release. Immunology 1988;64:307–310.
78. Siraganian R. Biochemical events in basophil or mast cell activation and mediator release. In: Middleton E Jr, Reed CE, Ellis E, Adkinson, NF, Jr, Yunginger JW, Busse WW, eds. Allergy Principles and Practice. 5th ed. St. Louis: Mosby-Year Book, 1998:204–227.
79. Schellenberg RR, Adkinson NF Jr. Assessment of the influence of irrelevant IgE on allergic sensitivity to two independent allergens. J Allergy Clin Immunol 1979; 63:15–22.
80. Witteman AM, Stapel SO, Perdok GJ, Sjamsoedin DH, Jansen HM, Aalberse RC, van der Zee JS. The relationship between RAST and skin test results in patients with asthma or rhinitis: a quantitative study with purified major allergens. J Allergy Clin Immunol 1996;97:16–25.
81. Stenius B, Wide L, Seymour WM, Holford-Strevens V, Pepys J. Clinical significance of specific IgE to common allergens. 1. Relationship of specific IgE against *Dermatophagoides* spp. and grass pollen to skin and nasal tests and history. Clin Allergy 1971;1:37–55.
82. Haahtela T, Jaakonmaki L. Relationship of allergen-specific IgE antibodies, skin prick tests, and allergic disorders in unselected adolescents. Allergy 1981;36:251–256.
83. Vanto T. Efficiency of different skin prick testing methods in the diagnosis of allergy to dog. Ann Allergy 1982;49:340–344.

84. Kelso JM, Sodhi N, Gosselin VA, Yunginger JW. Diagnostic performance characteristics of the standard Phadebas RAST, modified RAST, and Pharmacia CAP system versus skin testing. Ann Allergy 1991;67:511–514.
85. van der Zee JS, de Groot H, van Swieten P, Jansen HM, Aalberse RC. Discrepancies between skin test and IgE antibody assays: study of histamine release, complement activation in vitro, and occurrence of allergen-specific IgE. J Allergy Clin Immunol 1988;82:270–281.
86. van der Veen MJ, van Ree IL, Aalberse RC, Akkerdaas J, Koppelman SJ, Jansen HM, van der Zee JS. Poor biologic activity of cross-reactive IgE directed to carbohydrate determinants of glycoproteins. J Allergy Clin Immunol 1997;100:327–334.
87. Williams PB, Dolen WK, Koepke JW, Selner JC. Comparison of skin testing and three in vitro assays for specific IgE in the clinical evaluation of hypersensitivity. Ann Allergy 1992;68:34–45.
88. Niemeijer NR, Goedewaagen B, Kauffman HF, de Monchy JG. Optimization of skin testing. I. Choosing allergen concentrations and cutoff values by factorial design. Allergy 1993;48:491–497.
89. Niemeijer N, Fluks AF, deMonchy JGR. Optimization of skin testing. II. Evaluation of concentration and cutoff values, as compared with RAST and clinical history, in a multicenter study. Allergy 1993;48:498–503.
90. Murray AB, Milner RA. The accuracy of features in the clinical history for predicting atopic sensitization to airborne allergens in children. J Allergy Clin Immunol 1995;96:588–596.
91. Pastorello EA, Incorvaria C, Ortolani C, Bonini S, Canonica GW, Romagnani S, Tursi A, Zanussi C. Studies on the relationship between the level of specific IgE antibodies and the clinical expression of allergy: I. Definition of levels distinguishing patients with symptomatic from patients with asymptomatic allergy to common aeroallergens. J Allergy Clin Immunol 1995;96:580–587.
92. Nelson HS, Oppenheimer J, Buchmeier A, Kordash TR, Freshwater LL. An assessment of the role of intradermal skin testing in the diagnosis of clinically relevant allergy to timothy grass. J Allergy Clin Immunol 1996;97:1193–1201.
93. Report from the Committee on Insects. The discontinuation of Hymenoptera venom immunotherapy. J Allergy Clin Immunol 1998;101:573–575.
94. Vandenplas O, Delwiche JP, Evrard G, Aimont P, van der Brempt X, Jamart J, Delaunois L. Prevalence of occupational asthma due to latex among hospital personnel. Am J Respir Crit Care Med 1995;151:54–60.
95. Sampson HA. Adverse reactions to foods. In: Middleton E Jr, Reed CE, Ellis E, Adkinson, NF, Jr, Yunginger JW, Busse WW, eds. Allergy Principles and Practice. 5th ed. St. Louis: Mosby-Year Book, 1998:1162–1182.
96. Adkinson NF Jr. Drug Allergy. In: Middleton E Jr, Reed CE, Ellis E, Adkinson, NF, Jr, Yunginger JW, Busse WW, eds. Allergy Principles and Practice. 5th ed. St. Louis: Mosby-Year Book, 1998:1212–1224.
97. Nelson HS, Knoetzer J, Bucher B. Effect of distance between sites and region of the body on results of skin prick tests. J Allergy Clin Immunol 1996;97:596–601.
98. Vichyanond P, Nelson HS. Circadian variation of skin reactivity and allergy skin tests. J Allergy Clin Immunol 1989;83:1101–1106.

99. Paquet F, Boulet LP, Bedard G, Tremblay G, Cormier Y. Influence of time of administration on allergic skin prick tests response. Ann Allergy 1991;67:163–166.
100. Oppenheimer JJ, Nelson HS. Seasonal variation in immediate skin test reactions. Ann Allergy 1993;71:227–229.
101. Skassa-Brociek W, Manderscheid JC, Michel FB, Bousquet J. Skin test reactivity to histamine from infancy to old age. J Allergy Clin Immunol 1987;80:711–716.
102. Menardo JL, Bousquet J, Rodiere M, Astruc J, Michel FB. Skin test reactivity in infancy. J Allergy Clin Immunol 1985;75:646–651.
103. Sears M, Burrows B, Flannery E, Herbison GP, Holdaway MD. Atopy in childhood. I. Gender and allergen related risks for development of hayfever and asthma. Clin Exp Allergy 1993;23:941–948.
104. Friedhoff LR, Meyers DA, Marsh DG. A genetic-epidemiologic study of human responsiveness to allergens in an industrial population. II. The associations among skin sensitivity, total serum IgE, and age, sex, and the reporting of allergies in a stratified random sample. J Allergy Clin Immunol 1984;73:490–499.
105. Forastiere F, Agabiti N, Corbo GM, Dell'Orco V, Porta D, Pistelli R, Levenstein S, Perruci CA. Socioeconomic status, number of siblings, and respiratory infections in early life as determinants of atopy in children. Epidemiology 1997;8:566–570.
106. Turkeltaub PC, Gergen PJ. The risk of adverse reactions from percutaneous prick puncture allergen skin testing; venipuncture, and body measurements: data from the Second National Health and Nutrition Examination Survey 1976–80. J Allergy Clin Immunol 1989;84:886–890.
107. Valyasevi MA, Maddox DE, Li JT. Systemic reactions to skin tests at Mayo Clinic (abstr). J Allergy Clin Immunol 1998;101:S30.
108. Thompson M, Shearer D, Lockey R, Fox R, Ledford D. Systemic reactions to percutaneous and intradermal skin tests (abstr). J Allergy Clin Immunol 1998;101: S30.
109. Lockey RF, Turkeltaub PC, Olive CA, Baird-Warren IA, Olive ES, Bukantz SC. The Hymenoptera venom II. Skin test results and safety of venom skin testing. J Allergy Clin Immunol 1989;84:967–974.
110. Lockey RF, Benedict LM, Turkeltaub PC, Bukantz SC. Fatalities from immunotherapy and skin testing. J Allergy Clin Immunol 1987;79:660–677.
111. Allergen Standardization Committee requests reports on fatalities related to immunotherapy. Academy News, American Academy of Allergy, Asthma, and Immunology, June/July 1997:16.
112. The diagnosis and management of anaphylaxis. VII. Evaluation and management of patients with a history of anaphylaxis. J Allergy Clin Immunol 1998;101:S482–S485.
113. The diagnosis and management of anaphylaxis. VIII. Allergenic extracts and immunotherapy. J Allergy Clin Immunol 1998;101:S486–S487.

3

In Vitro Diagnostic Tests of IgE-Mediated Diseases

Robert G. Hamilton and Anne Kagey-Sobotka
Johns Hopkins University School of Medicine, Baltimore, Maryland

ABBREVIATIONS

ECP Eosinophil cationic protein
ELISA Enzyme-linked immunosorbent assay (two-site immunoassay

with allergen attached to a microtiter plate and enzyme-labeled detection antibody)

IEMA Immunoenzymetric assay (two-site immunoassay with antibody as a purified capture antibody and enzyme-labeled detection antibody)

IgE Immunoglobulin E

IRMA Immunoradiometric assay (two-site immunoassay with antibody as a purified capture antibody and radioiodinated detection antibody)

MBP Major basic protein from eosinophils

NAL Nonammoniated Latex

NCCLS National Committee on Clinical Laboratory Standards, Wayne, PA (body of academic, government, and manufacturing scientists who set laboratory standards)

RAST Radioallergosorbent test (two-site immunoassay with allergen attached to an allergosorbent medium and radioiodinated detection antibody for human IgE)

PST Puncture skin test

YJV Yellow jacket venom

The clinical immunology laboratory provides an array of analytical measurements that aid clinicians in the diagnosis, management, and epidemiological study of IgE-mediated diseases. After the discovery of IgE as a unique antibody isotype in the late 1960s, immunoassays were rapidly developed to quantify total serum IgE and allergen-specific IgE antibodies in human serum. During the subsequent 30 years, there have been marked improvements in the solid phase matrices, conjugate-labeling technology, and the availability of standardized reference reagents and more uniform data processing methods. These have led to more sensitive and specific assays for total and allergen-specific IgE antibody and other analytes that are useful in the diagnosis and management of individuals with type 1, or immediate-type, hypersensitivity.

This chapter focuses on methods for the detection and quantitation of IgE antibodies and their relative performance compared to in vivo tests. Assays for measuring vasoactive mediators (e.g., histamine) and markers of mast cell degranulation (e.g., tryptase) and eosinophilia (e.g., eosinophil cationic protein) are then discussed as alternative diagnostic and research methods. An inhibition format of the radioallergosorbent test (RAST) is reviewed within the context of measuring allergenic potency of skin test and immunotherapy vaccines. Two-site immunoenzymetric assays (IEMAs) for direct measurement of individual allergens in environmental specimens are presented as tools available for facilitating allergen avoidance by identifying allergen risks in home, school, and work environments. Finally, assays for research analytes that are used in the study of IgE-mediated diseases are reviewed briefly.

I. IN VITRO DETERMINATION OF IgE ANTIBODIES

The IgE antibody with defined allergen specificity is the single most important diagnostic analyte measured in the clinical immunology laboratory for assessing type 1 hypersensitivity. In 1968, the radioallergosorbent test was first introduced by Wide et al. for the detection of allergen-specific IgE antibody (1). As depicted in Figure 1, it used a cyanogen bromide-activated cellulose solid phase (paper disk) to which mixtures of proteins from one of several hundred known allergen sources were covalently bound. In this assay, the allergosorbent paper disk was inserted into a 12 × 75-mm plastic tube containing 0.1 mL of human serum. Antibodies specific for insolubilized proteins (allergens) then bound to the solid phase over a 16- to 18-h incubation period at room temperature. After a buffer wash to remove unbound proteins, bound IgE antibodies were detected with ^{125}I-labeled polyclonal antihuman IgE that is Fcε-specific. The amount of radioactivity bound to the allergosorbent after a final buffer wash was proportional to the amount of IgE antibody bound. Serum from nonallergic (negative) controls and highly allergic (positive) controls were analyzed in each assay to evaluate nonspecific binding and to provide a multipoint calibration curve from which semiquantitative estimates of IgE antibody were interpolated in arbitrary units.

This basic assay design has essentially remained unchanged. The quality of allergen components has improved as a result of optimizing the methods used in the extraction and quality control of allergens. New materials have enhanced the binding capacity and reduced the nonspecific binding properties of the solid phase matrix of allergosorbents. Various combinations of polyclonal and monoclonal anti-IgE detection antibodies have been developed to ensure maximal assay sensitivity and specificity for human IgE. Finally, calibration systems used in the newer commercial assays have adopted a generic ''heterologous interpolation'' method in which a total serum IgE curve (calibrated in international units of IgE per volume [IU/mL]) is used to convert allergen-specific IgE assay response data into quantitative dose estimates of IgE antibody. These changes have resulted in a ''second generation'' of immunoassays that display superior sensitivity and specificity and are more quantitative, reproducible, and automated than their earlier counterparts. This has also allowed the serological assay for IgE antibody to become more diagnostically competitive with its in vivo puncture skin test counterpart, even though the intradermal skin test still appears to possess an inherent advantage in terms of analytical sensitivity.

In spite of the convergence of the many commercial assays toward improved performance and common calibration schemes, the specific IgE antibody levels that are measured in the different assays cannot be considered interchangeable. Marked differences remain in the specificity of allergen that is present in the allergen-containing reagent. This results in detection in any given serum of a different population of allergen-specific IgE antibodies for an otherwise common

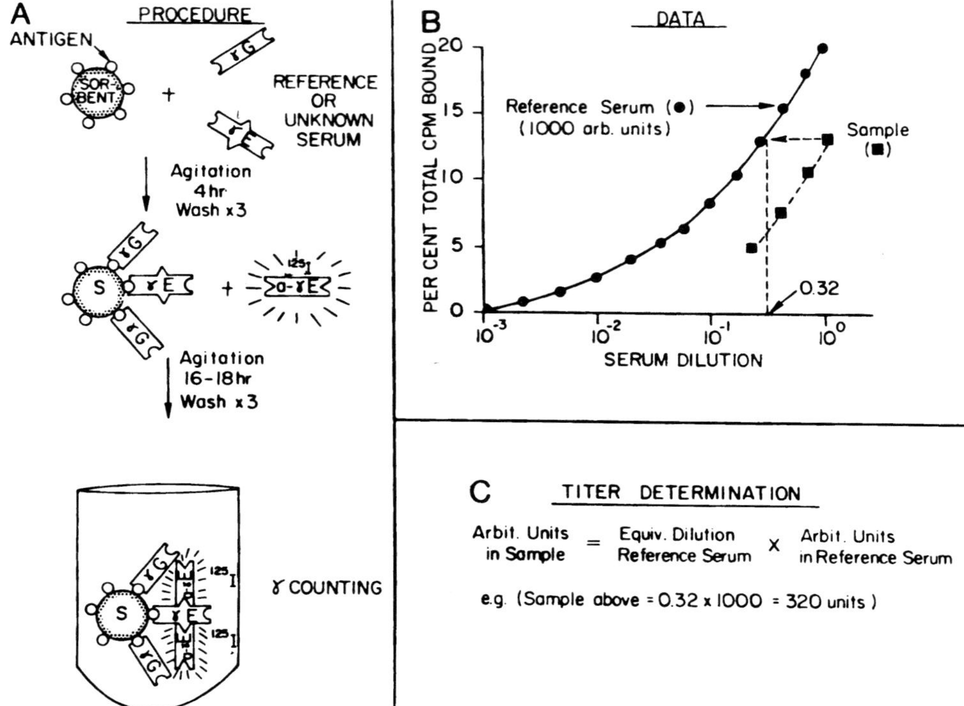

Figure 1 Schematic diagram of the radioallergosorbent test. In the first incubation, antigen-specific antibody of many isotypes (IgE, IgG) is bound from human serum with an allergosorbent. After buffer washes to remove unbound serum proteins, bound IgE antibody is detected with ^{125}I-labeled rabbit antihuman IgE detection antibody. The counts per minute (cpm) bound to the allergosorbent after a final buffer wash are proportional to the amount of specific IgE antibody in the original serum. Multiple dilutions of a reference serum (assigned 1000 arbitrary units) and the test serum are analyzed and their dose-response curves should dilute out in parallel. When the arbitrary units for the dilution of the test sample are determined by interpolation from the reference curve, the final titer or antibody estimate should be equivalent to each other when each dilution is corrected for its respective dilution factor. (From Ref. 24.)

allergen specificity. Because the overall quality of clinical IgE antibody assays remains dependent on the allergen-containing reagent, human IgE detection reagent, and the method of assay calibration, these technical aspects will be discussed individually.

A. Allergen-Containing Reagent

Both soluble (liquid phase, biotinylated) and insolubilized (solid phase, allergosorbent) allergens are used in current research and commercial IgE antibody assays. Hundreds of clinically important allergen vaccines have been prepared. A compendium of the allergen groups and purified allergens is presented in recent guidelines published by the NCCLS (2). These allergens are produced almost exclusively as mixtures of proteins that vary in their size (molecular weight), charge (isoelectric point), relative protein content, and immunogenicity or allergenic potency. The composition of an allergen received in the final serological assay reagent will vary as a function of (1) the season in which the raw material is collected; (2) the degree of difficulty in identifying the source material; (3) the presence of morphologically similar raw materials that can cause cross-contamination; and (4) proprietary differences among manufacturers in the extraction process used during allergen-reagent production. Prior to the use of allergen vaccines in allergosorbents, the manufacturer may ensure quality control by using isoelectrofocusing, sodium dodecyl sulfate-polyacrylamide gel electrophoresis (SDS-PAGE), crossed-immunoelectrophoresis, and immunoblotting. These methods are discussed in detail in Chapter 1. Moreover, once the allergen-containing reagent is prepared, remaining issues include stability during storage, heterogeneity of the human IgE antibody-containing individual or pooled sera used for quality control, and divergent criteria used by different manufacturers for acceptance of the finished allergen-containing reagent. These many variables guarantee that allergosorbents from different manufacturers will detect different populations of IgE antibodies for any given allergen specificity. Therefore, the NCCLS panel advises against comparing quantitative results from different commercial assays, even if they are designed to detect IgE antibody to the same allergen specificity. Appendix D in the NCCLS guideline (2) describes procedures that can be used to validate the specificity, stability, nonspecific binding, and binding capacity of commercial allergen-containing reagents.

B. Human IgE Detection Reagent

The labeled antihuman IgE detection reagent is a critical component because it confers the IgE specificity of the assay. This reagent must have restricted specificity for unique antigenic determinants on the ε-heavy chain of human IgE molecule. Equally important, it should exhibit no detectable cross-reactivity to human antigenic determinants on IgG, IgA, IgM, and IgD antibodies or to other human or animal serum proteins (e.g., albumin) that are present in the test or reference sera or are often added to buffer diluents used in the assays. Earlier techniques obtained polyclonal antihuman IgE Fc reagents from rabbits, sheep, and goats. In some cases, mixtures of monoclonal and polyclonal antibodies that are difficult to duplicate between manufacturers have superseded these reagents. There has also been a systematic transition from isotopic to nonisotopic labels that are coupled to the anti-IgE reagent. This conversion has improved the stability, enhanced safety, and lengthened the useful life of the detection reagents of IgE antibody assays. Manufacturers routinely use dilutional and competitive inhibition analyses with non-IgE immunoglobulins to confirm that their antihuman IgE reagent possesses no detectable cross-reactivity (e.g., $< 0.001\%$) to non-IgE human isotypes. These quality control methods are described in Appendix C of the NCCLS Guideline (2).

C. Assay Calibration

The newcomer to IgE assays will note the diversity of units that are used to report IgE antibody results. This diversity has resulted from the use of different reference reagents and calibration methods to convert assay response data into IgE antibody results. The NCCLS panel established consensus criteria for qualitative, semiquantitative, and quantitative IgE antibody assays (2).

In *qualitative assays*, IgE antibody levels are reported as nonreactive, negative, nondetectable, or absent; or reactive, positive, detectable, or present based on a predefined positive cutoff point or threshold. The manufacturers use a different balance of clinical and technical criteria to define this positive threshold level. A positive test result implies that the assay response signal exceeds the analytical threshold or reference serum level that has been set to achieve an arbitrary combination of detection limits and clinically defined specificity. It should also indicate the presence of IgE antibody specific for a particular allergen in the subject's blood. One illustration of a qualitative IgE antibody assay is the multiallergen screening test that uses a single reagent containing five or more allergens to detect IgE antibody to these allergen specificities in a single analytical measurement. These are complex assays due to the highly variable quantity and specificity of IgE antibody in the patient's serum and the many allergens that must all be represented in the multiallergen screening reagent. A second example of a qualitative assay is the dip stick test that detects IgE antibody specific for a single allergen specificity. The presence or absence of antibody is defined by visual assessment of color and intensity in relation to a positive control or reference IgE antibody dot or band.

Semiquantitative assays generate IgE antibody results in a series of increasing grades or classes (e.g., I to VI; low to high), a visually determined qualitative grading scheme (color chart), or an endpoint dilution at which the signal becomes negative (e.g., titer). These assays are not traceable to any common standard, and it is often difficult to detect a twofold change in IgE antibody when the test specimen is diluted twofold. Moreover, these assays often fail to meet the routine performance criteria for dilution recovery, parallelism, and linearity that are required in quantitative clinical assays.

Quantitative assays use the most advanced calibration methods available. Multipoint homologous (same specificity) or heterologous (different specificity) calibration curves define the assay's dose-response relationship (3). Due to the difficulty in obtaining large amounts of ''homologous'' human serum calibrators with IgE antibody for each of the hundreds of clinically important allergen specificities, most commercial assay manufacturers have adopted the heterologous calibration curve strategy. The earliest RAST, for instance, used a dose-response curve that was generated with four or five dilutions of a pooled reference serum containing birch pollen-specific IgE antibodies that bound to a birch allergosorbent. Response results (counts per minute bound) were interpolated from this multipoint curve into arbitrary PRU/mL (Phadebas relative units per milliliter). More recently, several IgE antibody assays have used a total serum IgE calibration curve that is generated simultaneously with the allergen-specific IgE portion of the assay. Because this calibration curve is traceable to the World Health Organization (WHO) 75/502 international human IgE standard, all manufacturers are currently able to cross-standardize their assay to a common reference preparation. Most commercial IgE antibody assays that report interpolated quantitative IU/mL estimates of antibody are subsequently cross-checked for accuracy by using a common secondary IgE reference preparation such as the United States Standard for Human Serum IgE (NIAID-NIH/BOB-FDA Cat A-699-001-500). Some laboratories also have chosen to convert the quantitative IU/mL IgE antibody result into mass units per volume using 2.4 or 2.44 as the conversion factor (1 IU/mL = 2.44 ng/mL). Immunoglobulin E antibody levels measured in patients' sera dilute out in parallel with this calibration system, and thus it appears that the total serum IgE heterologous reference curve is a generic solution to the problem of interlaboratory cross-standardization of IgE antibody assays.

II. SPECIMEN AND PATIENT SELECTION CONSIDERATIONS

Blood and environmental specimens (e.g., dust or air samples) are routinely evaluated in the clinical immunology laboratory. When a patient's clinical history is consistent with a diagnosis of immediate-type hypersensitivity, confirmatory tests such as those listed in Table 1 can be run on the patient's serum in the diagnostic laboratory. The allergist may choose to use the in vivo skin test as the primary confirmatory test because it provides rapid diagnostic information in the patient's own skin and it is highly sensitive. However, several clinical conditions can occur

Table 1 Analytes Measured in the Diagnostic Allergy Laboratory

Allergen-specific IgE
(multiallergen-specific IgE screen)
Total serum IgE
Allergen-specific IgG
Mast cell tryptase (α, β)
Eosinophil cationic protein
Urinary histamine
Indoor aeroallergens
Der p 1/Der f 1 (Domestic mite allergen)
Fel d 1 (Cat) allergen (*Felis domesticus*)
Can f 1 (Dog) allergen (*Canis familiaris*)
Bla g 1/Bla g 2 (Cockroach; *Blattella germanica*)
Mus m 1 (Mouse urinary protein)
Viable mold spores

in which in vitro assessment of specific IgE antibody in the blood may be preferred over a puncture or intradermal skin test. Young children or apprehensive adults often tolerate venipuncture better than a skin test. In the case of children with food allergies, Sampson and Ho have shown that certain levels of IgE antibodies in the blood can be highly predictive of clinical sensitivity to egg, milk, peanut, and fish, but not soy and wheat (4). Predefined levels of IgE antibody to these foods in the blood are highly predictive of a food allergy and can often eliminate the need for the tedious, double-blind, placebo-controlled food challenge. If the patient has extensive dermatographism or dermatitis that prevents proper interpretation of a skin test, in vitro detection of IgE antibody is a useful alternative. Premedication with antihistamines, tricyclic antidepressants, or topical corticosteroids is known to alter skin reactivity and can invalidate the skin test. If these medications cannot be withdrawn, a serological measurement may be the only alternative diagnostic evaluation possible. Finally, the venipuncture process is generally less likely than immediate hypersensitivity skin testing to produce a systemic reaction.

III. COMPARATIVE ANALYTICAL SENSITIVITY AND SPECIFICITY OF THE IN VIVO AND IN VITRO TESTS

The performance of both the skin test and the serological test are highly technique dependent. Therefore, direct comparison of the relative performance of these two diagnostic methods for IgE antibody is problematic. In general, there is a good correlation between the presence of IgE antibody in the skin and the blood. However, quantitative relationships between the amount of IgE antibody detected by skin test and immunoassay may vary widely as a function of the materials (skin testing devices), mode of allergen introduction into the skin (puncture or intradermal), and the reagents used by the investigator. As many as 25% of skin test-positive patients may have negative serological test results. These discrepancies appear to stem from issues concerning both analytical sensitivity and allergen-related specificity. In respiratory pollen allergy, there is a significant positive correlation between the quantity of IgE antibody as detected by either a PST or an in vitro analysis and the symptoms experienced during relevant natural aeroallergen exposure (5).

Natural rubber latex has been used as a model to examine the relationship between in vivo skin testing and in vitro immunoassay performance. In a recent multicenter study, 324 subjects were classified according to their clinical history as latex allergic (n = 134) and nonlatex allergic (n = 180). After informed consent, all subjects provided blood and were then skin tested with characterized nonammoniated latex (NAL) at 1100, and 1000 μg/mL concentrations prepared by Greer Laboratories (Lenoir, NC). A two-stage powdered latex glove provocation test was used to arbitrate the latex allergy status of the 15% of individuals who gave a positive latex allergy history, but who had a negative latex PST. Sera available from these study subjects were analyzed in the three Food and Drug Administration (FDA)-sanctioned natural rubber latex-specific IgE assays from Pharmacia-UpJohn (CAP System), Diagnostic Products Corporation (AlaSTAT), and Hycor (HyTECH). The Greer NAL puncture skin testing reagent produced a diagnostic sensitivity of 96% and specificity of 99%, at 100 μg/mL when compared to the subject's clinical history (6). The diagnostic sensitivity of the CAP System and AlaSTAT assays compared well to each other, but both were significantly lower than the sensitivity of the puncture skin test. Only approximately 75% of subjects defined as latex allergic by their clinical history and PST had a positive IgE anti-latex result in these two assays (7). The Hycor HyTECH assay, which uses a modified scoring system, displayed a higher sensitivity (90% versus history; 92% versus skin test), but a poorer specificity (68% versus history; 72% versus skin test). Of the available diagnostic methods for latex allergy, the PST provides the best balance of sensitivity and specificity.

IV. ELISA AND RAST INHIBITION ASSAYS

Competitive inhibition IgE antibody assays can be performed to quantify the amount of allergen in a source skin-testing allergen vaccine, a test vaccine prepared from a device (e.g., latex glove), or an environmental specimen (e.g., settled dust or air sample) (8). The RAST, and more recently, ELISA inhibition assays are performed either in a simultaneous or sequential addition mode. In the RAST inhibition assay, a test vaccine (e.g., 0.1 mL) is added to a plastic test tube containing allergen-specific human IgE antibody (e.g., 0.1 mL). In the simultaneous assay, the allergosorbent is added immediately to the mixture, whereas the sequential mode involves adding the allergosorbent 2–8 h after a preincubation of the antibody with soluble allergen. Once the allergosorbent is added, any soluble allergen in the test vaccine competes with the solid phase allergen for limited IgE antibody binding sites. When the binding reaction has achieved equilibrium (typically after 16–18 h), the allergosorbent is washed to remove unbound IgE antibody. Radioiodinated antihuman IgE is added in molar excess to bind IgE bound to the allergosorbent. After a final buffer wash, bound radioactivity is measured with a gamma counter. The amount of radioactivity bound is proportional to the amount of IgE antibody bound and inversely proportional to the allergen content in the test vaccine.

The ELISA inhibition assay is a minor modification of the RAST inhibition assay. Allergen is adsorbed onto plastic microtiter plate wells or tubes and antihuman IgE is labeled with an enzyme (e.g., horseradish peroxidase, alkaline phosphatase, or β-galactosidase). Caution should be exercised to ensure that all the relevant allergenic proteins are adsorbed onto the solid phase. After the final buffer wash, substrate appropriate for the enzyme is added. Color develops in proportion to the amount of enzyme bound, which itself is proportional to the amount of IgE antibody bound and inversely proportional to the amount of soluble allergen in the initial reaction mixture. The RAST and ELISA inhibition data are reported in arbitrary units of allergen per milliliter of vaccine depending on interpolation of the test vaccine's response (binding) levels from a dose-response curve generated with a reference allergen preparation. Because these inhibition assays tend to be highly variable, multiple replicates and dilutions of the reference and test vaccines are commonly evaluated to ensure valid results. These inhibition assays are useful in the quality control of vaccines prepared for skin testing (8). They also have been used successfully to quantify the amount of allergen extractable from devices such as natural rubber latex gloves, or environmental specimens such as house dust (9).

One important clinical application of the RAST inhibition assay has been as an adjunct test that facilitates the selection of Hymenoptera venom for immunotherapy (10). Extensive cross-reactivity is known to exist between yellow jacket (*Vespula*) and wasp (*Polistes*) venom proteins. Therefore, many seemingly positive skin and serological tests to *Polistes* venom are in fact due to the presence of IgE antibodies specific for cross-reactive YJV proteins. These cross-reactive antibodies can be identified by a competitive RAST inhibition assay in which the binding of a patient's anti-*Polistes* IgE to a *Polistes* venom allergosorbent is inhibited by preincubation of the serum with a molar excess of soluble (fluid phase) YJV. If complete (> 90%) inhibition is achieved, then all the IgE binding to the *Polistes* venom solid phase is known to cross-react with YJV. A patient with YJV cross-reactive anti-*Polistes* IgE does not require treatment with *Polistes* venom. This measurement may therefore prevent possible sensitization of the patient to wasp venom allergens, and it permits the allergist to optimize his or her venom immunotherapy regimen with yellow jacket or mixed vespid venom alone. This provides considerable savings to the patient (especially a child) in time, cost, and discomfort.

Attempts have been made to substitute a murine monoclonal or polyclonal rabbit, goat, or sheep antiserum into the inhibition assay in place of the human serum containing IgE antibody. The advantage of this substitution is the lower cost and greater inter-lot reproducibility of animal antisera for individual allergens. However, neither polyclonal nor monoclonal antisera match human IgE antibody-containing serum pools in their ability to detect complex mixtures of allergenic proteins in biological extracts. The limitation of the human serum as a reagent resides in its inter-lot heterogeneity that stems from the difficulty in obtaining large quantities of human serum for reagent pool production and the need to use undiluted human serum because of the typically low level of IgE antibody. Polyclonal/monoclonal antibody-based, two-site (capture and detection) IEMAs are attractive alternatives to human IgE-based competitive inhibition immunoassays for some allergens, such as domestic mites (Der p 1, Der f 1), cat (Fel d 1), dog (Can f 1), German cockroach (Bla g 1), and natural rubber latex (Hev b 1–7). IEMAs currently are used to assess indoor environments for contamination by individual aeroallergens (see below). The Hev b 1–7 assays may some day serve as the primary means for quantifying the level of allergenic protein in natural rubber gloves and other rubber-containing medical products.

V. BASOPHIL HISTAMINE RELEASE ASSAY

Basophils and mast cells have high-affinity IgE receptors ($Fc_{\varepsilon}RI$) on their surface and they contain histamine, a 110 Da biogenic amine, in granules that stain purple with basic dyes such as toluidine or alcian blue. Histamine is formed in these cells by cleavage of preformed histidine by histidine decarboxylase. Levels of histamine in mast cells and basophils range from 1–3 pg/cell. Allergen added in vitro to ''IgE-sensitized'' basophils in a suspension of washed leukocytes and calcium can cross-link IgE antibody, inducing the release of preformed histamine and the production of mediators such as leukotriene C_4 (LTC_4) from the metabolism of arachidonic acid. LTC_4 is secreted in concentrations nearly 100-fold less on a molar basis than histamine, but it possesses 100–6000 times greater potency for contracting smooth muscle than histamine. The release of histamine and LTC_4 from basophils by specific allergen cross-linking of IgE antibody on their surface correlates with the severity of clinical symptoms experienced by allergic individuals to defined antigens. For this reason, the basophil histamine release (BHR) assay has been considered a useful research assay that complements specific IgE antibody immunoassays and skin tests for evaluating the allergic status of individuals. Basophil histamine release has also been used to demonstrate IgE antibody immunoreactivity using normal leukocyte suspensions that are passively sensitized with IgE from the serum of patients with clinical symptoms (11). Finally, BHR assays using leukocytes from clinically defined allergic donors have been used in quality control of allergens for their stability, potency, and cross-reactivity.

Histamine has been measured in many body fluids (including plasma, urine, synovial fluid, tears, nasal secretions, and bronchial washings) and in skin chambers. After anaphylaxis, plasma histamine levels tend to peak 5 to 15 min after antigen challenge and return to baseline by 30 min. It has been difficult to use blood histamine levels as a clinical marker of mast cell or basophil degranulation, because plasma histamine only has a 2-min biological half-life. Moreover, coagulation, cell injury, or hemolysis from venipuncture, centrifugation, or improper storage can all produce artifactual elevations in plasma histamine. Because BHR assays require the use of whole blood, they have been limited to primary research analyses. A variety of bioassays, fluorometric assays, and radioenzymatic assays have been developed to measure histamine and methyl-histamine (Table 2). Of these, the automated fluorometric assay of Siraganian (12) has become the principal laboratory method for measuring histamine. In this method, histamine is extracted into *n*-butanol, back extracted with heptane in dilute acid, and complexed with o-phthalaldehyde (OPT) to produce a fluorescent product that is measured in a fluorometer. Sample volumes of 0.5–1 mL are evaluated and histamine can be measured from a dose-response curve ranging from 0.5–1000 ng/mL. One limitation of this method is the interference by serum proteins that aggregate and tend to produce spuriously elevated estimates of histamine. For this reason, the measurement of histamine in whole blood or serum greater than 10% requires acid precipitation or dialysis to remove protein prior to analysis. Details of the test procedures are presented elsewhere (13). Radioimmunoassays for histamine are also available, but the cost is generally prohibitive and the methods are not well standardized.

Urinary histamine also has been used as a measure of systemic histamine release. Approximately 50% of histamine is excreted as 1-methylimidazole-4-acetic acid. The remainder is excreted as imidazoleacetic acid (30%), 1,4 methyl-histamine (5%) and 2% nonmetabolized histamine. As the main metabolite, the concentration of 1-methylimidazole-4-acetic acid after normalization to urinary creatinine provides a quantitative marker for the endogenous release of histamine. Imidazolic acids can be measured by ELISA, radioimmunoassay, mass spectrometry, or gas chromatography. Some genitourinary tract bacteria can convert histidine to histamine, falsely elevating urinary histamine levels. Therefore, the normal range of urinary histamine and its metabolites is large.

Table 2 Assays for Histamine Measurement

Assay type	Substrate	Parameter measured	Strengths and limitations
Bioassay	Strips of ileum from sensitized guinea pig	Contractile response proportional to histamine concentration	Laborious, difficult to standardize, sensitive
Spectrophotometric assay	2,4-dinitrofluorobenzene	Monodinitrophenyl derivative of histamine formed	Sensitive to 5–10 ng/mL, interferences
Fluorometric assay (most widely used)—2 common methods	(a) o-phthalaldehyde (OPT) (b) Borosilicate glass; adsorption of histamine	(a) Creates fluorescent product with histamine at alkaline pH (b) Desorption with $HClO_4$, coupled to OPT	(a) Interfering substances, automated, 30 samples per hr, −0.5 to 100 ng/mL working range (b) Minimal interferences from serum
Radioenzymatic assay	^{14}C-adenosylmethionine	Enzyme transfer of ^{14}C methyl group to histamine to form ^{14}C-methylhistamine	Sensitivity to 30 pg/mL, complex, time consuming, little protein interference

VI. MAST CELL TRYPTASE ANALYSES

After activation, mast cells release a variety of mediators in addition to histamine (Table 3). The proteases present in a particular cell distinguish it as one of two mast cell types. The MC_{TC} cells contain tryptase, chymase, mast cell carboxypeptidase, and cathepsin G, whereas MC_T cells contain only tryptase (14). β-Tryptase is a neutral serine endoprotease that possesses trypsin-like substrate specificity and is stored in secretory granules (10–35 pg per mast cell) complexed to heparin. It is active as a tetramer and it converts to inactive monomers upon dissociation from heparin. Because negligible amounts of tryptase are present in basophils (0.04–0.05 pg per cell), tryptase is considered a specific marker of mast cell activation and is released along with histamine during degranulation. Importantly, tryptase is stable in the blood, remaining elevated for up to 4 h after release, whereas histamine is degraded rapidly. This makes tryptase a more reliable index

Table 3 Mediators Released from Activated Mast Cells

Biogenic amine
Histamine
Proteoglycans[a]
Heparin
Chondroitin sulfate E
Proteases[a]
Tryptase
Chymase
Mast cell carboxypeptidase
Cathepsin G
Fibroblast growth factor (bFGF)[a]
Newly formed mediators
Leukotriene C_4 (LTC_4)
Prostaglandin D_2 (PGD_2)
Cytokines
TNF-alpha
(IL) 4, 5, 6, 13[b]

[a] Primarily released from mast cells.
[b] Primarily released from basophils.

of mast cell activation. There are at least two tryptase genes on chromosome 16 that code for α-tryptase and β-tryptase, which show 92% homology at the mRNA and presumably the protein level. The actions of tryptase have not been completely defined. Active β-tryptase can cleave and inactivate fibrinogen, and it can generate C3a from C3. The biological functions of tryptase are discussed elsewhere (14).

A variety of isotopic and nonisotopic immunoassays have been developed to measure tryptase in serum and plasma. In one commercially available immunoenzymetric assay (15), monoclonal capture antibody (clone G5) binds to linear epitopes of predominantly β-tryptase. After a buffer wash, bound protease is detected with goat IgG antitryptase and enzyme-conjugated anti-goat IgG. The analytical sensitivity of this assay is 2.5 ng of tryptase per milliliter in serum or plasma. Other monoclonal antibodies such as clone B12 bind to both β-tryptase and α-protryptase. Assays using this antibody measure both α and β forms of tryptase and they permit an assessment of the total tryptase concentration in the blood.

From a clinical point of view, β-tryptase is normally less than 1 ng/mL in the serum of healthy individuals using the G5 antibody-based immunoassay. After hypotensive anaphylaxis, β-tryptase levels can rise to a maximal level (≥

5 ng/mL) by about 1 h, and they decline with a half-life of 2 h. The serum levels of β-tryptase correlate with the severity of hypotension after insect sting-induced anaphylaxis. β-Tryptase levels higher than 10 ng/mL in postmortem blood samples reflect significant predeath mast cell activation and suggest mast cell-dependent anaphylaxis as the cause of death.

VII. EOSINOPHILS AND SUBSTANCES DERIVED FROM EOSINOPHILS

Eosinophil infiltration has been demonstrated in lung biopsies and bronchial lavage fluids collected from reaction sites in individuals with mild to moderate asthma. The number of eosinophils in the lung correlates with the degree of airway hyperresponsiveness and asthma severity (16). Eosinophils contain granule-associated proteins such as MBP that are thought to induce epithelium destruction in asthma. When activated, they also release ECP, a highly basic protein that is thought to be cytotoxic, inducing membrane damage and killing of parasites. Major basic protein and ECP can be used as in vivo markers of eosinophil activation because they can be detected in serum, sputum, and bronchial lavage fluid. Both MBP and ECP are measured by immunoassays. Levels of ECP in the serum of 100 healthy adults ranged from 2.3–15 ng/mL (geometric mean = 6.0 ng/mL) using a commercially available ECP assay (Pharmacia-UpJohn). Major basic protein remains a research analyte because no commercial immunoassays are available.

VIII. QUANTITATION OF INDOOR AEROALLERGENS

There are three modes of managing allergic disease: allergen avoidance, pharmacotherapy, and immunotherapy. Of these, avoidance or the separation of the allergen from the allergic patient is probably the most effective, best tolerated, and least expensive approach. Domestic (dust) mites, pets, insects, rodents, and molds all produce potent aeroallergens that are present in home, school, and work environments. They represent sources of allergen exposure that can induce allergic symptoms and increase sensitization in genetically predisposed individuals. To facilitate avoidance of these allergens, it is often necessary to establish their presence and quantity and ultimately demonstrate their removal after remediation of the particular environment.

An environmental assessment has been developed to quantify indicator aeroallergens for each of these allergen groups in the fine settled dust of indoor home, school, and work environments. The decision to perform a dust analysis begins with a patient's clinical history and confirmatory skin test or serology to show that the individual's allergic symptoms are related to one or more indoor aeroallergens. These symptoms may begin upon a move into a new home or after extensive remodeling that exposes allergen sources in an existing home. The allergic symptoms can intensify as indoor allergens accumulate and the patient's sensitivity increases. In addition to allergen content, other factors can alter the symptoms experienced by the patient. These include the type of residence (e.g., age, location, and number of inhabitants in the home), the environmental temperature and humidity, the type of furniture and carpet in the home, the type of home cooling/heating system, and the number of pets in the home. Similar considerations are appropriate for school and work environments. For instance, higher temperatures (> 23 °C) and humidity ($> 70\%$) foster the growth of molds and domestic mites.

A. Domestic Mites

Four species of domestic mite (Pyroglyphidae) are present in most North American homes: *Dermatophagoides pteronyssinus, D. farinae, D. microcercas*, and *Euroglyphus maynei. Blomia tropicalis*, a glycyphagid mite, is found in tropical and subtropical climates, including some homes in the southern United States. Of these, fecal material (20 μm average particle diameter) from *D. pteronyssinus* and *D. farinae* represent more than 90% of the potent allergens that have been detected in fine house dust throughout North America (17). Mites reportedly produce up to 200 times their own weight in feces during their 2–3.5-month life span. Mattresses, carpets, and upholstered furniture are locations where mites breed while they consume human skin and animal dander. Group 1 *Dermatophagoides* allergens (Der p 1, Der f 1) are structurally homologous proteins (25,000 MW, pI = 4.5–7.1), and they serve as useful indicator molecules in settled dust for the presence of their respective species (*D. pteronyssinus* and *D. farinae*). Two-site immunoenzymetric assays for these major mite allergens can quantify the relative amounts of *Dermatophagoides* allergen in an environment. A level of 2000 ng of allergen per gram of fine dust is approximately equivalent to 100 mites per gram of dust (18). Der p 1 or Der f 1 quantities of 400, 2000, and 10,000 ng per gram of fine dust are the levels assigned for identifying very low, low, and moderate to high risk levels of mite allergen exposure, respectively, for inducing sensitization and allergic symptoms. Combined Der p 1 and Der f 1 levels less than 2000 ng/g of dust are desirable for the indoor environment and are considered low risk for allergen sensitization.

B. Animals—Pets

Many animals can contribute to the allergen burden of the home, school, or work environments. Cats, dogs, guinea pigs, hamsters, rabbits, rats, and mice all produce dander, saliva, and urine that contain potent allergens capable of inducing allergic symptoms. The domesticated cat (*Felis domesticus*) is the most common household pet in the United States. Different breeds of cats produce the same potent 35 kD protein (Fel d 1) in their sublingual mucous salivary gland and hair root sebaceous glands (19). Fel d 1 adheres tenaciously to carpets, upholstered furniture, and dust particles from 2–10 μm. Twenty weeks or more are needed after cat removal from the home for levels of Fel d 1 to decline to levels comparable with homes that have no cats (20). Levels of Fel d 1 identify the presence of a cat in the environment. Fel d 1 quantities of 50, 8000, and 80,000 ng per gram of fine dust are the levels assigned for identifying very low, low, and moderate to high risk, respectively, for sensitization and the induction of symptoms in cat-allergic individuals.

The domestic dog (*Canis familiaris*) is the second most popular indoor pet. Dog dander vaccines contain more than 20 protein bands that have been identified as potential allergens. Some allergens appear to be breed-specific, whereas others may cross species (21). Can f 1 allergens may share comparable allergen (action) level thresholds with Fel d 1, but this has yet to be confirmed in a clinical study.

Mice and rats produce potent allergens that induce occupational asthma and rhinitis in laboratory animal workers and inner city children. The group 1 mouse allergen (Mus m 1) is produced in the salivary gland and liver. This 17.8-kD protein is excreted into the urine, where it constitutes approximately 80% of the urinary protein. No risk ranges have been established for Mus m 1. Two potent rat allergens have been identified in rat urine, saliva, and pelt. Rat n 1.01 (20–21 kDa) and Rat n 1.02 (16–17 kDa) are thought to be prealbumin and α_2-euglobulin, respectively. These allergens can be measured only in select research laboratories, and risk ranges for these allergens have not been established.

C. Insects—Cockroaches

Eight of the more than 50 varieties of cockroaches are considered clinically important in the United States. *Blattella germanica* is considered the metropolitan cockroach, with a high percentage of domestic mite allergic individuals in urban areas being skin test-positive to German cockroach allergen. Bla g 1 (25 kD) and Bla g 2 (36 kD) can be measured as indicators for the presence of a cockroach infestation. The presence of any detectable cockroach allergen in house dust indicates the risk for increased sensitization or symptoms within that environment.

D. Mold

There are two approaches for the assessment of mold content in the indoor environment. The first strategy evaluates the quantity of viable mold spores in the environment that can produce individual colonies on a microbiological plate containing medium from which mycelia can visibly grow (22). A small sample of fine settled dust (e.g., 5 mg in PBS-Tween) is plated aseptically onto a microbiological culture plate containing Sabouraud's dextrose agar with selected antibiotics (penicillin, streptomycin, and gentamycin). Larger dust specimens will produce too many colonies, causing overcolonization of the plate. Plates are incubated in an inverted position for 1–2 days at room temperature, and the number of viable mold colonies is quantified at 24 h and corrected for sample weight to viable colonies per gram of fine dust. At present, risk ranges are not available. Colony counts greater than 10,000 per gram may be considered sufficiently high to identify homes where environmental intervention such as mildew removal, control of indoor humidity and HEPA filtration of air may be appropriate. The correlation between allergic symptoms and the measured viable mold spore colony count is poor because four molds (*Cladosporium, Alternaria, Penicillium*, and *Aspergillus*) are found in most indoor environments in different relative amounts. Induction of an individual's symptoms depends on the specificity of his or her own IgE antibody and the degree to which he or she is exposed to the relevant mold allergens. Although speciation of the mold in the dust may theoretically be useful, it is rarely performed because it is tedious, expensive, and often difficult to ascertain if the dust specimen is representative of the total environment to which the individual is exposed.

A second approach to environmental mold spore assessment is based on the assumption that all mold spores (viable and nonviable) are clinically important. An air sampler deposits mold spores onto a silicone-greased film, a glass slide, or a moving paper tape, and the spores are subsequently stained and microscopically examined. The different types of mold spores are quantified morphologically on the basis of their distinct shapes, sizes, and staining patterns. Interpretation of the total mold content of indoor environments is commonly provided in comparison to the outdoor reference environment. This total mold spore evaluation is performed less frequently inasmuch as many allergists ascribe to the concept that identification of viable mold spores is clinically more important than identifying nonviable mold spores.

IX. IN VITRO DETERMINATION OF IgG ANTIBODIES

There was a period when the induction of high levels of IgG "blocking" antibodies was believed to be the primary mechanism by which immunotherapy provided protection from systemic reactions and symptom relief. The concept of IgG antibody scavenging allergen and preventing from cross-linking IgE on the surface of the mast cell and basophil has been shown in recent years to be too simplistic. Immunoglobulin G antibody measurements are performed to document an exposure of an individual to an immunizing dose of antigen. In selected cases, it can serve as a useful indicator of the effectiveness of various antigen doses used to induce a specific IgG response in immunotherapy. The role of IgG antibody in immunotherapy-induced symptom relief remains controversial; however, one group continues to believe that allergen-specific IgG antibody measurements can be useful in monitoring individuals who are receiving venom immunotherapy. In a 1992 study, Golden et al. performed 211 insect sting challenges in 109 patients during a 4-year period to investigate the clinical significance of venom-specific IgG antibody levels (23). Individuals on immunotherapy for 4 years demonstrated a reduced risk of systemic symptoms from 16% to less than 1.6% with IgG antibody levels higher than 3 μg/mL. The IgG antivenom levels had no predictive value in subjects who had been on immunotherapy for more than 4 years. The conclusion was that low venom-specific IgG levels are associated with an elevated risk of treatment failure during the first 4 years of immunotherapy with yellow jacket or mixed vespid venom. Currently, sting challenge studies are being performed to reexamine the usefulness of serological markers such as venom-specific IgG antibodies in predicting those who remain protected even after stopping venom immunotherapy. The assay methods used to quantify IgG antivenom in serum are analogous to those used in the quantification of IgE antibodies, except a labeled anti-IgG detection reagent is used. Details of these assays, their standardization, and quality control are discussed elsewhere (24).

X. NEWER ANALYTES

A variety of research analytes that are readily measured by flow cytometry are used to study the phenotype, recruitment, accumulation, and activation of eosinophils, basophils, mast cells, and T cells during a human allergic inflammatory reaction. One group of analytes consists of the cell adhesion molecules that are divided into the integrins (e.g., intercellular adhesion molecule-1 [ICAM-1] and vascular cell adhesion molecule-1 [VCAM-1]), immunoglobulin-like structures, selectins, and sialylated carbohydrate counter-ligands for selectins (25). In microtiter plate-based assays, the adhesion molecules or monolayers of cells from vascular endothelium, epithelium, or cell lines that express the specific adhesion molecules are immobilized on a plastic surface (overnight at 4°C). Specificity of these assays is verified using antagonists such as adhesion molecule blocking antibodies.

Cytokines were once thought to be produced only by lymphocytes. They constitute another group of molecules that are of interest to the research immunologist because they are present in inflammatory foci and some are involved in IgE production and eosinophil survival. Although many cytokines are reportedly made by human mast cells, basophils, and eosinophils, most of these studies involve in situ hybridization and cytochemical methods that are difficult to interpret. Moreover, cytokine production has not been documented in many of these studies. Rodent (and perhaps human) mast cells produce tumor necrosis factor (TNF)-α and human basophils produce large quantities of both interleukin (IL)-4 and IL-13. Human eosinophils contain messenger RNA for IL-5, and under certain conditions, they may secrete IL-5 protein. Measurements of mRNA involve technically rigorous isolation and amplification methods only available in research settings. Cytokine protein measurements can be performed in a research setting using commercially available solid-phase enzyme immunoassays that are described elsewhere (13).

XI. SALIENT POINTS

1. Human IgE antibody of a defined allergen specificity is the most clinically useful analyte that can be measured by the clinical immunology laboratory for the diagnosis of human allergic disease.
2. Whether measured in vivo by skin test or in vitro in serum by RAST or by basophil histamine release assays, the presence of significant IgE antibody supports a diagnosis of type 1 hypersensitivity.
3. Immunoglobulin E antibody specificity is useful in defining the allergen group(s) that may elicit clinical allergy symptoms.
4. Although different serological IgE antibody assays use similar components (allergen-containing reagent, human IgE detection reagent, and calibration schemes), the quality of these reagents and techniques varies greatly among assays, precluding direct comparison of reported IgE antibody results between assays.
5. The multiallergen screen (e.g., Phadiatop) is a qualitative test that detects IgE antibody to the majority of allergen specificities that elicit aeroallergen-related disease. As such, it is the single most useful in vitro test for excluding IgE-mediated disease when the clinical history is questionable.
6. Enzyme-linked immunosorbent assays and RAST inhibition assays are used to quantify the amount of allergen in a fine dust specimen or an allergen vaccine, and to select the appropriate venom(s) for inclusion in a Hymenoptera venom immunotherapy regimen.
7. In the management of the allergic patient, direct quantitation of allergen levels in an individual's home, school, or work environment can identify an allergen exposure problem and aid the clinician in assessing the success of allergen avoidance and control measures.

8. Tryptase is a reliable marker of mast cell activation that remains elevated up to 4 h after its release.
9. Histamine, ECP, adhesion molecules, and a variety of cytokines are examples of research analytes that can aid in the study of the mechanisms involved in the induction of IgE-mediated responses, recruitment of inflammatory cells, and the induction of mediator release from mast cells and basophils.

REFERENCES

1. Wide L, Bennich H, Johansson SGO. Diagnosis by an in vitro test for allergen specific IgE antibodies. Lancet 1967; 2:1105–1109.
2. Matsson P, Hamilton RG, Adkinson NF Jr, Esch R, Homburger HA, Maxim P, Williams PB. Evaluation methods and analytical performance characteristics of immunological assays for human immunoglobulin E (IgE) antibodies of defined allergen specificities. NCCLS Approved Guideline 1997; 17:24.
3. Butler JE, Hamilton RG. Quantitation of specific antibodies: methods of expression, standards, solid phase considerations and specific applications. In: Butler JE, ed. Immunochemistry of Solid Phase Immunoassays. Boca Raton: CRC Press, 1991: 173.
4. Sampson HA, Ho DG. Relationship between food-specific IgE concentrations and the risk of positive food challenges in children and adolescents. J Allergy Clin Immunol 1997; 100:44–51.
5. Johansson SGO, Foucard T. IgE in immunity and disease. In: Middleton E Jr, Reed CE, Ellis EF, eds. Allergy: Principles and Practice. St. Louis: CV Mosby Company, 1978:551–554.
6. Hamilton RG, Adkinson NF Jr, and Multi-Center Latex Task Force. Diagnosis of natural rubber latex allergy: multi-center latex skin testing efficacy study. J Allergy Clin Immunol 1998; 102:482–490.
7. Hamilton RG, Biagini RE, Krieg EF, and Multi-Center Latex Task Force. Diagnostic performance of FDA-cleared serological assays for natural rubber latex-specific IgE antibody. J Allergy Clin Immunol, 1999; 103:773–779.
8. Yunginger JW, Swanson MC. Quantitation and standardization of allergens. In: Rose NR, Conway de Macario E, Folds JD, Lane HC, Nakamura RM, eds. Manual of Clinical Laboratory Immunology. Washington DC: American Society for Microbiology, 1997:868–874.
9. Bronzert CT, Wisenauer JA, Adkinson NF, Hamilton RG. Quantitation of latex allergen in rubber gloves. J Allergy Clin Immunol 1994; 93:306.
10. Hamilton RG, Wisenauer JA, Golden DBK, Valentine MD, Adkinson NF Jr. Selection of Hymenoptera venoms for immunotherapy based on patient's IgE antibody crossreactivity. J Allergy Clin Immunol 1993; 92:651–659.
11. Levy D, Osler A. Studies on the mechanisms of hypersensitivity phenomena. XIV. Passive sensitization in vitro of human leukocytes to ragweed pollen antigen. J Immunol 1966; 97:203–212.

12. Siraganian RP. An automated continuous flow system for the extraction and fluorometric analysis of histamine. Anal Biochem 1974; 57:383–394.
13. Schroeder JT, Kagey-Sobotka A. Assay method for measurement of mediator and markers of allergic inflammation. In: Rose NR, Conway de Macario E, Folds JD, Lane HC, Nakamura RM, eds. Manual of Clinical Laboratory Immunology. Washington, DC: American Society for Microbiology, 1997:899–907.
14. Duff Hogan A, Schwartz LB. Markers of mast cell degranulation. Methods 1997; 13:43–52.
15. Schwartz LB, Sakai K, Bradford TR, Ren SL, Zweiman B, Worobec AS, Metcalfe DD. The alpha form of human tryptase is the predominant type present in blood at baseline in normal subjects and is elevated in those with systemic mastocytosis. J Clin Invest 1995; 96:2702–2710.
16. Bochner BS, Undem BJ, Lichtenstein LM. Immunological aspects of allergic asthma. Annu Rev Immunol 1994; 12:295–335.
17. Tovey ER, Chapman MD, Platts-Mills TAE. Mite feces are a major source of house dust allergens. Nature 1981; 290:592–593.
18. Lind P, Inemann L, Brouvez M. Demonstration of species specific sensitization to major allergens of *Dermatophagoides* species by solid phase adsorption of human IgE antibodies. Scand J Immunol 1987; 25:1–10.
19. Leitermann K, Ohman JL. Cat allergen I: biochemical antigenic and allergenic properties. J Allergy Clin Immunol 1984; 74:147–52.
20. Wood RA, Chapman MD, Adkinson NF Jr., Eggleston PA: The effect of cat removal on allergen content in household dust samples. J Allergy Clin Immunol 1989; 83: 730–734.
21. Hamilton RG, Eggleston PA. Environmental allergen analyses. Methods 1997; 13: 53–60.
22. Hamilton RG, Chapman MD, Platts-Mills TAE, Adkinson NF Jr. House dust aeroallergen measurements in clinical practice. A guide to allergen free home and work environments. Immunol Allergy Pract 1992; 14:96–112.
23. Golden DBK, Lawrence ID, Hamilton RG, Kagey-Sobotka A, Valentine MD, Lichtenstein LM. Clinical correlation of the venom specific IgG antibody level during maintenance venom immunotherapy. J Allergy Clin Immunol 1992; 90:386–393.
24. Hamilton RG, Adkinson NF Jr. Immunological tests for diagnosis and management of human allergic disease: total and allergen specific IgE and allergen specific IgG. In: Rose NR, Conway de Macario E, Folds JD, Lane HC, Nakamura RM, eds. Manual of Clinical Laboratory Immunology. Washington, DC: American Society for Microbiology, 1997:881–892.
25. Bochner BS, Sterbinsky SA, Saini SA, Columbo M, MacGlashan DW Jr. Studies of cell adhesion and flow cytometric analyses of degranulation, surface phenotype and viability using human eosinophils, basophils and mast cells. Methods 1997; 13: 61–68.

4

Diagnostic Tests for Urticaria and Angioedema

Allen P. Kaplan
Medical University of South Carolina, Charleston, South Carolina

I. INTRODUCTION

The diagnosis of urticaria and angioedema is always dependent upon a detailed history that elicits a description of the hives or swelling, including the items listed below:

1. How long has urticaria or angioedema been present?
2. What is the shape and size of the lesions—circular, linear, serpiginous, or other shapes? Is the lesion a few millimeters in diameter, the size of a dime, nickel, quarter, or half-dollar, or are there giant hives that are 3 in. or more in diameter?
3. Particular characteristics: Is the border clear? Are the lesions pruritic, painful, or burning? Are black and blue marks associated with them? Do they lead to scar formation and if so, is it part of the healing process or is it due to the trauma of scratching?

4. Where are urticarial lesions located—face, scalp, trunk, extremities, palms, soles?

5. How long do individual lesions last? Are they typically gone in less than 2 h or do they last more than 4 h? 24 h? 48 h?

6. Is there swelling of the lips, tongue, throat, hands, feet, genitalia? Is there swelling of the cheeks or eyes? When swelling occurs, is it symmetrical or asymmetrical? How long does it last? Are individual areas normal by 24 to 72 h? Is there any permanent swelling? Is the skin over the areas of swelling normal in appearance or is there always an associated hive?

7. Any family history of hives or swelling?

8. Any personal or family history of thyroid disorder or connective tissue disease (e.g., systemic lupus erythematosus or vasculitis)?

9. Are hives or swelling prompted by physical stimuli—touching cold objects; touching warm or hot objects; hives when swimming; pruritic hives associated with exercise, sweating, hot showers, or anxiety; itching and hives with light exposure? Will window glass prevent light-dependent hives? Does scratching create hives? Is there a predilection for hives about pressure points from tight garments (belt, brassiere, elastic)? Does walking cause foot swelling, hammering cause hand swelling, sitting cause buttock swelling? Does water cause hives independent of temperature?

10. Are hives associated with use of medication, either one used regularly or sporadically? Is this association reproducible? If all suspected medications are discontinued, does urticaria or angioedema cease?

11. Are hives associated with foods? Is it reproducible? Will a minute amount of the food cause an episode or is a large quantity needed? Are one or two foods suspected, three to five foods, or is there a very long list of suspected foods? If suspected foods are eliminated, does urticaria or angioedema cease? Have special diets been tried and, if so, what was the outcome?

The diagnosis of a physically induced hive should be considered if there is evidence that one of the aforementioned stimuli can precipitate hives or swelling (item 9 above) or if individual lesions tend to disappear within 2 hours. The major exception is pressure-induced urticaria, which is synonymous with delayed pressure urticaria and, by definition, occurs 4–6 h after the stimulus is applied, with individual lesions lasting from 4 to 36 h. As a group, tests for these disorders involve in vivo provocations.

II. IN VIVO TESTING

A. Ice Cube Test

This test is performed by placing an ice cube for 5 min on the forearm of a patient suspected of having cold urticaria. The site is wiped dry and observed for 10

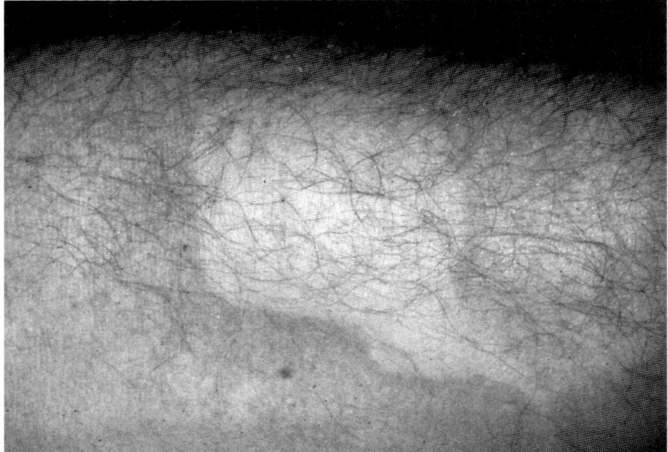

Figure 1 Positive ice cube test in a patient with cold urticaria. The confluent wheal and flare reaction is characteristic. The hive extends where ice water dripped down the patient's forearm.

min (1,2). The cube is held steady so as not to elicit urticaria in a dermatographic person. The normal response observed is a reddened area where the ice cube was applied that gradually fades. A positive test results in wheal formation, which usually begins along the periphery of the ice application site and fills in so that an elevated area the shape of the ice cube is seen (Fig. 1). The erythema may be more pronounced at the periphery and may last more than 10 min. Smaller wheals within the challenge site that has been challenged are considered positive. Some advocate an ice cube test of 10 min, which may give a slightly higher yield of positive tests. The challenged site is often pruritic, but this is variable. A rare form of cold urticaria, called localized cold urticaria, is associated with cold-induced hives restricted to certain sites, such as the face and neck only (3). In such cases the test must be performed at the site suggested by the history, along with some other area that serves as a negative control.

B. Local Heat Challenge

This is a test for local heat urticaria (hives) occurring at the site of application of a warmed object to the skin. The best method is to fill a test tube with water warmed to 44 °C and then apply the test tube to the person's arm or back for 5 min. The site is then observed for increasing redness and wheal formation for another 10 min. A positive test yields hives limited to the area where the test tube was applied (4).

C. Generalized Heat Urticaria (Cholinergic Urticaria)

The test for cholinergic urticaria is best performed in a warmed room so that exercise will readily cause perspiration. Because the initial urticarial lesions can be subtle, it is important to begin by examining the skin on the face, neck, chest, and back for any blemishes, rash, or acneiform lesions. The patient should wear a ''sweat suit'' and jog in place for 10–15 min or exercise on an exercise bicycle for the same period. It is important that sweating is induced by the challenge. Exercise should be stopped and the skin examined during the 10–15 min, particularly if the subject begins to complain of generalized pruritus. Most subjects will become hot and flushed during this exercise and a positive test is dependent upon the identification of small punctate urticarial lesions a few millimeters in diameter that are surrounded by a prominent flare, usually beginning about the neck and upper chest and spreading to involve the face, abdomen, and extremities (Fig. 2). Because lesions sometimes are seen first on the extremities, the progression may be variable. As time passes, more urticarial lesions are seen, even after exercise is stopped, and they may coalesce to form larger, more obvious wheals. It is wise, therefore, to stop the exercise once a positive test is discerned. Although systemic reactions have not been reported, confluence of lesions with prominent angioedema occasionally results. A negative test should require a minimum of 10 min, and preferably 15 min, of exercise. This assumes a healthy, reasonably conditioned person, with no cardiac, pulmonary, or neuromuscular disorder.

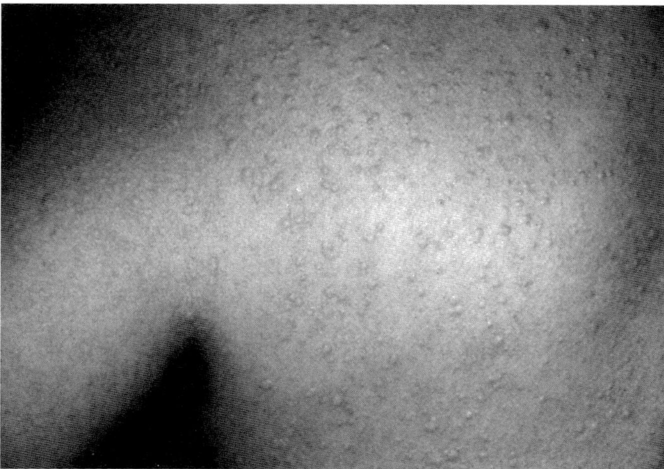

Figure 2 Punctate urticarial lesions characteristic of cholinergic urticaria. The episode was precipitated by having the patient run in place for 15 min in a room heated to 80 °F.

D. Dermatographism

This test, the simplest of those for physically induced hives, involves scratching the skin with a sharp object (often a finger nail or tongue blade is sufficient to elicit a response). A linear wheal and flare response is seen within 1 to 3 min (5). The appearance of a wheal and not simply erythema is critical. When the skin is stretched a white line is visible and clearly elevated (i.e., a ridge is felt) when the skin is lightly palpated perpendicular to the hive. More formalized tests for dermatographism use a spring-loaded dermographometer that can be used to apply stimuli of varying pressure. The pressure required to produce a wheal of 2 mm in width with surrounding erythema is determined (6). A pressure of 500 g/cm^2 is used for screening.

E. Pressure-Induced Urticaria

Pressure symptoms may occur in association with chronic urticaria, usually at the site of tight garments. If it is clear that spontaneous urticarial lesions are occurring, pressure testing is not essential. However, some patients have an uncommon, severe disorder in which symptoms are strictly pressure-induced and formal testing of such patients is desirable. Lesions occur many hours after the pressure stimulus is applied and the disorder may be synonymous with delayed dermatographism in which stroking the skin yields a linear hive 4–6 h later. It is difficult to standardize a test for this disorder and a few approaches have been advocated. In one, a shoulder bag containing a 15-lb weight is hung from one shoulder for 15 min (7). The shoulder is observed for the ensuing 12 h. Positive reactions consist of hives or swelling that typically peak in severity between 4 and 8 h later. Graded pressure devices (8) that apply accurate, pinpoint pressures varying from 48–234 g/mm^2 allow semiquantitation of patient sensitivity.

F. Solar Urticaria

This disorder consists of types I–V, depending on the wavelength of light, which precipitates symptoms (9,10), as well as type VI, which is due to ferrochetalase deficiency (11). The latter is a familial disorder (hereditary protoporphyria) with autosomal dominant inheritance (12). Type I solar urticaria is due to ultraviolet light exposure and causes urticaria wherever there is exposure. Because ordinary window glass filters out ultraviolet light, a critical determination is whether urticaria occurs indoors with sun exposure but with windows shut. Types II–V solar urticaria occur due to differing wavelengths of light within the visible spectrum. They can all be specifically diagnosed in only a few research centers where light of defined wavelengths can be directed at the patient's forearm for 1–5 min. The area is observed for the appearance of urticaria for the ensuing 20 min. If hereditary protoporphyria is suspected, one can determine protoporphyrin IX in erythrocytes, plasma, or stool. Also, common gene mutations have been identified that include intron/exon splicing errors resulting in deletions or missense mutations with amino acid replacements or early polypeptide chain termination. Research methods using molecular biology can help identify the specific genetic abnormality (12).

G. Aquagenic Urticaria

In this instance hives are due to water exposure. Tests for cold urticaria or localized heat urticaria done with ice water or warmed water within tests tubes will be negative, whereas water of any temperature applied to the patient's arm will form hives promptly.

H. Other

Systemic cold urticaria is a disorder in which exposure to cold yields severe generalized urticaria (under clothing too). The ice cube test is negative, but sitting in a cold room for 5–15 min will cause hives. The patient must be checked frequently and removed to ambient temperature as soon as a positive symptom is observed because anaphylactoid reactions can occur (13).

Cold-dependent dermatographism is a disorder in which a dermatographic response is obtained if the skin is first chilled. Hives are more common in winter and tend to be linear. The ice cube test for cold urticaria is negative, and a test for dermatographism is negative or weakly positive. Chilling the skin (e.g., sitting in a cold room) and then testing for dermatographism yields a strikingly amplified response (Fig. 3) (13).

Cold-induced cholinergic urticaria is a disorder in which exercise-induced hives are seen only when the person is systemically chilled. Thus, exercise-induced hives occur most commonly in winter or in a cold environment and are not associated with sweating or hot showers. The ice cube test for cold urticaria, a systemic cold challenge for systemic cold urticaria, and exercise challenge for typical cholinergic urticaria are negative. Exercise in a cold environment, however, yields hives that resemble the rash of cholinergic urticaria (14).

I. Some Difficult Distinctions

1. A patient has hives associated with swimming. It can be due to cold urticaria, cholinergic urticaria, or both. Do an ice cube test *and* an exercise challenge.

2. A patient gets hives on the left arm while it is hanging outside the driver's window. Distinguish local heat urticaria (warmed test tube test) from solar urticaria. Hives while seated at the beach can be due to the light (solar urticaria) or to heating the skin (local heat urticaria), unless it is so hot that the person is sweating and has generalized heat (cholinergic) urticaria. Separate tests for each are necessary.

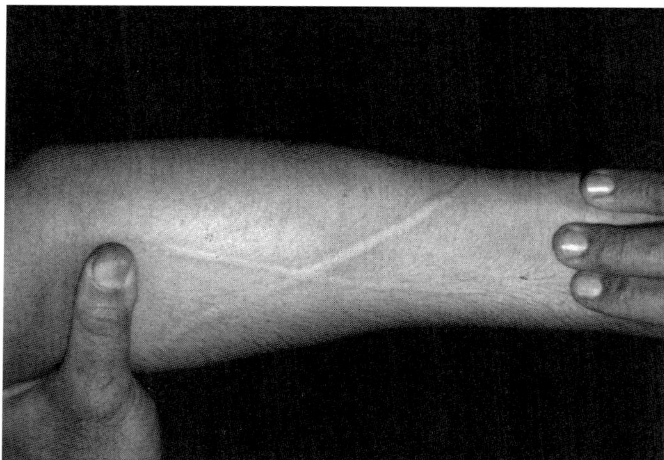

Figure 3 Linear hive forming an "X" where the patient was scratched after being seated in a cold room for 10 min. Scratching at room temperature yields a minimally positive test.

3. A patient reports hives due to exercise and either hot or cool showers. An ice cube test and an exercise challenge are both positive, suggesting combined cold urticaria and cholinergic urticaria. A test for dermatographism is also strikingly positive. A cold challenge by placing one hand in very cold water (a research test for histamine release in cold urticaria) (2) is negative, and an exercise challenge with profuse sweating is negative if all clothing but a bathing suit (bikini for women) is worn. The correct diagnosis is very severe dermatographism with hives due to drops of water hitting the skin in the shower, and clothing rubbing along the skin while exercising, and moving the ice cube a little during the test for cold urticaria.

III. IN VITRO METHODS

A. Methacholine Skin Test

This is an intracutaneous injection with methacholine that can be used to verify a diagnosis of cholinergic urticaria (15). Methacholine, 100 μL (1 mg/mL) is injected and the area is observed for 15 min. Because methacholine is a vasodilator, everyone develops a red spot at the injection site. A series of punctate urticarial lesions at a distance (1–3 cm) from the injection site represents a positive test. A positive test is observed only in severe cases of cholinergic urticaria so that many would be missed if this were used as a diagnostic test (16).

B. Thyroid Function Tests (Antithyroid Antibodies)

There is an association between chronic urticaria and Hashimoto's thyroiditis (17,18), particularly in women. Thus all patients with chronic urticaria (continual hives for more than 8 weeks) should have a complete battery of thyroid function tests. However, the patient may be euthyroid, inasmuch as the association is really with the presence of antithyroid antibodies (i.e., antimicrosomal antibodies and antithyroglobulin antibodies). The former are probably the most critical. Some patients may present with a history of hypothyroidism and may already be taking thyroid supplementation. If thyroid function has been recently assessed, it may only be necessary to determine antithyroid antibodies. Patients who are positive for antibodies but are euthyroid should have their thyroid function tested annually because many will slowly develop hypothyroidism.

The association represents one of the first observations to suggest that a substantial percentage of patients with chronic urticaria have an autoimmune disorder involving the skin.

C. Erythrocyte Sedimentation Rate, ANA

A subset of patients with chronic urticaria may have associated arthralgias and myalgias. Some of these are due to periarticular urticarial lesions or angioedema, but without a true synovitis. The distinction may be difficult. Because a small fraction of patients with chronic urticaria can have a cutaneous vasculitis (less than 1%) or a systemic connective tissue disorder such as a systemic lupus erythematosus, an erythrocyte sedimentation rate and ANA should be obtained. Neither test is appropriate as a screening test for chronic urticaria patients in the absence of symptoms of an underlying collagen-vascular disease, because the yield is extremely low. Many chronic urticaria patients have a positive ANA of 1:160 or less with speckled pattern. This requires no further evaluation if urticaria or associated thyroid disorder is the only symptom or sign of disease. An ANA higher than 1:160 with a homogeneous pattern may require further screening testing and consultation with a rheumatologist. A significant elevation of sedimentation rate in association with chronic urticaria with arthralgia and myalgias requires a skin biopsy to rule out a cutaneous vasculitis and determination of C4 and C3 levels.

D. Screening for Hepatitis B, Epstein-Barr Virus

Acute urticaria can be associated with a serum-sickness like presentation (i.e., fever, urticaria, lymphadenopathy, proteinuria [30%], arthralgias, or arthritis), which can be caused by drugs or viruses, particularly during the prodrome phase of hepatitis B and the early stages of infectious mononucleosis. Thus new-onset urticaria presenting with this constellation of symptoms or with exposure to either virus should be assessed for the presence of hepatitis B antigen and antibody (immunoglobulin [Ig] M, IgG) and also for Epstein-Barr (EB) virus or anti-EB virus antibody titer to early and nuclear antigen determinants. Inasmuch as these are immune complex-mediated disorders, a C4 and C3 determination, and a C1q binding assay or Raji cell assay for circulating immune complexes may be revealing.

E. Food Skin Testing, Radioallergosorbent Test

Patients with acute urticaria or intermittent urticaria (but not chronic urticaria) may have allergic reactions to foods. Usually the patient has identified one or two foods that are suspect and, if eliminated from the diet, urticaria should subside. Chronic urticaria patients may suspect large numbers of foods are contributory, but hives remain as individual foods or groups of foods are eliminated from the diet. Typically all of these suspicions turn out to be incorrect.

Percutaneous skin tests or radioallergosorbent test (RAST) for foods may be used to determine whether a food allergy is possible. They can confirm cases of acute urticaria because of foods or may assist in the diagnosis of acute urticaria or unexplained intermittent urticaria. Also, RAST testing is available for some foods and condiments for which skin testing reagents have not been developed.

The double-blind, placebo-controlled challenge with food capsules (19) is the most reliable method for determining whether an adverse reaction (in this case urticaria or angioedema) is due to a food.

IV. SKIN BIOPSY

The histopathology of chronic urticaria consists of a nonnecrotizing perivascular infiltration with mononuclear cells and variable numbers of eosinophils (20). Immune complex or local complement depositions are rarely seen. If one eliminates patients with physically induced hives, then this type of histology is seen in more than 95% of patients with acute or chronic urticaria (Fig. 4) (21). Thus routine skin biopsy for patients with chronic urticaria is not recommended and in general is not helpful with regard to specific diagnosis or approach to therapy. There are a variety of circumstances, outlined below, in which a biopsy may be indicated.

1. When the patient is poorly responsive to therapy with maximal doses of antihistamines and low-dose alternate day steroids (22). A variant histological presentation of neutrophilic urticaria (23) in which neutrophils are unusually abundant tends to be more difficult to treat. The vascular integrity is maintained, and this does not represent a cutaneous vasculitis.
2. A patient with known connective tissue disease who now presents with urticaria. In this instance a cutaneous vasculitis (leukocytoclastic angiitis or cutaneous necrotizing venulitis) may be seen with leukocytoclasis, neutrophil predominance, disruption of vascular integrity and, in some instances, deposition of immunoglobulin and complement (24,25).
3. A patient with chronic urticaria in whom arthralgias, myalgias, or frank

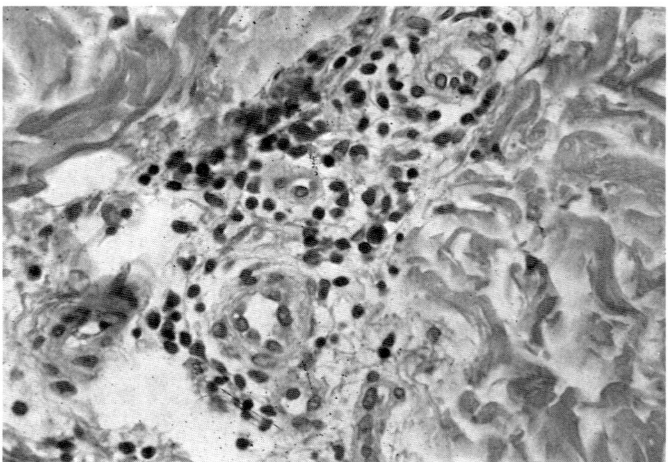

Figure 4 Skin biopsy of a patient with chronic urticaria demonstrating a nonnecrotizing perivascular infiltrate that is predominantly mononuclear.

arthritis is seen, has episodes that are associated with fever, or has an elevated sedimentation rate or a significantly positive ANA. Note that patients with systemic lupus or Sjögren's syndrome can have chronic urticaria of an autoimmune type that is indistinguishable from typical chronic urticaria, or they may present with a cutaneous vasculitis.

4. If it is difficult to distinguish between urticaria and a dermatitis with discrete areas of involvement or two rashes that may be present simultaneously. Here skin biopsy can assist in making the proper diagnosis.

5. Where systemic mastocytosis is suspected. The patients usually have symptoms of dermatographism and have pigmented macules or slightly elevated papules that may urticate with stroking, indicative of urticaria pigmentosa. A significantly increased number of mast cells on skin biopsy is consistent with this disorder (26). Elevated blood tryptase levels are present, particularly when anaphylactoid episodes occur. A variant with telangiectasia (telangiectasia macularis eruptiva perstans) requires biopsy confirmation.

V. EXPERIMENTAL TESTS

A. Chronic Urticaria

An autologous skin test can be performed for patients in whom chronic urticaria is suspected. Blood is drawn, serum is obtained, and 20 μL is injected into the patient's forearm, as for a standard intradermal skin test. The area is examined for production of a wheal and flare reaction (27). A positive test is indicative of autoantibodies triggering histamine release from cutaneous mast cells. The prevalence of positive reactions is uncertain, but it was originally reported to be as high as 30%. Of these, a small number are attributed to IgG anti-IgE antibodies (28,29), and the remainder appear due to IgG anti-IgE receptor antibody (27–29). The skin test is a simple office procedure, but is more difficult to interpret than routine intradermal skin tests because many nonspecific, weakly positive reactions occur. Thus only very strong positive reactions are reliable. This approach has been supplanted by other research methods.

A more reliable method is to determine histamine release after incubation of patient serum with blood basophils (30) or cutaneous mast cells (31). This method is positive in 35–45% of patients, depending on the report cited (32,33). Most of the positive tests are due to IgG antibodies directed to the α-subunit of the high affinity IgE receptor, which is present in both basophils and mast cells.

Another approach is to test sera by immunoblot analysis. A preparation of the cleaved α-subunit (molecular weight is 30–34 kD) is subjected to sodium dodecyl sulphate (SDS) gel electrophoresis, transferred to nitrocellulose, and the sera to be tested are applied. If IgG antibody directed to the α-subunit is present, it binds and can be detected with a labeled anti-IgG that yields a blue-brown color on development (34). This is not a quantitative binding assay but it yields a ''yes'' or ''no'' answer regarding the presence of the antibody (Fig. 5). It does not indicate whether the antibody is functional. When functional analysis using basophils or mast cells is combined with immunoblotting, 45–50% of patients with chronic urticaria have an autoimmune origin for their chronic urticaria (35). It is hoped that an enzyme-linked immunosorbent assay (ELISA) method using the α-subunit will be developed and available commercially for quantitative estimates of the presence of the antibody.

B. Hereditary and Acquired C1 Inhibitor Deficiency

It appears that bradykinin is the mediator of the swelling characteristic of C1 inhibitor deficiency (36), and that complement activation is a parallel phenomenon. However, the changes in complement protein levels and function are particularly useful in terms of diagnostic testing. It has been shown that the plasma protein from which bradykinin is derived, high-molecular-weight kininogen (HK), is cleaved during episodes of swelling. This can be assessed by an immunoblot of patient's serum, using a labeled anti-HK antibody. Native HK has a molecular weight of 115 kD in nonreduced SDS gels, but cleaved HK migrates as a 96-kD band. This difference is readily discerned by immunoblot.

Patients with C1 inhibitor (C1 INH) deficiency present with angioedema, including laryngeal edema and bowel wall edema. Abdominal attacks of cramp-

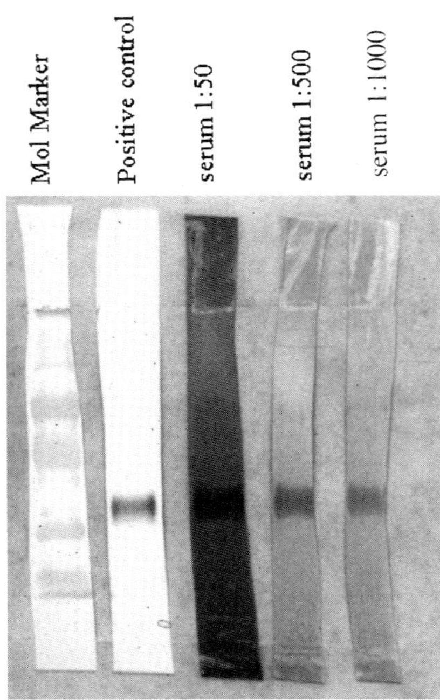

Figure 5 Immunoblot analysis of serum of patient with chronic urticaria tested at 1:50, 1:500, and 1:1,000 wt/vol dilutions (lanes 3–5). Molecular weight markers are shown at the far left, followed by a positive control of a rabbit monoclonal antibody directed to the α subunit of the high affinity IgE receptor. A broad band at molecular weight 33,000 kD is seen at all dilutions of the patient's serum with nonspecific staining eliminated at 1:500 and 1:1000 dilutions.

ing and diarrhea can resemble an acute abdomen (37). The hereditary disorder is transmitted with a dominant pattern of inheritance. About 85% of patients have a deficient (i.e., low level) of C1 INH and 15% synthesize a dysfunctional protein but may have normal or increased blood C1 INH levels (38,39). The diagnosis is most easily made by a C4 determination. Patients with idiopathic angioedema, a far more common disorder, have normal C4 levels, whereas patients with hereditary angioedema (with rare exceptions) have a diminished C4 level even when they are asymptomatic. Once swelling begins, the C4 level decreases to 0, and the C2 level diminishes. If C4 is found to be low, a quantitative assay for C1 INH is done. If it is abnormally low, a diagnosis of hereditary angioedema is confirmed. If it is normal or elevated, a functional C1 INH must be ordered. This will be abnormal in those patients who synthesize a dysfunctional protein. Be-

Table 1 Distinctions Among Types of C1 INH Deficiency

	Hereditary angioedema	Acquired C1 INH deficiency (depletion)	Autoimmune C1 INH deficiency
C1q	N	↓	N
C4	↓	↓	↓
C1 INH	85% ↓ 15% Normal or ↑	↓	↓ molecular weight
Functional C1 INH	↓	↓	↓
Family History	+	—	—

cause all patients have a single normal gene, a 50% C1 INH level would be expected, but hypermetabolism of the normal C1 INH yields a far lower value (40) and angioedema is seen when the level of normal protein is less than 25%.

Acquired C1 INH deficiency is associated with B-cell lymphoma (41) and connective tissue disorders (42). There is depletion of C1 INH due to immune complex activation of C1 or, in the case of B cell lymphoma, IgG antibody directed against idiotypic antigens of the immunoglobulin on the cell surface (43). When C1r and C1s are activated, each binds to the C1 INH, and the complexes are cleared from the circulation. If utilization exceeds synthesis, C1 INH depletion results. This disorder typically is unassociated with any family history of angioedema (although a hereditary angioedema patient with a new mutation would present similarly), and it has a low level of C1q in addition to a low C4 and diminished C1 INH level. Lastly, there is a much less common form of acquired C1 INH deficiency in which an IgG antibody is directed to C1 INH (44). The C1 INH is readily digested by enzymes to which it is bound (C1r, C1s, factor XIIa, kallikrein), but these enzymes are not inactivated and they digest the C1 INH. The result is a depleted level of C1 INH, which is cleaved to a lower molecular weight form. There is normal C1q, low C4 and C1 INH, and a C1 INH band of 96 kD upon SDS gel electrophoresis, rather than the usual 105-kD band. The distinctions among the various forms of C1 INH deficiency are summarized in Table 1.

VI. SALIENT POINTS

1. There are specific tests that can be performed in the office for each type of physically induced urticaria. They should be pursued when a suggestive history is obtained or when individual urticarial lesions last less than 2 hours.

2. A skin biopsy typically reveals no abnormality in physically induced hives, with the exception of delayed-pressure urticaria. A nonnecrotizing perivascular infiltrate consisting primarily of mononuclear cells and variable numbers of eosinophils or neutrophils characterizes chronic urticaria and is distinct from a true cutaneous vasculitis (leukocytoclastic angiitis) in which immunoglobulin and complement deposition also may be seen.
3. Twenty-four percent of patients with chronic urticaria have associated antithyroid antibodies, even if they are euthyroid.
4. The latest data regarding the pathogenesis of chronic urticaria suggest the presence of an IgG antibody directed to the α-subunit of the IgE receptor.
5. C1 inhibitor deficiency can be either hereditary (85% with decreased protein and 15% with a dysfunctional protein) or acquired. The latter includes patients in whom C1 inhibitor is consumed by massive complement activation, or it can be due to an autoimmune disorder in which antibody is directed to the C1 inhibitor protein.

REFERENCES

1. Houser DD, Arbesman CE, Ito K, Wicher K. Cold urticaria: immunologic studies. Am J Med 1970;49:23–33.
2. Kaplan AP, Gray L, Shaff RE, Horakova Z, Beaven MA. In vivo studies of mediator release in cold urticaria and cholinergic urticaria. J Allergy Clin Immunol 1975;55:394–402.
3. Kurtz AS, Kaplan AP. Regional expression of cold urticaria. J Allergy Clin Immunol 1990;86:272–273.
4. Grant JA, Findlay JR, Thueson DO, Fine DP, Krueger GG. Local heat urticaria/angioedema: evidence for histamine release without complement activation. J Allergy Clin Immunol 1981;67:75–77.
5. Garafolo J, Kaplan AP. Histamine release and therapy of severe dermatographism. J Allergy Clin Immunol 1981;68:103–105.
6. Kaur S, Greaves M, Eftekhari N. Factitious urticaria (dermographism): treatment by cimetidine and chlorpheniramine in a randomized double-blind study. Br J Dermatol 1981;104:185–190.
7. Sussman GL, Harvey RP, Schocket AL. Delayed pressure urticaria. J Allergy Clin Immunol 1982;70:337–342.
8. Estes SA, Yung CW. Delayed pressure urticaria: An investigation of some parameters of lesion induction. J Am Acad Dermatol 1981;5:25–31.
9. Sams WM, Epstein JH, Winkelmann RK. Solar urticaria. Investigation of pathogenic mechanisms. Arch Derm 1969;99:390–397.
10. Harber LC, Holloway RM, Wheatley VR, Baer RL. Immunologic and biophysical studies in solar urticaria. J Invest Dermatol 1963;41:439–443.

11. Bottomley SS, Tanaka M, Everett MA. Diminished erythroid ferrochetalase activity in protoporphyria. J Lab Clin Med 1975;86:126–131.
12. Sellers VM, Dailey TA, Dailey HA. Examination of ferrochetalase mutations that cause erythropoietic protoporphyria. Blood 1978;91:3980–3985.
13. Kaplan AP. Unusual cold induced disorders: cold-dependent dermatographism and systemic cold urticaria. J Allergy Clin Immunol 1984;73:453–456.
14. Kaplan AP, Garofalo J. Identification of a new physically induced urticaria: cold induced cholinergic urticaria. J Allergy Clin Immunol 1981;68:438–441.
15. Kaplan AP, Beaven MA. In vivo studies of the pathogenesis of cold urticaria, cholinergic urticaria, and vibration induced swelling. J Invest Dermatol 1976;67: 327–332.
16. Commens CA, Greaves MA. Tests to establish the diagnosis in cholinergic urticaria. Br J Dermatol 1978;98:47–51.
17. Leznoff A, Josse RG, Denberg J, Dolovich J. Association of chronic urticaria and angioedema with thyroid autoimmunity. Arch Dermatol 1983;119:636–640.
18. Leznoff A, Sussman GL. Syndrome of idiopathic chronic urticaria and angioedema with thyroid autoimmunity: a study of 90 patients. J Allergy Clin Immunol 1989; 87:66–71.
19. Bock SA, Atkins FM. Patterns of food hypersensitivity during sixteen years of double-blind, placebo-controlled food challenges. J Ped 1990;117:561–567.
20. Natbony SF, Phillips ME, Elias JM, Godfrey HP, Kaplan AP. Histologic studies of chronic idiopathic urticaria. J Allergy Clin Immunol 1983;71:177–183.
21. Elias J, Boss E, Kaplan AP. Studies of the cellular infiltrate of chronic idiopathic urticaria: Prominence of T lymphocytes, monocytes, and mast cells. J Allergy Clin Immunol 1986;78:914–918.
22. Kaplan AP. Urticaria and angioedema. In: Kaplan, AP, ed. Allergy, 2nd ed. Philadelphia: WB Saunders, 1997:573–592.
23. Toppe E, Haas N, Henz BM. Neurophilic urticaria: clinical features, histological changes and possible mechanisms. Br J Dermatol 1998;138(2):248–253.
24. Soter NA, Austen KF, Gili I. The complement system in necrotizing angiitis of the skin. Analysis of complement component activities in serum of patients with concomitant collagen-vascular diseases. J Invest Dermatol 1974;63:219–226.
25. Mackel SE, Jordon RE. Leukocytoclastic vasculitis. A cutaneous expression of immune complex disease. Arch Dermatol 1982;118:296–301.
26. Bianchine PJ, Metcalfe DD. Systemic mastocytosis. In: Kaplan, AP, ed. Allergy. Philadelphia, PA: Churchill Livingstone, 1997:854–875.
27. Gratten CEH, Boon AP, Eady RAJ, Winkelmann RK. The pathology of the autologous serum skin test response in chronic urticaria resembles IgE-mediated late phase reactions. Int Arch Allergy Appl Immunol 1990;93:198–204.
28. Gruber BL, Baeza ML, Marchese MJ, Agnello V, Kaplan AP. Prevalence and functional role of anti-IgE autoantibodies in urticarial syndromes. J Invest Derm 1988; 90:213–217.
29. Gratten CEH, Francis DM, Hide M, Greaves MW. Detection of circulating histamine releasing autoantibodies with functional properties of anti-IgE in chronic urticaria. Clin Exp Allergy 1991;21:695–704.
30. Zweiman B, Valenzano M, Atkins PC, Tanus T, Getsy JA. Characteristics of hista-

mine releasing activity in the sera of patients with chronic urticaria. J Allergy Clin Immunol 1996;98:89–98.

31. Niimi N, Francis DM, Kermani F, O'Donnell BF, Hide M, Kobza-Black A, Winklemann RK, Greaves MW, Barr RM. Dermal mast cell activation by autoantibodies against the high affinity IgE receptor in chronic urticaria. J Invest Derm 1996;106: 1001–1006.
32. Hide M, Francis DM,Gratten CEH, Hakimi J, Kochan JP, Greaves MW. Autoantibodies against the high affinity IgE receptor as a cause of histamine release in chronic urticaria. N Engl J Med 1993;328:1549–1604.
33. Tong LJ, Balakrishnan G, Kochan JP, Kinet J-P, Kaplan AP. Assessment of autoimmunity in patients with chronic urticaria. J Allergy Clin Immunol 1997;99:461–465.
34. Fiebiger E, Hammerschmid F, Stingl G, Maurer D. Anti $Fc_eR1\alpha$ autoantibodies in autoimmune-mediated disorders. Identification of a structure-function relationship. J Clin Invest 1998;101:243–251.
35. Ferrer M, Kinet J-P, Kaplan AP. Comparative studies of functional and binding assays for IgG anti Fc_eR1_α (α subunit) in chronic urticaria. J Allergy Clin Immunol 1998;101:672–676.
36. Fields T, Ghebrehiwet B, Kaplan AP. Kinin formation in hereditary angioedema plasma: Evidence against kinin-derivation from C2 and in support of ''spontaneous'' formation of bradykinin. J Allergy Clin Immunol 1983;72:54–60.
37. Frank MM, Gelfand JA, Atkinson JP. Hereditary angioedema: The clinical syndrome and its management. Ann Intern Med 1976;84:580–593.
38. Donaldson VH, Harrison R, Rosen FS, Bing DH, Kindness G, Conan J, Wagner CJ, Awad S. Variability in purified dysfunctional C1-inhibitor proteins from patients with hereditary angioneurotic edema: functional and analytic gel studies. J Clin Invest 1985;75:124–132.
39. Kramer J, Katz Y, Rosen FS, Davis III AE, Strunk RC. Synthesis of C1 inhibitor in fibroblasts from patients with type I and type II hereditary angioneurotic edema. J Clin Invest 1991;87:1614–1620.
40. Quastel M, Harrison R, Cicardi M, Alper CA, Rosen FS. Behavior in vivo of normal and dysfunctional C1 inhibitor in normal subjects and patients with hereditary angineurotic edema. J Clin Invest 1983;71:1041–1046.
41. Gelfand JA, Boss GR, Conley CL, Reinhart R, Frank MM. Acquired C1 esterase inhibitor deficiency and angioedema: A review. Medicine 1979;58:321–328.
42. Sheffer AL, Austen KF, Rosen FS, Fearon DT. Acquired deficiency of the inhibitor of the first component of complement. Report of five additional cases and commentary on the syndrome. J Allergy Clin Immunol 1985;75:640–646.
43. Geha RS, Quinti I, Austen KF, Cicardi M, Sheffer A, Rosen FS. Acquired C1-inhibitor deficiency associated with antiidiotypic antibody to monoclonal immunoglobulins. N Engl J Med 1985;312:534–540.
44. Malbran A, Hammer CH, Frank MM, Fries LF. Acquired angioedema: Observation on the mechanism of action of autoantibodies directed against C1 esterase inhibitor. J Allergy Clin Immunol 1988;81:1199–1204.

5

Ocular Allergic Diseases: Differential Diagnosis, Examination Techniques, and Testing

Marc Dinowitz, Ronald Rescigno, and Leonard Bielory
UMDNJ–New Jersey Medical School, Newark, New Jersey

The eye is a common site for the development of allergic inflammatory disorders. Ophthalmologists and allergists frequently encounter allergic diseases of the eye in their general practice. Although the eye may be the only organ system involved in an allergic reaction, typically there also exists a systemic allergic component. Even so, ocular signs and symptoms often are the most prominent features of the entire allergic response (1,2).

The differential diagnoses of conditions presenting with a red eye include allergic disorders and a variety of other ocular abnormalities, some of which can produce profound visual loss if not treated appropriately. The signs and symptoms associated with these conditions often overlap, and it can be difficult to differentiate one ocular disease from another. Therefore, an understanding of ophthalmologic examination techniques and diagnostic procedures can help a health care provider make an accurate diagnosis of ocular allergy.

This chapter provides a review of the various forms of allergic inflammation and focuses on the clinical characteristics that help to differentiate allergic disorders, both from each another and from other ocular conditions. The technique for the use of a direct ophthalmoscope in ocular examination is also outlined. Finally, various procedures and tests used to formulate the diagnosis and treatment of ocular allergy are discussed.

I. MANIFESTATIONS OF OCULAR ALLERGY

The clinical presentation of ocular surface allergic disorders is varied and depends, in part, on the immunologic mechanism involved and the specific ocular tissues affected. Based on these differences, the most common differential diagnoses of allergic ocular disease can be divided into allergic conjunctivitis, vernal keratoconjunctivitis, atopic keratoconjunctivitis, giant papillary conjunctivitis, contact allergy, and dry eye (Fig. 1A–C).

Seasonal allergic conjunctivitis is the most common form of allergic conjunctivitis and accounts for approximately one half of all cases seen (1,3). Sea-

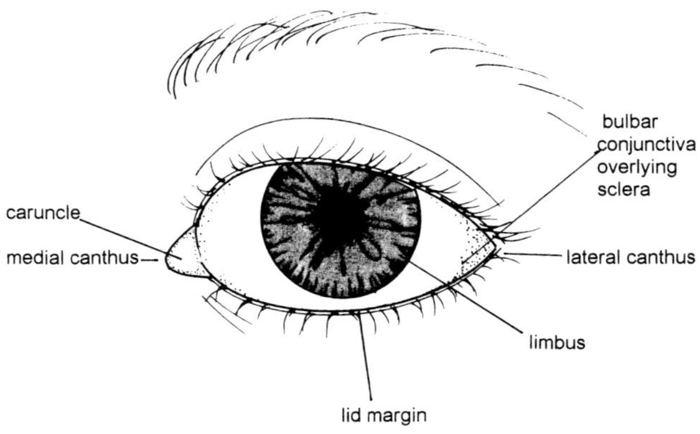

Figure 1 Gross anatomy of the eye (A) Frontal view. (B) Frontal view with eversion of lower eyelid. (C) Sagittal view.

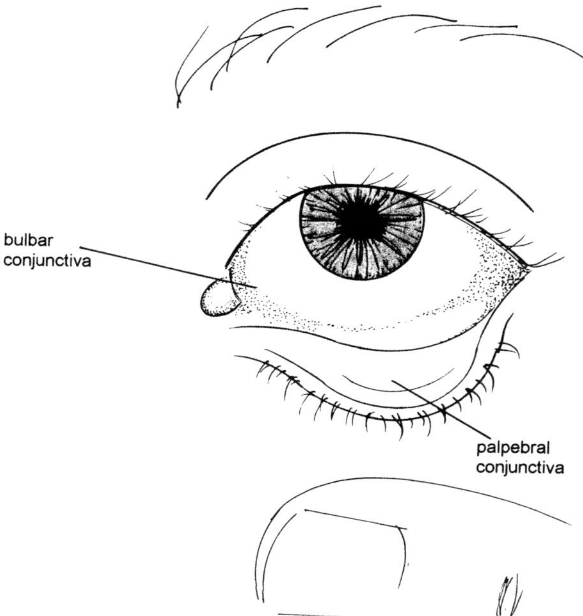

B

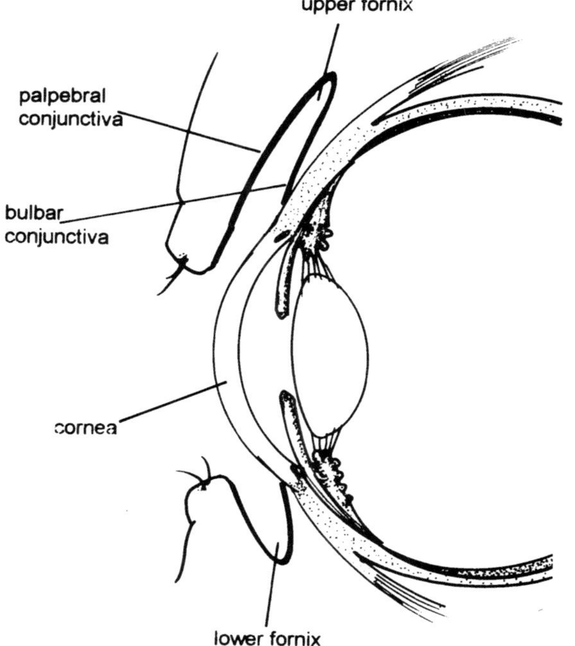

C

Figure 1 Continued

sonal onset of symptoms tends to be related to the appearance of specific airborne pollen allergens, including trees, grasses, or weeds. The immediate hypersensitivity reaction characteristic of this disorder is initiated after these specific allergens react with immunoglobulin (Ig) E attached to mast cells in the conjunctiva. Typical symptoms include tearing, itching, burning, red eyes, sneezing, and runny nose. Associated ocular discharge is usually scant or watery. Although ocular signs are often mild, the conjunctiva takes on a pale, boggy appearance that evolves into diffuse areas of papillae (small vascularized nodules). These papillae tend to be most prominent on the superior palpebral conjunctiva. Involvement of the cornea is rare. Occasionally, dark circles beneath the eyes (''allergic shiners'') are present as a result of localized venous congestion (1,3,4–6).

Less severe signs and symptoms are seen in a related disorder called **perennial allergic conjunctivitis**. Like seasonal allergic conjunctivitis, this disorder exhibits the classic IgE/mast cell-mediated hypersensitivity to airborne allergens. Instead of sensitivity to grass or weed pollens, however, patients with perennial allergic conjunctivitis usually are more sensitive to common household allergens such as dust mites, animal dander, and possibly, cockroach (3).

The ocular reaction seen in both seasonal allergic and perennial allergic conjunctivitis resolves quickly once the offending allergen is removed. The diagnosis of these disorders can be made by taking a detailed history from the patient. Both eyes are typically affected simultaneously and a family history of hay fever or atopy may be elicited. The diagnosis can often be confirmed by Giemsa staining of conjunctival scrapings taken from the inner surface of the upper or lower lid (see procedure, described below). Polymorphonuclear cells with eosinophils or eosinophilic granules seen with Giemsa stain typically support the diagnosis of seasonal allergic or perennial allergic conjunctivitis (1,3,4,6).

Treatment of seasonal allergic or perennial allergic conjunctivitis centers initially on avoidance of the offending agent. Depending on the severity of the patient's signs and symptoms, pharmacological therapy may be used. In addition to cool compresses and artificial tears, oral or topical antihistamines, topical cromolyn, and topical nonsteroidal anti-inflammatory drugs (NSAIDS) may be used (1,3–7).

Vernal keratoconjunctivitis is a mast cell/lymphocyte-mediated allergic disorder that mainly affects young men between 3 and 20 years of age. Onset is between ages 11 and 13 years. This condition is seasonally recurrent and chronic in nature, occasionally lasting up to 10 years. Symptoms include severe itching, foreign body sensation, photophobia, eyelid spasm, blurred vision, and copious amounts of thick ropy mucous discharge. Clinically, two forms of the disease are seen, depending upon whether the palpebral or limbal conjunctiva is affected. These two forms may occur singly or simultaneously in the disease process. The classic feature of vernal keratoconjunctivitis is giant papillae (cobblestones) found on the upper palpebral conjunctiva. Papillae along the limbal conjunctiva are more common in black patients and are typically described as thickened, gelatinous nodular masses with neighboring whitish inclusions (Horner-Trantas dots). These dots represent focal aggregations of epithelial cells and eosinophils (1,3,6,8). The masses and dots are seen most often at the superior limbus. Diffuse areas of punctate corneal epithelial defects can occur in some cases. These defects are best appreciated with a cobalt blue light after the instillation of topical fluorescein dye (see procedure, described below). In severe cases, these superficial punctate defects may progress to epithelial ''shield ulcers,'' which often develop centrally in the cornea slightly above the visual axis (1,3,6,8,9). A shield ulcer is a large area of denuded corneal epithelium similar in appearance to a corneal abrasion. On rare occasions, abnormal corneal steepening (keratoconus) may develop from frequent rubbing of itchy eyes (1,3,6,10).

The diagnosis of vernal keratoconjunctivitis is made clinically. The signs and symptoms associated with this disorder are straightforward and can be revealed after a detailed history from the patient. The majority of patients with this illness live in warm, dry climates. In addition, a personal or family history of seasonal allergies, asthma, and other atopic diseases is often elicited. Like seasonal allergic and perennial allergic conjunctivitis, vernal keratoconjunctivitis is associated with Giemsa-stained conjunctiva showing eosinophils (1,3,6,9,10).

An important part of the therapy for vernal keratoconjunctivitis begins with patient education. Patients must be made aware that this condition is chronic, tends to be seasonal, and has the potential for serious ocular sequelae. As with seasonal allergic conjunctivitis, initial treatment plans rely on cool compresses and artificial tears for comfort measures. Topical antihistamines, NSAIDS, and cromolyn can be used to control itching and relieve discomfort. Individuals who remain symptomatic after this initial therapy are sometimes prescribed topical pulse corticosteroids. Topical steroids should be reserved for those patients with moderate to severe discomfort because of their significant ocular side effects (11). On rare occasions, surgical excision of giant papillae may be necessary. In patients with persistent epithelial defects, bandage soft contact lenses can be helpful (1,3,6–8).

Atopic keratoconjunctivitis is a mast cell/lymphocyte-mediated ocular disorder known to occur in patients who have or have had atopic dermatitis. Patients with this disease often have an inherited tendency to develop hypersensitivity to specific allergens. Although the specific cause of atopic keratoconjunctivitis is unknown, both immediate and delayed hypersensitivity to specific allergens is thought to play a role (1,3,6). This disorder usually occurs in men and presents in the late teens or early 20s, with a peak incidence near the fifth decade of life. Symptoms are not seasonal and are generally more severe than seasonal allergic conjunctivitis or vernal keratoconjunctivitis. Patients with this disorder have bilateral involvement and complain of chronic itching, burning, photophobia, tearing, a thick ropy discharge, and chronic redness. Affected patients show eczematoid changes of their eyelids typified by erythema, induration, maceration, and scaling (blepharitis). As a result of such chronic inflammation, plugging of the meibomian gland orifices may develop, leading to a deficient precorneal tear film and the signs and symptoms of dry eye. In addition, chronic inflammation may cause redness and edema of the conjunctiva. The inferior fornix and palpebral conjunctiva are the regions most often affected, and conjunctival scarring in the inferior fornix may occur in severe disease. Corneal involvement is common and presents as punctate epithelial defects. In rare cases, persistent epithelial defects and ulcers may occur.

Atopic keratoconjunctivitis is associated with a number of other ocular conditions, including herpes simplex keratitis, cataract, and keratoconus (1,3). Herpes simplex keratitis in these patients may be severe, with frequent recurrences and persistent epithelial defects. Cataracts are frequently bilateral and symmetric, and may require extraction if vision deteriorates.

Atopic keratoconjunctivitis can be simple to diagnose. Patients with this disorder usually have had undiagnosed red, itchy eyes for many years. These patients may have many other nonocular problems including pruritus, chronic and relapsing dermatitis, and a variety of other atopic diseases (i.e., asthma, urticaria, eczema, rhinitis). The appearance of the eyelids and the periorbital area easily differentiates this disorder from seasonal allergic conjunctivitis. In contrast to vernal keratoconjunctivitis, this disorder primarily involves the inferior palpebral conjunctiva and is characterized by small papillae. Of note, Giemsa-stained conjunctival scrapings in atopic keratoconjunctivitis usually show fewer and less degranulated eosinophils as compared with other ocular allergies (1,3,4,6,10).

The goals of treating atopic keratoconjunctivitis focus on avoidance of potential allergens, relief of symptoms, and prevention of associated ocular complications. Like other ocular allergic disorders, cool compresses, antihistamines, and artificial tears can provide significant relief from itching. Topical steroids administered in pulse fashion often are needed to control the significant degree of keratitis and conjunctival inflammation that may occur (1,3,6,7). Treatment of associated ocular conditions should be initiated at time of diagnosis. Lid scrubs, warm compresses, and oral antibiotics may help curb severe blepharitis and meibomian gland dysfunction. Preservative-free lubricant drops and ointments may be needed to relieve dry eye. In those patients with concurrent herpetic infection, topical antiviral therapy may be indicated. However, patients with atopic keratoconjunctivitis and active herpes simplex keratitis cannot be started on topical steroids along with antiviral therapy. Although pulse steroids may help the ocular allergy, they can worsen the herpetic keratitis and associated ocular infection (1). Once ocular inflammation is under reasonable control, cataract extraction and/or corneal transplant can be considered if necessary. Overall, the treatment of atopic keratoconjunctivitis is extremely difficult compared to other forms of ocular allergy (3).

Giant papillary conjunctivitis is most often associated with contact lens wear (particularly extended-wear soft contact lenses), but may also occur in patients with ocular prostheses or exposed monofilament sutures in contact with the conjunctiva (1,3,6,12). The main feature of this disorder is the development of large papillae on the upper palpebral conjunctival surface, usually 1 mm in diameter or larger. Although the exact etiology of this disorder is unknown, two main theories have been postulated: (1) mechanical trauma to the upper palpebral conjunctiva secondary to poor contact lens design, and (2) antigen-antibody reaction in the upper palpebral conjunctiva secondary to antigen deposition on the contact lens surface (3,6). Regardless of etiology, most patients with this disorder complain of itching, increased mucous production, slight blurring of vision, conjunctival redness (injection), foreign body sensation, and contact lens intolerance. Clinical signs of giant papillary conjunctivitis usually follow the onset of symptoms by several days to weeks.

The diagnosis of giant papillary conjunctivitis can easily be made when a contact lens wearer presents with typical symptoms and enlarged papillae on the upper palpebral conjunctiva. If this disorder is in its early stages, minimal (if any) pathology may be seen. As a consequence, it is possible for giant papillary conjunctivitis to be confused with many other ocular disorders, including seasonal allergic conjunctivitis and toxic reactions to contact lens care products. With disease progression, however, conjunctival injection and thickening, giant papillae, and scarring often develop. Whereas the clinical and histologic features of this disorder most closely resemble those seen in vernal keratoconjunctivitis, the papillae seen in this disorder are more evenly distributed, flatter, and smaller (1,3,6,8,12).

The best method for diagnosing giant papillary conjunctivitis involves examination of the upper palpebral conjunctival surface (see procedure, described below). The upper palpebral conjunctival surface is best viewed after performing lid eversion (Fig. 2A). Topical fluorescein viewed with cobalt blue light helps to outline any papillae, especially in the early stages of this disorder when only small papillae may be present (Fig. 2B) (3). Unlike other ocular allergies, giant papillary conjunctivitis is associated with abnormal conjunctival accumulations of mast cells, basophils, and eosinophils (6).

The goal of therapy for giant papillary conjunctivitis is to enable patients to continue wearing contact lenses. This disorder is reversible and can be cured by eliminating contact lens wear. However, this solution is usually unsatisfactory to the patient. Topical antihistamines, cromolyn, and a contact lens "vacation" may be curative. Good lens hygiene and the use of disposable contact lenses are almost always curative (1,3,6,7,12).

Contact allergies involving the ocular surface and eyelids occur most commonly after using a variety of topical ophthalmic medications, contact lens solutions, and cosmetics. Contact allergies may occur acutely or have delayed onset.

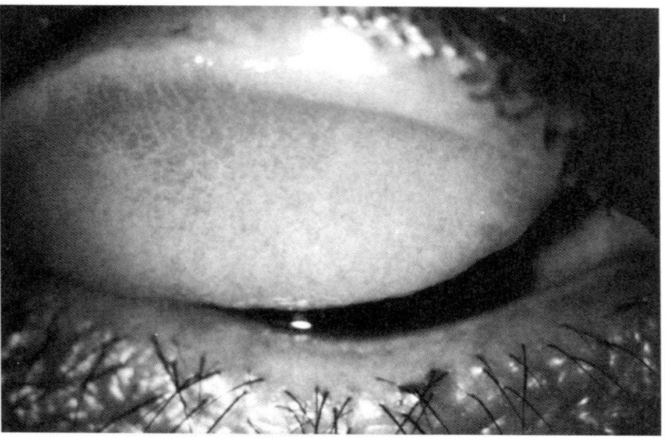

A

B

Figure 2 Slit-lamp view of giant papillae. Upper palpebral conjunctiva viewed after lid eversion. (A) Direct white illumination without fluorescein staining. (B) Cobalt blue light after instillation of fluorescein dye.

Acute reactions are classically IgE mediated and occur within several minutes after exposure to the allergen. Papillae and edema of the conjunctiva, watery ocular discharge, and eyelid erythema and swelling may result. Typical symptoms include severe itching, burning, and occasional photophobia. In general, the amount of ocular involvement in acute contact allergies may vary depending on the offending agent involved. In contrast to acute reactions, delayed hypersensitivity reactions are cell mediated and include an initial sensitization period followed by a delay period of 24–72 h before expression. The most common culprit agents are topical cholinergic medications, sulfonamides, aminoglycosides, neomycin, phenylephrine, and thimerosal (1,3,6). A red and inflamed eye with erythema, scaling, and thickening of the eyelid skin and margin may result. Typical symptoms include burning and irritation, but little or no itching.

A careful history is crucial to the diagnosis of contact allergy. It is important to question patients regarding the use of all medications, including over-the-counter products, prescription drugs, and ''homemade'' preparations. Giemsa-stained conjunctiva in acute contact allergies demonstrate eosinophils. In contrast, Giemsa-stained conjunctiva in delayed contact allergies do not show eosinophils.

Treatment of contact allergy involves identification and discontinuation of the offending agent. Cool compresses and preservative-free lubricating ointments or drops may help to minimize and control inflammation. Topical antihistamines and a short course of pulsed topical steroids may be useful if conjunctival signs and symptoms are particularly severe. To date, desensitization techniques have not proven helpful (1).

Dry eye is a frequent manifestation of ocular allergic disease. It is sometimes difficult to differentiate correctly between patients with dry eye and those with more serious pathology, including ocular allergy. The reason for this difficulty is that several ocular conditions are known to mimic the symptoms of dry eye, including blepharitis and viral or allergic conjunctivitis (13). True dry eye develops from decreased tear production, increased tear evaporation, or an abnormality in specific components of the aqueous, lipid, or mucin layers that comprise the tear film (2,6,14,15). Although dry eye may result from intrinsic tear pathology, it is frequently associated with other ocular disorders, such as ocular allergy and chronic blepharitis, and systemic diseases, including fifth or seventh nerve palsies, collagen vascular disease, Sjögren's syndrome, vitamin A deficiency, pemphigoid, and trauma. Dry eye is also associated with many pharmacologic agents, including antihistamines, anticholinergics, and some psychotropics (2, 6,14,15). Symptoms of dry eye are vague and include foreign body sensation, easily fatigued eyes, dryness, burning, ocular pain, photophobia, and blurry vision. Symptoms may be worse late in the day after prolonged use of the eyes or exposure to environmental conditions.

The diagnosis of dry eye can be made after a detailed history and examination. Dandruff-like flakes, lash collars, telangiectasia, and thickening of the eyelid margin are suggestive of blepharitis (Fig. 3), a known cause of dry eye. Typical conjunctival findings include mild to moderate injection, redundancy, thickening, and swelling. The tear film frequently reveals increased debris and a tear film meniscus height of 0.1 mm or less. Corneal pathology may be significant and includes an irregular corneal surface light reflex, punctate epithelial defects, or mucous thread formation on the surface.

A variety of simple tests and stains can be used to confirm the presence

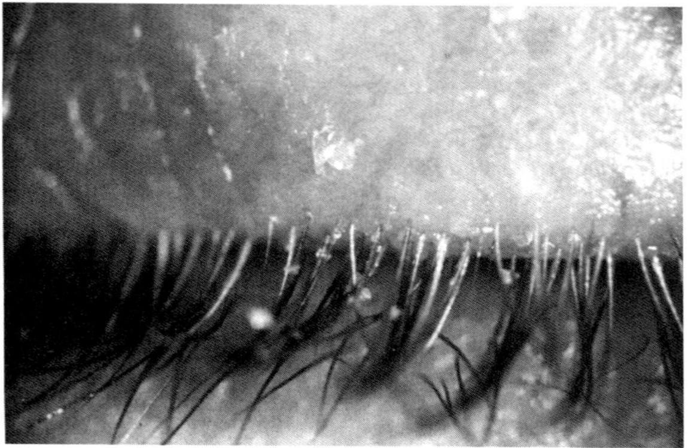

Figure 3 Upper eyelid margin. Note the dandruff-like flakes (scurf), lash collars, thickening, and telangiectasia consistent with blepharitis.

of dry eye. The Schirmer and vital staining tests, including fluorescein and rose bengal, are the most useful for diagnosing dry eye (see procedures, described below) (13,14). The Schirmer test quantitatively measures the amount of tears produced by the lacrimal gland. Fluorescein dye stains denuded corneal and conjunctival epithelium and is known to pool in surface irregularities. It is typically used to demonstrate tear film meniscus height, punctate epithelial defects in the cornea, and tear film breakup time (TBUT) (14,15). In contrast to fluorescein, rose bengal stains devitalized, degenerated, and dead epithelial cells of the cornea and conjunctiva (Fig. 4). In dry eye disease, rose bengal stains the conjunctiva more than the cornea, with the nasal conjunctiva staining more intensely than the temporal conjunctiva (16).

The treatment of dry eye is multifactorial. Tear substitutes (solutions and ointments) are the initial treatment modalities for this disorder. Whereas ointments tend to remain in the eye longer than drops, their usefulness is limited because they may blur vision. Exacerbating conditions, such as ocular allergy and blepharitis, must be treated before the patient can experience relief. Blockage of the canalicular system (tear drainage system) in the eyelid with cautery or punctal plugs can be helpful in those patients whose symptoms are not relieved with frequent use of tear supplements (6,14,15).

II. DIFFERENTIAL DIAGNOSIS OF OCULAR ALLERGY

The differential diagnoses of conditions presenting with a red eye include allergic disorders as well as many other ocular diseases. Signs and symptoms associated

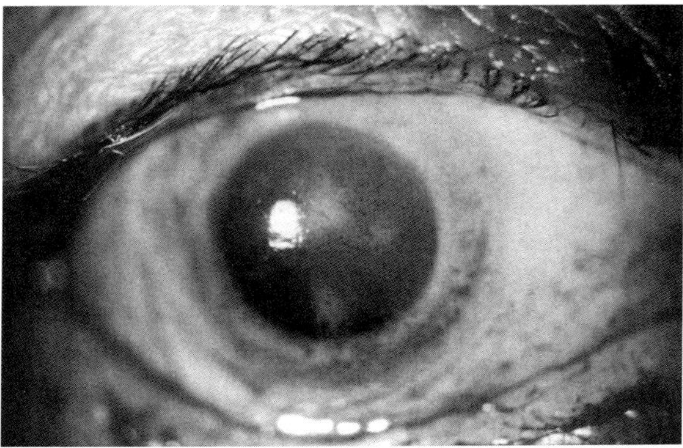

Figure 4 Rose bengal stain of ocular surface. Note the increased punctate staining of the cornea and inferonasal conjunctiva consistent with dry eye.

with these many conditions frequently overlap and may be confusing to differentiate. Although the most typical causes of a red eye are considered ''benign'' and do not threaten vision, several potentially serious disorders can cause permanent visual loss if they are not accurately diagnosed and treated. Therefore, an understanding of the most common causes of a red eye is critical to avoid the potential pitfalls associated with misdiagnosis.

Diagnosis or referral to an ophthalmologist is made only after a detailed history and physical examination. The history should include an accurate description of symptoms, time and rapidity of onset, associated signs, medications, allergies, and so on. A detailed and descriptive patient history is critical and often provides reasonable insight into the diagnosis even before the ocular examination is begun.

Non–vision-threatening causes of red eye include subconjunctival hemorrhage, ocular allergy, infectious conjunctivitis, blepharitis, dry eye, and corneal abrasion (6,17,18). The complaints of patients with such entities include burning, itching, a scratchy sensation, eyelid tenderness, or ocular discharge. A history of burning is very nonspecific and usually is not a definitive sign of specific ocular disease (18). Itching suggests an allergic etiology, especially if it is accompanied by a thick, ropy discharge. A scratchy sensation is indicative of corneal/conjunctival foreign body, corneal abrasion, or dry eye. Purulent ocular discharge is associated with bacterial conjunctivitis. Patients with this disorder often complain of matted eyelids that stick together, especially in the early morning hours. Watery ocular discharge and a painful preauricular lymph node are characteristic of viral conjunctivitis. This disorder is extremely contagious and often follows an upper respiratory infection.

Vision-threatening causes of red eye are diverse and include acute angle closure glaucoma, uveitis, herpes keratitis, corneal ulcers, and scleritis. These disorders are associated with symptoms of ocular pain, blurred vision, and photophobia (17,18). In the presence of these symptoms, it is important to exclude a history of trauma, recent eye surgery, or contact lens wear before the ocular examination.

The **ocular examination** begins with the eyelids and lashes. Evidence of lid margin erythema, telangiectasia, thickening, scaling, or lash collars should be noted.

The sclera and conjunctiva are examined next. The presence of injection should be noted immediately. Characteristics of injection can pinpoint the diagnosis. Subconjunctival hemorrhage often develops suddenly after coughing, sneezing, or straining, and results from the spontaneous rupture of a conjunctival or episcleral capillary. It is characterized as a focal area of solid redness surrounded completely by normal white sclera. It is usually painless, frequently resolves on its own, and does not warrant an ophthalmology consultation, except in the presence of trauma (17,18). The redness of scleritis develops gradually over a few days and is associated with several rheumatologic conditions, particularly rheumatoid arthritis and Wegener's granulomatosis. Signs and symptoms of scleritis include moderate to severe ocular pain, tender and inflamed conjunctiva, and thickened and injected sclera. Early referral to an ophthalmologist is warranted in this condition. Circumcorneal injection (ciliary flush) is described as a ring of redness that completely encircles the edge (limbus) of the cornea. This injection is usually a hallmark of serious ocular pathology that requires immediate ophthalmologic evaluation (18).

The cornea is examined next. A corneal opacity, seen as a whitish infiltrate, is a sign of a bacterial corneal ulcer, which requires immediate evaluation by an ophthalmologist because of the significant possibility of perforation (17). Diffuse corneal haze, which can significantly alter the view of the iris, is a sign of corneal edema. This edema occurs in acute angle closure glaucoma attacks, necessitating urgent ophthalmologic evaluation. Fluorescein and rose bengal stains help to differentiate between punctate epithelial defects (diffuse punctate staining), herpes simplex keratitis (dendrite-shaped staining) and abrasion (large solid area of staining seen after trauma).

Examination of pupil size can be helpful when formulating the diagnosis of red eye. In iritis, the affected pupil is usually smaller and sluggish. In acute angle closure glaucoma attacks, the pupil is usually mid-dilated and sluggish or fixed.

Treatment of red eye can be initiated once an accurate diagnosis is made. All cases of suspected angle closure glaucoma, iritis, scleritis, and bacterial corneal ulcer require immediate ophthalmologic consultation. Any patient with vision-threatening signs and symptoms should be referred immediately to an ophthalmologist (6,17,18). Although treatment of particular disorders may warrant the use of topical steroids, it is unwise to do so without an evaluation by an ophthalmologist (17). Topical steroids have significant ocular side effects and may actually worsen many disorders, especially if misdiagnosed initially.

III. TECHNIQUES OF OPHTHALMIC EXAMINATION

A few specific ophthalmologic examination techniques help to formulate the differential diagnosis of ocular allergic diseases. An acceptable ''basic'' examination of the eye requires only a few simple items, including a visual acuity Snellen chart or card, an occluder, a pocket penlight, a magnifying lens, fluorescein strips, rose bengal, a cotton-tipped applicator, and a direct (hand-held) ophthalmoscope with a cobalt blue filter (19).

Physical examination of the eye begins with a careful and thorough overview of the entire patient as he or she enters the examination room. Attention should focus on abnormalities in facial features, skin complexion, and physical disabilities. Typical facial and skin features that often provide clues to diagnosis include forehead and eyelid vesicular eruption of herpes zoster; malar rash of systemic lupus erythematosus; enlarged parotid glands and extreme dryness of the lips associated with Sjögren's syndrome and sarcoidosis; and dermatological changes of rosacea associated with dry eye and blepharitis. In addition to the face and skin, a patient's extremities (especially the hands) can provide clues to the diagnosis. Examples include flexion contracture deformities of rheumatoid arthritis and Raynaud's phenomenon associated with scleroderma.

The formal ocular examination begins with assessment of the patient's visual acuity. *Visual acuity must be assessed and documented prior to any examination or procedure*. The Snellen chart or card is the tool used most often by physicians to measure a patient's visual acuity objectively. The chart is situated 20 feet from the patient under adequate, diffuse light without glare. By convention, visual acuity is expressed as a fraction, with 20/20 being normal. Each eye should be tested separately with the aid of an occluder (19).

The physical examination of the eye starts with the lids and lashes, followed by sclera and conjunctiva, and then cornea and precorneal tear film. A pocket penlight is helpful in providing a source of diffuse illumination. A hand-held magnifying lens helps to provide an adequate magnified view of the external ocular structures. A simple yet highly diagnostic aid that combines the importance of illumination and magnification into one piece of equipment is the direct ophthalmoscope (Welch Allyn, Skaneateles Falls, NY) (19–21). The direct ophthalmoscope is a hand-held instrument that consists of a handle, a headpiece with a light source, and a peephole with a range of built-in lenses and filters. Desired magnification is obtained by "plus" (convex) and "minus" (concave) lenses that can be easily selected by twirling the Rekoss disk found on the side of the ophthalmoscope headpiece. Some ophthalmoscopes have color-coded and numerically labeled lenses, making the distinction between plus (green) and minus (red) lenses simple. A "plus 10" lens (or greater) is typically used during the examination because it provides an adequate level of magnification (20). The cobalt blue filter can be selected by twirling the flat dial on the front of the ophthalmoscope headpiece. This filter produces a blue hue against the intense green color of instilled fluorescein dye. The cobalt blue filter works best with the ophthalmoscope rheostat turned to maximum illumination, as tolerated by the patient (20).

Direct ophthalmoscopy is performed using the eye that corresponds to the patient's eye being examined (Fig. 5). When examining a patient's left eye, the examiner's left eye should be used (21). Traditionally, the patient's right eye is examined first.

The eyelids and lashes are best evaluated with white light and diffuse illumination. The direct ophthalmoscope rheostat is usually set to maximum intensity, as tolerated by the patient. A "plus 10" lens is used to obtain an ideal magnified view of the fine lid and lash structures. The inferior eyelid should be examined first, followed by the superior eyelid. A thorough examination of the lid structures can be accomplished by gradually moving the ophthalmoscope light beam (in a sweeping motion) from lateral to medial across the lid/lash surface. It is important to keep the lid margin and lash structures in direct view to assess the presence of pathology (19,20,22–24).

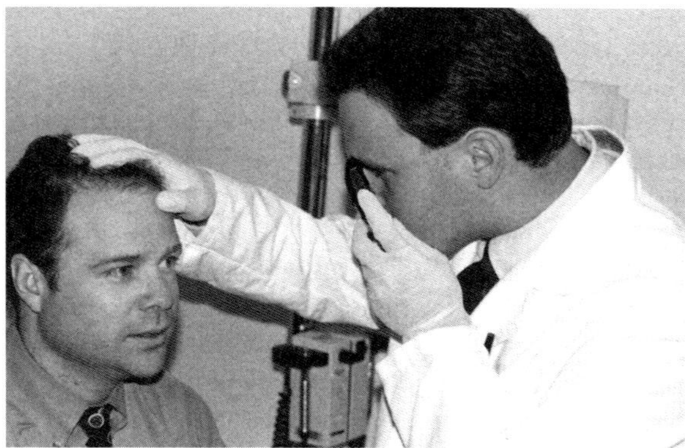

Figure 5 Direct ophthalmoscopy technique. The physician is using his left eye to perform direct ophthalmoscopy as the patient's left eye is examined.

Examination of the conjunctiva is performed in a stepwise fashion; the palpebral conjunctiva is examined first, followed by the limbal, then the bulbar conjunctiva. The conjunctiva is examined with diffuse white light illumination at maximal light intensity, as tolerated by the patient (19). A detailed view of the conjunctiva is often obtained with a ''plus 10'' or ''plus 12'' lens.

Examination of the inferior palpebral conjunctiva and fornix is straightforward. With the patient looking down, the skin below the lower lid is pressed with a cotton-tipped applicator and gently pulled downward. The patient is asked to ''look up,'' allowing the inferior fornix to prolapse outward and come into direct view. The superior palpebral conjunctiva is best appreciated after lid eversion (Fig. 6A) (19,24,25). A two-handed technique is suggested. As the patient ''looks down,'' the upper lid is gently pulled away from the globe by grasping the eyelashes. A cotton-tipped applicator is placed horizontally at the upper lid crease. As the upper eyelid is gently pulled down and out, the applicator stick is lightly dragged downward against the upper eyelid in the plane of the patient's face. This maneuver causes the upper eyelid to fold directly over the applicator stick without causing the patient any discomfort. The cotton applicator is withdrawn and the upper eyelid is held in place against the eyebrow (Fig. 6B). The upper eyelid is released and the patient is asked to ''look up'' once the examination is complete. This technique enables the upper eyelid to return to its natural resting position against the globe. A lid retractor may be needed in a few select cases where the lids are difficult to evert.

The limbal and bulbar conjunctiva are evaluated with diffuse white light with maximum illumination, as tolerated by the patient. Denuded and damaged epithelial cells of the conjunctiva are best appreciated after the instillation of fluorescein and rose bengal, respectively (see procedure, described below).

The cornea is examined by direct frontal illumination with diffuse white light. A detailed view of the cornea is obtained with a ''plus 10'' or ''plus 12'' lens dialed into the ophthalmoscope headpiece. On occasion, the ophthalmoscope is held near the temporal limbus with the light beam shined tangentially across the front of the eye toward the nose (23). This view can demonstrate many corneal disturbances that often go unnoticed with direct frontal illumination. Denuded and damaged epithelial cells of the cornea can be detected with fluorescein and rose bengal, respectively.

The precorneal tear film and TBUT are best evaluated with a cobalt blue filter after instillation of fluorescein dye (13,14,23). The patient is asked to blink several times to spread the fluorescein evenly over the entire corneal surface. The TBUT is a quantitative measure of tear film stability and is defined as the period between opening of the eyes and the first appearance of a defect (black spot) seen in the green fluorescein layer. Twenty seconds is the average TBUT in a normal eye (reference range, 15–35 seconds). An abnormal tear film is sug-

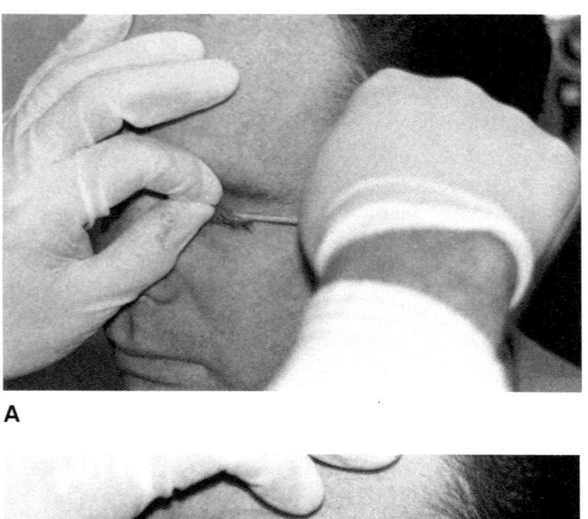

A

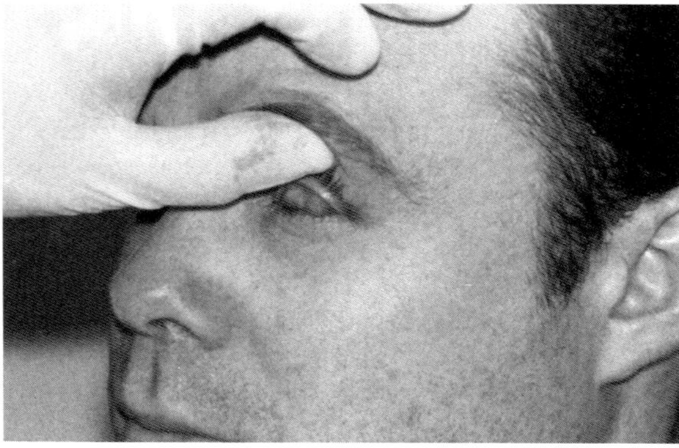

B

Figure 6 (A) Lid eversion technique showing position of examiner's hands and proper placement of cotton-tipped applicator. (B) Lid eversion technique showing upper palpebral conjunctiva. By holding the upper lid in place against the patient's eyebrow after performing lid eversion, an ideal view of the upper conjunctiva is easily obtained.

gested by a TBUT less than 10 seconds (13,14,23). Patients with classic dry eye symptoms often have a TBUT of 3 seconds or less (13,14).

The height of the tear meniscus between the inferior lid margin and the globe is also examined with a cobalt blue filter after instillation of fluorescein dye. A slightly concave tear meniscus should be free of debris, mucous strands, or sediment. A normal tear meniscus height is about 0.3–0.5 mm. A tear meniscus height of 0.1 mm or less is consistent with a tear film abnormality (14).

The gross measurement of intraocular pressure is determined by palpating the eye through a patient's closed lids. Although this technique may not help detect subtle differences in intraocular pressure, it will help to determine the extremely low or high pressures that often are signs of potentially serious ocular pathology. A normal eye can be slightly indented by direct palpation through the lid. In sharp contrast, an eye with acute angle closure frequently cannot be indented by direct palpation because it is extremely hard. Of note, it is always advisable to palpate a patient's normal eye first (or your own eye) to gain a better understanding of what a normal eye feels like (17).

IV. OPHTHALMIC PROCEDURES AND TESTING

As supplements to a detailed and thorough history and physical examination, there are several additional procedures and tests that help in confirming a diagnosis of ocular allergy. More importantly, these various testing modalities help differentiate the many disorders that mimic allergic disorders of the eye.

The **Schirmer tear test** (Alcon Laboratories, Inc., Fort Worth, TX) is the most commonly used and easily performed test for the evaluation of dry eye (14,15,26). It is a quantitative measurement of tear production by the lacrimal gland. Tear production is assessed by the amount of wetting seen on a folded strip of sterile filter paper after it is placed into the conjunctival sac. The patient is seated with the room lights dimmed. The patient is asked to ''look up'' as the lower eyelid is gently pulled downward. Excess moisture and tears are dried along the eyelid margin and conjunctiva using a sterile cotton-tipped applicator. The *rounded* end of the test strip is bent at the notch about 90–120° before opening the sterile paper packaging. The bent end of the strip is hooked into the conjunctival sac at the junction of the middle and lateral one third of the lower eyelid margin (Fig. 7). The patient's eyes remain closed throughout the examination. The test strips are removed from each eye after 5 minutes. The length of the moistened area from the notch to the *flat* end of the sterile strip is measured using a millimeter ruler or the scale imprinted on the test strip package (14,15,26).

The Schirmer I test (without anesthesia) measures both basal and reflex tearing. Without topical anesthesia, the filter paper provides a stimulus for local irritation that causes reflex tearing above and beyond the basal tearing rate. A measurement of 5 mm or less of wetting after a 5-minute interval is considered abnormal in the Schirmer I test (14,15,26). The Schirmer II test (with anesthesia) measures only the basal secretion of tearing and is performed as outlined above, but after topical anesthesia is instilled. The amount of tear production in the Schirmer II test most closely approximates the basal tearing rate because the anesthesia blunts the irritation and resultant reflex stimulus caused by the filter

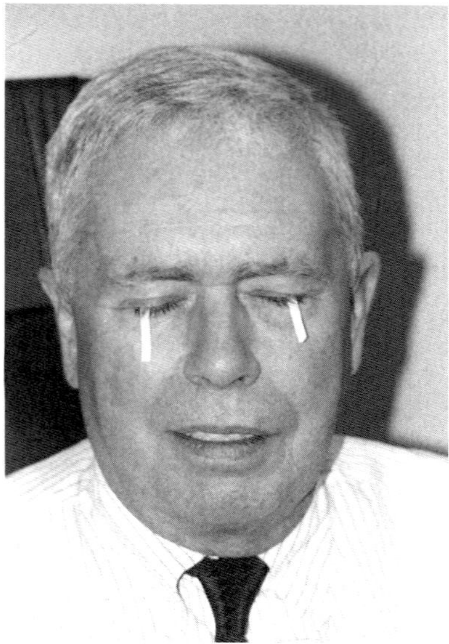

Figure 7 Schirmer test. Schirmer test strips are placed into the conjunctival sac at the junction of the middle and lateral one third of the lower eyelid margin. The cornea should not be touched during placement of the strips since this may cause patient discomfort.

paper in the conjunctival sac. A measurement of 3 mm or less of wetting after a 5-minute interval is considered abnormal in the Schirmer II test (14,15,26).

Fluorescein is a water-soluble dye used to examine the cornea, conjunctiva, corneal tear film, and TBUT (14,18,22,24,26). Fluorescein dye stains denuded areas of epithelium and pools into surface irregularities of the cornea and conjunctiva. It is placed into the eye either with a sterile fluorescein sodium ophthalmic strip (Fluor-I-Strip, Ayerst Laboratories, Inc., Philadelphia, PA) or with a dropper in liquid form. A cobalt blue filter is needed to appreciate best the fluorescein staining pattern of the conjunctiva and cornea. This filter produces a blue hue against the intense green color of the fluorescein dye. Fluorescein instillation begins by moistening the end of a Fluor-I-Strip with a drop of sterile water. The skin below the lower lid margin is gently pulled downward as the patient is asked to "look up." The moistened strip is placed into the inferior conjunctival sac at the fornix close to the punctum. The patient is asked to close his or her lids tightly over the strip to assure adequate instillation of the dye. The strip is removed and the patient is asked to blink several times to spread the fluorescein uniformly and evenly over the entire corneal and conjunctival surface (14,18,22,24,26). Of note, soft contact lenses must be removed prior to fluorescein instillation to prevent their permanent staining. At least 1 hour must pass after completion of the examination before the lenses can be replaced in the eyes.

Rose bengal (RoseGlo, Wilson Ophthalmic Corp., Mustang, OK), a red aniline dye, also permits an excellent view of the ocular surface (6,14,16,18,26). Rose bengal is a derivative of fluorescein. However, it differs significantly from fluorescein because it does not stain the precorneal tear film; it stains only dead and degenerating (not denuded) epithelium of the conjunctiva and cornea. Rose bengal also stains mucous particles, strands, filaments, and plaques more vividly than does fluorescein, making it a better diagnostic aid in the evaluation of the conjunctiva and tear film (6,14,16,18,26). Rose bengal is sometimes difficult to obtain commercially because many drug companies find marketing it to be unprofitable. Therefore, many physicians rely on their local pharmacy to supply them with a ''custom-made'' supply of 1% rose bengal ophthalmic solution (26).

Rose bengal is instilled into the eye either with a sterile rose bengal ophthalmic strip (RoseGlo) or with a dropper in liquid form. The technique of rose bengal instillation is similar to that of fluorescein. Rose bengal may cause a significant amount of discomfort after it is instilled into the conjunctival sac. The liquid form of rose bengal tends to cause more discomfort than the strip form. The irritation appears to be directly proportional to the amount of staining seen on the ocular surface. Therefore, this discomfort may be considerable in patients with severe epithelial damage or tear film dysfunction (6,14,16,18,26). It is possible to alleviate some of this discomfort by instilling only a small fraction of a drop into the eye. This is done by placing only a small portion of a drop onto the wooden end of a cotton-tipped applicator and then touching the applicator to the inferior conjunctival sac. Special care must be taken when instilling rose bengal because it can stain facial skin and clothing easily.

In addition to the Schirmer and vital staining tests, there are many procedures and techniques that can help to evaluate the morphology and condition of the ocular surface. Common techniques include ocular surface smears and cultures, scraping, biopsy, and cytology. To perform these tests in an office setting, it is recommended that a ''procedures kit'' be prepared and fully stocked with gloves, sterile cotton-tipped applicators, topical anesthesia, lid specula, precleaned glass microscope slides, fixative for smears, scalpels and Kimura spatulas, and fresh solid (blood, chocolate, and Sabouraud's dextrose agars) and liquid (thioglycolate broth) media (Fig. 8) (27).

Smears and cultures of the lid margin and conjunctiva are usually taken prior to obtaining corneal cultures. The ophthalmic pattern of plating has been used for many years and is now considered a ''standard.'' Horizontal streaks denote conjunctival specimens, ''R'' and ''L'' letters represent lid specimens, and ''C'' streaks denote corneal specimens (27).

Conjunctival cultures are obtained using a sterile cotton-tipped applicator moistened in thioglycolate broth. Moistened swabs are preferred as they pick up

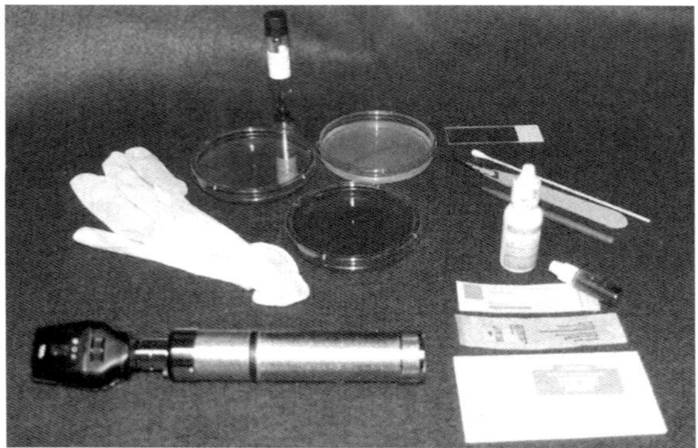

Figure 8 Equipment used in ophthalmologic examinations and procedures. Clockwise, from bottom left: direct ophthalmoscope, gloves, fresh solid and liquid media, glass slides, cotton-tipped applicator, scalpel, Kimura spatula, topical anesthetic, rose bengal stain, fluorescein dye, and Schirmer test strips.

and release bacteria better than do dry swabs. The lower palpebral conjunctiva is lightly wiped with the applicator stick for 5 seconds as the patient is asked to look upward. The sample is inoculated onto each of the agar plates using horizontal streaks. The cotton applicator is then placed into the thioglycolate broth and twirled several times. The wooden portion of the applicator stick is broken off, leaving the cotton-tipped swab in the sterile broth. Finally, all cultures are incubated under appropriate conditions (27).

Eyelid cultures are also obtained using a sterile cotton-tipped applicator moistened in thioglycolate broth. The base of the eyelashes and affected lid margins are lightly rubbed for at least 5 seconds. The surface of all agar plates are inoculated using ''R'' or ''L'' streaks to denote the right or left lids, respectively. The applicator swab is then placed in the thioglycolate broth and twirled several times. The wooden portion of the applicator stick is broken off, leaving the cotton-tipped swab in the sterile media. Lastly, all cultures are incubated under appropriate conditions (27).

Corneal cultures are obtained with the aid of a slit-lamp. Therefore, it is recommended that physicians in general practice not take corneal cultures without first consulting an ophthalmologist. The cornea is anesthetized and a lid speculum is inserted to prevent potential contamination by the eyelashes as the culture is taken. Betadine 5% solution is instilled and allowed to air dry. Specimens from both the leading edge and the base of the ulcer are taken using firm strokes with a scalpel blade or Kimura spatula (VISITEC, Sarasota, FL). The surface of all agar plates are inoculated using ''C'' strokes. The scalpel or spatula is then placed in the thioglycolate broth and twirled several times. All cultures are then incubated under appropriate conditions (25,27).

Conjunctival scrapings are taken with a Kimura spatula from the site of maximal disease, preferably during the active stage. Topical anesthesia is instilled. The epithelial surface of the conjunctiva is gently, but firmly, scraped in a horizontal motion with the Kimura spatula, taking care not to cause any bleeding. The scrape should be at least 2–3 mm from the lid margin to avoid potential contamination. The sample is spread on the center of a precleaned glass slide. The slide is fixed immediately and Gram or Giemsa stain applied. The slide is viewed by light microscopy (27).

Conjunctival biopsies are obtained with the aid of surgical forceps, scissors, and high-temperature electrocautery (SOLAN, Xomed Surgical Products, Inc., Jacksonville, FL). Health care providers should not perform conjunctival biopsies without first consulting an ophthalmologist. Topical anesthesia is instilled. A few millimeters of conjunctiva is gently grasped and lifted with surgical forceps. The desired specimen is snipped off in one smooth motion with surgical scissors. The specimen is immediately placed in 10% formalin (for light microscopy) or 2% buffered glutaraldehyde (for electron microscopy). If fixatives are unavailable, the specimen can be placed on a Telfa pad for immediate delivery to the pathology department. High-temperature electrocautery is occasionally used for hemostasis once the specimen is removed. The eye is patched overnight and the conjunctival wound heals on its own without the placement of surgical sutures.

In **impression cytology**, ocular surface cells are removed, stained, and examined by light microscopy. Separate 4 × 6-mm strips of acetate filter paper are used to obtain an impression of the ocular surface. The filter is pressed against the conjunctiva using a glass rod and then gently removed with a lifting motion. Surface epithelial and goblet cells adhere to the filter paper as it is removed, making an impression of the ocular surface. The filter paper is fixed, Giemsa stained, and cover slipped. The specimen is examined by light microscopy. The use of topical anesthesia is not recommended because it is known to alter cellular morphology, thereby creating erroneous results (28,29).

Brush cytology is a new technique being used by some practitioners. In contrast to impression cytology, this technique uses a special disposable nylon brush. The conjunctiva is scraped by several gentle rotations of the brush under direct slit-lamp observation. Collected material is smeared on a slide, fixed, stained, and cover slipped. The specimen is examined by light microscopy. While investigations with this technique continue, brush cytology is becoming more popular than impression cytology because it is more efficient at removing surface cells and is easier and less expensive to perform (30).

Ocular provocation testing can be likened to ''skin testing'' of the eye. Known quantities of specific allergen are instilled onto the ocular surface and the resulting allergic response is measured. The visible changes in the conjunctiva are typically viewed with a slit-lamp under high magnification. Mediator release and cellular infiltration are easily measured in tear samples and conjunctival tissue after a biopsy is performed (31). Although this technique is not routinely used in the clinical setting by ophthalmologists, it is important in the research laboratory and pharmaceutical industry, especially in the development of new drugs against ocular allergies.

V. CONCLUSION

Allergic inflammatory disorders are encountered frequently by the general practitioner. Unfortunately, the differential diagnoses of conditions that mimic ocular allergy are somewhat exhaustive and include a variety of vision-threatening and benign disorders. Furthermore, the signs and symptoms associated with these various conditions often overlap and are frequently difficult to differentiate. Only with a complete and thorough understanding of differential diagnoses, examination techniques, and diagnostic procedures can health care providers make expedient and accurate diagnoses of ocular allergic disorders.

VI. SALIENT POINTS

1. Coordination of ocular allergy care between the primary care provider, allergist, and ophthalmologist is essential.
2. An acceptable ''basic'' examination of the eye includes a Snellen chart or card, an occluder, fluorescein strips, rose bengal solution, a cotton-tipped applicator, and a direct ophthalmoscope with a cobalt blue filter.
3. Visual acuity must be assessed and documented before performing any examination or procedure.
4. The assessment of ocular allergy begins with evaluation of the lids and lashes, followed by sclera and conjunctiva, and then the cornea and precorneal tear film.
5. The direct ophthalmoscope is a simple yet highly diagnostic tool that provides the illumination and magnification essential for adequate ocular examination.
6. The differential diagnosis of red eye includes allergic disorders and a variety of other ocular abnormalities, some of which can produce profound visual loss. A comprehensive ocular history and examination are absolutely essential to differentiate between these disorders.
7. Topical ophthalmic steroids may have significant ocular side effects and can worsen many disorders. Their usage is unwise without first consulting an ophthalmologist.

8. Several procedures can help to confirm the diagnosis of ocular allergy, including the Schirmer test, fluorescein and rose bengal stains, and ocular surface smears, cultures, scrapings, biopsies, and cytology.

ACKNOWLEDGMENT

This work was supported, in part, by an Unrestricted Grant from Research to Prevent Blindness, Inc., and by the Lions Eye Research Foundation of New Jersey. The authors gratefully acknowledge Ms. Maxine Wanner, Director of Ophthalmic Imaging, and Mr. Michael Lazar for their superb photography; Ms. Catherine Horan for her outstanding illustrations; Dr. William Grant (retired) for his encouragement and dedication to teaching; and Dr. Jessica Perrone for her patience, love, and unconditional support.

REFERENCES

1. Friedlander MH. Conjunctivitis of allergic origin: clinical presentation and differential diagnosis. Surv Ophthalmol 1993;38:105–114.
2. Rothenhaus TC, Polis MA. Ocular manifestations of systemic disease. Emerg Med Clin North Am 1995;13:607–629.
3. Donshik PC, Ehlers WH. Clinical immunologic diseases. In: Smolin G, Thoft RA, eds. The Cornea: Scientific Foundations and Clinical Practice. New York: Little, Brown, and Company, 1994:347–364.
4. Abelson M, Schaefer K. Conjunctivitis of allergic origin: immunologic mechanisms and current approaches to therapy. Surv Ophthalmol 1993;38:115–132.
5. Bielory L, Friedlander M, Fujishima H. Allergic conjunctivitis. Immunol Allergy Clin North Am 1997;17:19–32.
6. External Disease and Cornea. Basic and Clinical Science Course, Section 8. San Francisco: American Academy of Ophthalmology, 1996.
7. Stock EL, Bielory L. Treatment of ocular allergy. Immunol Allergy Clin North Am 1997;17:75–88.
8. Lee Y, Raizman MB. Vernal conjunctivitis. Immunol Allergy Clin North Am 1997; 17:33–52.
9. Dinowitz K, Trocme SD. Ocular manifestations of immunologic and rheumatologic inflammatory disorders. Curr Opin Ophthalmol 1993;4:106–112.
10. LaVene D, Halpern J, Jagoda A. Loss of vision. Emerg Med Clin North Am 1995; 13:539–560.
11. Dinowitz K, Aldave AJ, Lisse JR, Trocme SD. Ocular manifestations of immunologic and rheumatologic inflammatory disorders. Curr Opin Ophthalmol 1994;5:91–98.
12. Donshik PC, Ehlers WH. Giant papillary conjunctivitis. Immunol Allergy Clin North Am 1997;17:53–74.

13. Toda I, Shimazaki J, Tsubota K. Dry eye with only decreased tear, but is sometimes associated with allergic conjunctivitis. Ophthalmology 1995;102:302–309.
14. Constad WH, Bhagat N. Keratitis sicca and dry eye syndrome. Immunol Allergy Clin North Am 1997;17:89–102.
15. Wright M, Baljean D. Diagnosis and treatment of dry eyes. Practitioner 1997;241: 210–216.
16. Feenstra RP, Tseng SC. What is actually stained by rose bengal? Arch Ophthalmol 1992;110:984–993.
17. Duguid, G. Red eye: avoid the pitfalls. Practitioner 1997;241:188–195.
18. Hara JH. The red eye: diagnosis and treatment. Am Fam Physician 1996;54:2423–2430.
19. Wilson FM, ed. Practical Ophthalmology–A Manual for Beginning Residents. San Francisco: American Academy of Ophthalmology, 1996.
20. Luff A, Elkington A. Better use of the ophthalmoscope. Practitioner 1992;236:161–165.
21. Spalton DJ, Hitchings RA, Holder GE. Methods of ocular examination. In: Spalton DJ, Hitchings RA, Hunter PA, eds. Atlas of Clinical Ophthalmology. London: Wolfe Publishing, 1994:19–21.
22. Barr DH, Samples JR, Hedges JR. Ophthalmologic procedures. In: Roberts JR, Hedges JR, eds. Clinical Procedures in Emergency Medicine. Philadelphia: W. B. Saunders Company, 1991:997–1018.
23. Gaston DK. The slit lamp biomicroscope in the contact lens examination. J Ophthalmic Nurs Technol 1994;3:82–85.
24. Knoop K, Trott A. Ophthalmologic procedures in the emergency department—Part III: slit lamp use and foreign bodies. Acad Emerg Med 1995;2:224–230.
25. Santen SA, Scott JL. Ophthalmic procedures. Emerg Med Clin North Am 1995;13: 681–701.
26. Stulting RD, Waring GO. Diagnosis and management of tear film dysfunction. In: Leibowitz HM, ed. Corneal Disorders: Clinical Diagnosis and Management. Philadelphia: W. B. Saunders Company, 1984:445–465.
27. Brinser JH, Weiss A. Laboratory diagnosis in ocular disease. In: Tasman W, Jaeger EA, eds. Duane's Clinical Ophthalmology. New York: Lippincott-Raven Publishers, 1996:1–14.
28. Holly FJ. Diagnostic methods and treatment modalities of dry eye conditions. Int Ophthalmol 1993;17:113–125.
29. Nelson JD. Ocular surface impressions using cellulose acetate filter material. Ocular pemphigoid. Surv Ophthalmol 1982;27:67–69.
30. Yagmur M, Ersoz C, Ersoz TR, Varinli S. Brush technique in ocular surface cytology. Diagn Cytopathol 1997;17:88–91.
31. Anderson DF. The conjunctival late-phase reaction and allergen provocation in the eye. Clin Exp Allergy 1996;26:1105–1107.

6

Intranasal Disease and Provocation

Donnie P. Dunagan and John W. Georgitis
Wake Forest University, Winston-Salem, North Carolina

I. INTRODUCTION

The eyes are described by poets as being the windows to the soul. If that is so, then the nasal cavity is the window to the body. The nose is a highly accessible tool for observing the intricate details of the human immunological and vascular systems, especially as they relate to chronic rhinitis conditions. By examining the nasal mucosa and collecting secretions, the clinician or researcher can investigate normal physiological conditions and the allergic elements: the early phase, late phase, and chronic response. There are numerous methods developed to characterize and quantify nasal responses. The clinician can use some of these techniques whereas others are intended only for research purposes. This chapter will review three common procedures used in the evaluation of allergen-induced changes in the nose: the nasal smear, nasal provocation, and rhinomanometry. Each of these procedures is easily tolerated by the patient and can be performed in either the office or laboratory setting. Invaluable objective information is obtained regarding improvement and modification of the underlying inflammatory process. Each of these procedures will be reviewed, along with indications for the test, a discussion of the technique, and expected responses for patients with and without nasal disease.

II. NASAL SMEAR

A. Introduction

Allergic rhinitis symptoms are an indirect response to mediators produced by activated inflammatory cells residing within the nasal mucosa and submucosa. In the allergic response, allergens bind to surface-bound IgE antibodies, resulting in mast cell activation. Cellular activation causes immediate release and subsequent production of inflammatory mediators such as histamine, platelet activating factor, leukotrienes, and prostaglandins. These mediators in turn cause an acute inflammatory reaction called the early allergic response. Both preformed and newly produced mediators promote the recruitment to the site of additional inflammatory cells (eosinophils, neutrophils, basophils and lymphocytes). These cells continue the inflammatory process as the late phase response. The eosinophil is the primary inflammatory cell identified in allergic rhinitis, but lymphocytes, neutrophils, mast cells, and basophils are also present. Accurate identification of these cells assists the physician in correctly diagnosing the condition and selecting appropriate therapy. In the research setting, techniques for evaluating cellular components of nasal secretions give further insight into the pathogenesis and pathophysiology of allergic and nonallergic rhinitis. The nasal smear provides one means of identifying inflammatory cells in the nasal mucosa and the secretions. The Hansel stain, described by F. K. Hansel in 1953, is a rapid, easily performed technique used to identify the primary cellular components of nasal secretions (1). Over time, other diagnostic methods have been developed. This section will discuss nasal sampling techniques, staining techniques, cell evaluation, the clinical relevance of the diagnostic findings, and the expected changes with therapy.

B. Nasal Smear Sampling

Several methods are available to obtain specimens for microscopic evaluation, and each has distinct advantages and disadvantages (Table 1) (2). One of the oldest and easiest methods is simply to have the patient blow his or her nose onto a piece of plastic wrap or waxed paper. The expelled secretions are then transferred to a microscopic slide for staining. Alternatively, secretions may be

Table 1 Methods for Obtaining Nasal Cellular Samples

Expelled secretions
Nasal swab
Nasal brushing
Nasal scraping
Imprinting
Nasal lavage
Mucosal biopsy

obtained by gently rubbing a cotton swab across the middle and inferior turbinates. Both methods are well tolerated by patients, but samples represent only the surface characteristics of the nose. Methods such as nasal scraping, imprinting, and nasal brushing provide much more detail regarding cellular changes at the epithelial level. The brushing technique involves the insertion and retrieval of a small plastic brush between the nasal septum and the inferior turbinate. Imprinting is done by placing a paper on the mucosal surface, peeling it off, and transferring it to a glass microscopic slide for review. Nasal scrapings are obtained by scraping the lining of the middle third of the inferior turbinate with a small curetting instrument. The brushing, imprinting, and scraping methods are alternatives for obtaining specimens in certain patients with absent or diminished nasal secretions. Mild irritation, insignificant local pain, and minor bleeding can occur with these methods, but they generally are well tolerated by patients. Other techniques for obtaining cellular samples include nasal lavage and nasal biopsy. The nasal lavage method is performed by placing 5 mL of normal saline into the nasal cavity with the head slightly tilted backward. Lavage fluid is then obtained as the patient leans his or her head forward to allow the fluid to drain into a collection reservoir. This method can be repeated several times to increase the yield. Pooled secretions are then centrifuged to concentrate the cellular components. The nasal mucosal biopsy gives the classic tissue specimen for cytological evaluation but has limited clinical application due to patient discomfort, requirement of a topical anesthetic, and the risk of bleeding. Nasal biopsies are not done routinely and are best left for complicated cases that require extensive tissue sampling with intact histological features.

C. Staining Techniques

Numerous staining methods are available. The one used depends on the cells to be examined or the ease of a particular staining procedure. The Hansel stain, often referred to as the "1-min method," is easily performed in the office and

Table 2 Staining Techniques and Primary Cells Identified

Hansel's—eosinophils
Wright's—basophils
Wright-Giemsa—eosinophils/neutrophils/basophilic cells
Papanicolaou—epithelial cells/nuclear and cytoplasmic changes
Toluidine Blue—basophilic cells
Leishman's—eosinophils
Alcian Yellow—mast cells
Randolph's—eosinophils
Alcian Blue—basophilic cells
May-Grunwald—neutrophils

primarily demonstrates eosinophils and neutrophils (3). Other staining methods are listed in Table 2 (4). The steps for performing the Hansel stain and Wright's stain are presented in Appendices 1 and 2.

D. Examination of Smear

Each prepared slide should first be examined with a microscope under low power (100×) to determine the areas of cellularity and overall adequacy of the specimen. Areas are then examined under oil immersion (1000×). Interpretation of the cellular components can be performed using both quantitative and qualitative analysis (5). Quantitative analysis involves determining the number of specific cells per 10 high-power fields (HPF) examined. Qualitative analysis is more subjective and estimates the cell number per high power field. Both methods are demonstrated in Table 3.

Cellular constituents of nasal secretions and mucosa vary depending on the presence of inflammation and the specific inflammatory response. Major cellular components include eosinophils, neutrophils, mast cells/basophils, lymphocytes, and epithelial cells. Eosinophils (Fig. 1a) are 9 to 12 μm in diameter, usually have a peripherally located, bi-lobed or indented nucleus, and they feature an abundance of positively charged granules that eosin stains bright pink or red. Neutrophils (Fig. 1b) are generally 10 to 12 μm in diameter, contain abundant basophilic cytoplasm, and have a heterochromatic nucleus. Basophilic-staining cells include both mast cells and basophils. Basophils are smaller than both neutrophils and eosinophils with diameters of approximately 8 to 10 μm. Their name is derived from the numerous intensely staining, bluish cytoplasmic granules. Mast cells have a variable shape but are usually 9 to 12 μm in diameter. They have numerous cytoplasmic granules and exhibit thin elongated folds in their

Table 3 Analysis of Cellular Components of Nasal Smear

	Quantitative Analysis	
Grade	Eosinophils, Neutrophils/10 HPFs	Basophils, Mast Cells/10 HPFs
0	0–1.0	0–0.3
1+	1.1–5.0	0.4–1.0
2+	6.0–15.0	1.1–3.0
3+	16.0–20.0	3.1–6.0
4+	>20.0	>6.0

	Qualitative Analysis
Grade	Eosinophils, Neutrophils, Basophils, Mast Cells/HPF
0	No cells seen
1+	Few cells seen
2+	Moderate number of cells seen
3+	Many cells seen
4+	Large number of cells seen

Abbreviation: HPF, high power field.

plasma membranes. Lymphocytes are small cells (7–9 μm) containing relatively large nuclei and little cytoplasmic volume.

E. Interpretation of Results

Nasal smears obtained from normal control individuals generally are acellular except for occasional epithelial cells, neutrophils, and rare bacteria. Smears from patients with perennial and seasonal allergic rhinitis are characterized by a predominance of eosinophils and basophilic staining cells (6,7). Eosinophilic concentrations are much greater during pollen season and can be induced by repeated allergen challenge (8). Eosinophils may also be seen in the disorder, nonallergic rhinitis with eosinophilia (NARES). Neutrophil influx is primarily associated with rhinosinusitis secondary to infection but also can be seen in such disorders as irritant rhinitis (exposure to irritating dusts, odors, and gases). Neutrophils can accompany eosinophils in patients with allergic rhinitis (9). In those patients with infectious rhinitis, specific organisms such as bacteria or fungi are occasionally observed with the stain and may give insight into a specific causative agent. In isolated viral rhinitis, the epithelial cells may take on a relatively characteristic morphological change referred to as ciliocytophthoria (increased shedding of ciliated cells). The nuclei of these virally infected epithelial cells show pyknosis

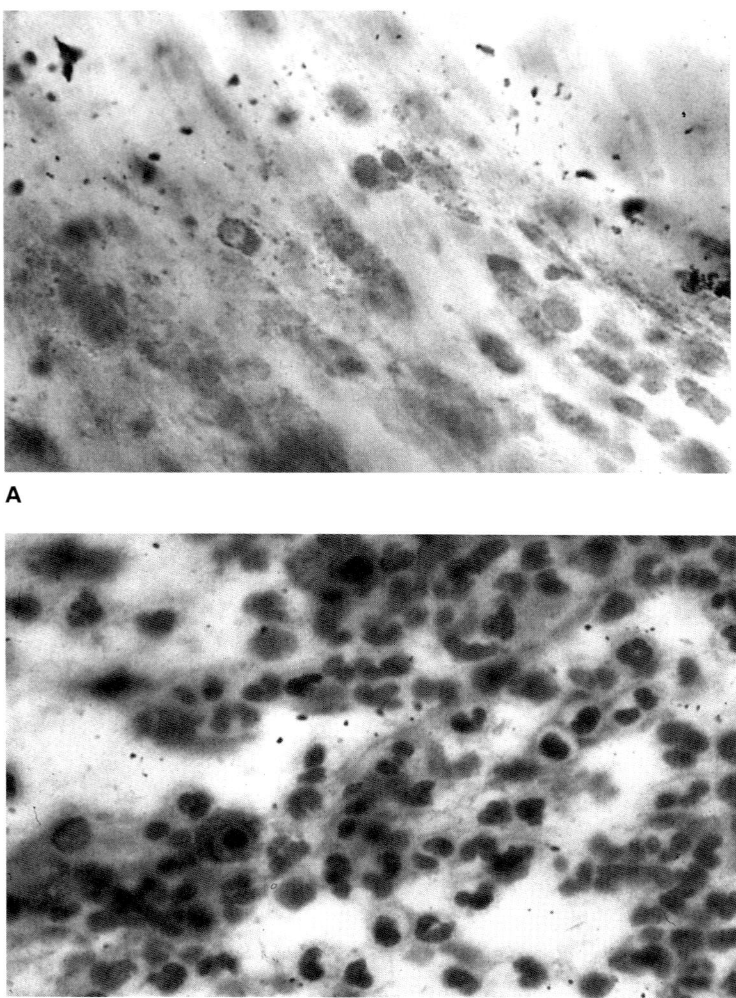

Figure 1 (A) Nasal smear using Hansel's stain, which highlights the eosinophils, blue nucleus with red cytoplasmic granular staining. (B) Nasal smear using Wright-Giemsa stain, which demonstrates bilobed nucleus with blue cytoplasm.

(condensation and reduction of the cell or cell nucleus), hyperchromasia (more intense staining of nucleus or cytoplasm), and chromatin clumping, while the whole cell may separate into a ciliated tuft portion and a proximal nucleated portion (10).

Many of the therapeutic options available for the treatment of allergic rhinitis have been demonstrated to modify the inflammatory response present in the nasal secretions and mucosa. Cromolyn sodium has been shown to decrease the influx of eosinophils into the nasal mucosa but not mast cells when used on a regular basis (11). Topical corticosteroids significantly reduce the number of eosinophils, basophils, and neutrophils in allergic rhinitis patients. In patients undergoing nasal provocation with allergen, pretreatment with nasal corticosteroids will prevent the influx of eosinophils and neutrophils associated with the late phase response (12). Prolonged topical corticosteroid therapy also has been demonstrated to modify metaplastic characteristics observed in severely inflamed epithelium. In addition, some clinical studies have demonstrated that H_1 receptor antagonists inhibit inflammatory mediator release and eosinophilic and neutrophilic cell influx during natural pollen exposure and allergen nasal provocation (13). Studies evaluating the effects of immunotherapy on the influx of inflammatory cells into the nasal secretions and mucosa have not been as well characterized. Two studies have demonstrated that immunotherapy reduces the number of eosinophils and basophilic cells in patients with allergic rhinitis (14,15). In patients with suspected bacterial sinusitis and rhinitis, treatment with antibiotic therapy will reduce the number of neutrophils and bacteria as the infection resolves.

III. NASAL PROVOCATION

A. Introduction

Allergic rhinitis results from the repeated exposure of allergens to the nasal mucosa. Recurrent exposure produces an ongoing chronic inflammatory response that eventually requires the patient to seek medical therapy. The initial inflammatory responses after allergen exposure are mucosal edema, increased blood flow, release of inflammatory mediators, and influx of proinflammatory cells. This process occurs almost daily in patients with both seasonal and perennial allergic rhinitis due to continued allergen exposure. Nasal provocation enables duplication of the acute process under controlled clinical conditions. Chemical compounds and/or allergens are introduced into the nasal cavity with subsequent initiation of the acute and, frequently, the late phase inflammatory response. Methods for quantifying the provocation response may include: counting the number of sneezes, measuring the volume of secretions, identifying the inflam-

Table 4 Indications and Contraindications to Nasal Provocation

Indications
Confirm a clinical diagnosis
Simulate a clinical response
To identify a specific antigen causing symptom
Reproduce a component of an effector pathway
The patient is unconvinced of his/her allergies
Test the efficacy of drug therapy
Contraindications
Acute mucosal inflammation of the nose or paranasal sinuses
Previous anaphylactic reaction
Suspicion of a high degree of sensitivity indicated by history, skin testing or RAST
Uncertainty of allergen dose being delivered
Pregnancy
Severe underlying cardiopulmonary disease
Recent nasal surgery

Abbreviation: RAST, radioallergosorbent testing.

matory cells present, or systematically measuring the inflammatory mediators present in the secretions. Indications and relative contraindications for nasal provocation are listed in Table 4 (16,17).

Using nasal provocation, significant advances have been made in the understanding of airway pathophysiology in nonallergic and allergic patients. Even though most work has been performed in the nose, similar inflammatory responses occur in the lower airways and help in our understanding of asthma. This section will review some of the basic techniques involved in nasal provocation, including introduction of allergen, measurement of symptoms, collection of secretions, tissue sampling, and measurement of physiological changes.

B. Challenge Material

Nasal provocation involves the placement of a particular allergen into the nasal cavity and observation of the subsequent clinical response. The first documented nasal challenge was performed in 1873 when Blackley described the development of classic hay fever symptoms after applying pollen to his own nasal mucosa (18). Modern nasal provocation is performed with immunological (i.e., allergens) and nonimmunologic (i.e., histamine, methacholine, capsaicin, or cold air) stimuli. Table 5 lists some of the common stimuli used for nasal challenge. Provocation with allergen (e.g., ragweed pollen) helps to evaluate the roles of specific IgE antibodies and mast cell activation in allergic rhinitis. Nonimmunologic stimuli are used to study the general reactivity of the nasal mucosa. Histamine, metha-

Table 5 Challenge Agents Used in Nasal Provocation

Immunological Agents
Allergens
Pollens
Mold spores
Animal danders
House dust vaccines
House dust mite
Nonimmunological Agents
Mast cell mediators
Histamine
Prostaglandin D2
Leukotrienes
Kinins
Cholinergics
Methacholine
Carbachol
Irritants
Ammonia
Ozone
Sulfur dioxide
Tobacco smoke
Cold air
Neural
Capsaicin

choline, and external stimuli such as cold air can induce symptoms similar to allergic rhinitis. These stimuli can bypass the immunoglobulin (Ig) E-associated activation of mast cells, yet they cause mast cell degranulation with production of symptoms indistinguishable from allergen-induced allergic rhinitis. The particular agent used during nasal challenge is based on the indications for testing and the desired outcome variable (e.g., measurement of inflammatory mediators after ragweed pollen challenge). If an allergen is to be used as the provocative agent, the patient should have demonstrated prior IgE specificity to the allergen either by skin testing or in vitro testing.

C. Delivery Systems for Deposition of Stimulus

Challenge material can be delivered to the nose by a variety of techniques: pump spray, paper disk, powder inhalation, or lavage solution. Nasal provocation is generally performed with either dry or liquid preparations. Dry pollen may be given as an intact whole grain, defatted or nondefatted pollen, or lyophilized powdered pollen. These substances are sniffed by the subject or introduced directly into the nasal cavity with spoons, spatulas, bulb syringes, dry-powder inhalers, or suspension cylinders. Limitations with the dry powder challenge have been the ability to obtain adequately distributed material throughout the nasal mucosa and possible inhalation of smaller particles into the lower airway. Liquid vaccines are more commonly used and are applied by dropper, pipette, air/oxygen-driven nebulizers, atomizers, paper disk, and hand-held metered-dose nebulizers such as those commercially used for such medications as topical nasal corticosteroids. Most of these methods, excluding disk, dropper, and pipette, allow for a wide dispersion of challenge material throughout the nasal mucosa. The disk and pipette delivery methods allow for the placement of a high concentration of stimulus to a localized area of the nasal cavity. One of the major limitations of using a fluid-based delivery system for nasal challenge is the possibility of obtaining false positive results. In some instances, the diluent solution by itself causes changes in mucosal edema or alterations in nasal resistance, which might be interpreted as a positive response. Performing appropriate control challenges with the delivery diluent solution can minimize this problem. Nasal provocation should always be performed with serial concentrations of challenge material, starting at a low concentration and increasing to the highest, using the desired nasal response or maximal test dose as the endpoint for the challenge. In general, testing with increasing fivefold dilutions will result in convenient and safe determination of nasal reactivity (19).

D. Evaluation of Response to Nasal Provocation Challenge

The nasal response to provocation is limited to sneezing, itching, changes in nasal secretions, increases in nasal obstruction, alterations in nasal blood flow, and influx of inflammatory mediators and cells. Systemic reactions such as generalized urticaria, angioedema, or anaphylaxis have not been reported during nasal provocation. Measurements of these responses obviously vary from subjective to very specific, objective measures.

1. Measuring Symptoms

Symptoms occurring after challenge include sneezing, itching, and congestion. One of the easiest ways to quantitate symptomatic responses to challenge is for the patient to grade his or her symptoms on a specific numerical scale. Others have found that greater sensitivity can be obtained by the use of a visual analog scale (16). Sneezes can easily be counted for a set period after challenge. Most authors agree that the measurement of symptoms can be clinically helpful but should always be accompanied by more objective measurements.

2. Obtaining and Measuring Nasal Secretions

There are several methods for measuring the volume of nasal secretions, yet the results tend to be imprecise. One simple method is to collect any secretions that drain from the patient's nose while he or she leans forward for 10 to 15 min after nasal challenge. Another simple technique is to have the patient blow into preweighed handkerchiefs to obtain estimates of the volume produced. Alternatively, secretions can be removed by suction devices, filter paper, washed, or even lavaged from the nose. It is important that the method chosen for secretion collection does not result in nonspecific mucosal irritation, thereby causing nonallergenic production of inflammatory mediators or cellular influx. This assurance is accomplished by repeated challenges with control or diluting solutions followed by accurate documentation of responses.

3. Nasal Congestion

Mucosal swelling within the limited space of the nasal cavity produces the symptom of nasal congestion. The most important factor affecting mucosal swelling is localized vascular changes, although increased secretions also contribute to congestion. The degree of congestion that can be measured subjectively or by direct visualization is highly variable and unreliable. Objective measurements of congestion include nasal peak flow, rhinomanometry, acoustic rhinometry, rhinostereoscopy, and computed tomography. Rhinomanometry, which measures nasal airflow and differential pressure, is probably the most frequently performed physiological test. Nasal peak flow is simple to perform but highly effort dependent and involves measuring the peak inspiratory or expiratory nasal airflow with a modified peak flow device. Peak flows tend to correlate well with other measurements of resistance, but they are inconsistent even in the same patient. Rhinostereoscopy uses a precise surgical microscope to make direct and noninvasive topographical measurements of the nasal mucosa. Acoustic rhinomanometry is a newer technique that evaluates nasal obstruction by analyzing reflected sound waves introduced through the nares. This technique is generally easy to perform, is noninvasive, and does not require patient cooperation like many of the other procedures. Although none of these procedures is absolutely perfect, most have sensitivities between 80% and 95%. The procedure chosen to measure nasal congestion should enable reproducible results for a given patient and be one with which all laboratory personnel or clinicians are comfortable.

4. Testing of Obtained Samples

Secretions and cells collected during the challenge can undergo a multiplicity of tests. The limitations are primarily the total volume of secretions collected, the volume required for specific test, and the laboratory facilities available. Most research has dealt primarily with inflammatory mediators such as histamine, leukotrienes, prostaglandins, tryptases, and kinins (20–22). These are a few of the mediators documented to increase during allergen challenge, but others probably could be measured in the nasal secretions. Pretreatment with antihistamines, mast cell stabilizers, or corticosteroids in turn can alter these mediator responses.

Quantification and characterization of inflammatory cells after nasal provocation can be performed in several ways. Either biopsy or nasal scrapings can procure tissue samples. Biopsies are usually obtained from the anterior portion of the inferior turbinates because this site is easily accessible. Nasal scrapings are generally better tolerated than nasal biopsy. However, they do not allow one to evaluate the nasal mucosa below the epithelial layer. Nasal smears, expelled secretions, nasal brushings, and nasal lavage can all be used to obtain cellular material for cytological evaluation, but they do not provide any information about epithelial surface integrity or submucosal appearance. Both the nasal smear and the expelled secretion are easy methods for obtaining cell samples but they tend to be complicated by variable yields. These two methods may not reflect the total inflammatory response that occurred in the nasal mucosa and submucosa (23). Nasal brushing has the advantage of collecting well-preserved cells, which can be easily quantified. Nasal lavage allows the investigator to collect inflammatory mediators in addition to large numbers of cells (24). A combination of the above procedures is more likely to result in a satisfactory collection of both cells and tissue material.

E. Clinical Usefulness of Nasal Provocation

Nasal provocation has been used for many years as a tool to study numerous aspects of the allergic nasal response. Despite its extensive use in the research laboratory setting, its clinical indications tend to be more limited and underutilized by the practicing physician. There are many patients with histories compatible with allergic rhinitis, yet they demonstrate equivocal skin testing or serum IgE radioallergosorbent test (RAST) titers. In this patient population, nasal provocation allows for direct observation of nasal response to a specific allergen. In most patients, detailed measurement of the production of inflammatory mediators is not necessary. Onset of rhinorrhea, sneezing, and nasal congestion during nasal provocation would indicate that the patient has an allergic response to the applied antigen. Further testing with different antigens also can be used to determine the presence or absence of specific allergen sensitivity.

One of the most promising clinical applications of nasal provocation is measurement of the effectiveness of a specific therapy. Nasal provocation using allergens should be performed prior to initiation of the therapy. Measurements of responses such as number of sneezes, quantification of rhinorrhea, and both subjective and objective determinations of nasal congestion should be obtained for a known allergen. Repeated testing can be performed after initiation of specific therapy such as immunotherapy, nasal corticosteroids, topical mast cell stabilizers, and antihistamines. For example, the clinician should consider adjusting or supplementing the medical regimen for a patient with little subjective improvement and no change in nasal provocation response after repeat challenge. However, the clinician may opt either to continue or to simplify the medical regimen if the patient displays significant clinical improvement or no symptoms on repeat provocation. As methods for the delivery of challenge material improve and simpler techniques for objective measurement of nasal response become available, nasal provocation may become a technique commonly used to determine the causes of allergic rhinitis and to measure clinical response to treatment.

IV. RHINOMANOMETRY

A. Introduction

Nasal congestion is one of the primary complaints for which patients seek medical attention, but it is difficult to quantitate without objective criteria. Symptoms vary greatly among patients and correlate poorly with objective measurements of nasal obstruction (25–27). As mentioned above, rhinomanometry measures nasal air flow and pressure differences between the anterior nares and posterior pharynx. Because air flows from an area of high pressure to an area of low pressure, pressure gradients and flow measurements may be used to calculate nasal resistance. This section will review nasal mechanics and the clinical indications and applications for measuring nasal airflow and resistance with rhinomanometry.

B. Physiology of Rhinomanometry

A brief description and review of nasal resistance, pressure-flow relationships, and methods for resistance calculation is necessary to understand rhinomanometry. Nasal airway resistance contributes approximately two thirds of the total airway resistance (28). Primary sites of nasal obstruction to airflow include the nasal vestibule, the nasal valves, and the nasal turbinates (Fig. 2). The nasal valves are the locations of minimal cross-sectional area of the nares and contribute most to total nasal resistance. Nasal resistance is highest during infancy, decreases with age, and is primarily controlled by the engorgement of the venous vessels in the middle and inferior turbinates (29,30).

Airflow through the anterior nares and nasal vestibule is initially laminar, yet with increased rates of flow becomes turbulent and nonlaminar. During any given breath, nasal airflow is a combination of both laminar and nonlaminar flow.

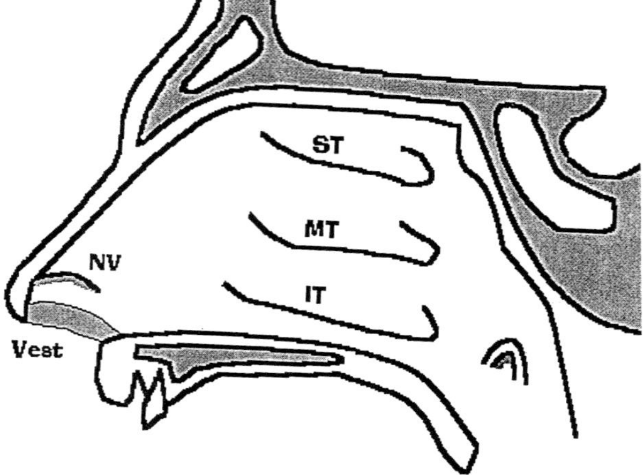

Figure 2 Cross section of nasal cavity. Vest = nasal vestibule, NV = nasal valve, IT = inferior turbinate, MT = middle turbinate, ST = superior turbinate.

If nasal air flow remained laminar, the pressure and flow relationship would be linear and could easily be expressed using Ohm's law:

$$R_n = \frac{\Delta p}{V}$$

R_n = nasal resistance
Δp = differential pressure
V = flow

Turbulent airflow is crucial for the cleansing and warming of inspired air, but it makes the relationship between air flow and pressure nonlinear. Thus, calculation of total resistance is more difficult. During rhinomanometry, dynamic measurements of pressure/flow relationship with inspiratory and expiratory maneuvers are plotted along an X/Y axis as shown in Figure 3. Increases in nasal airway resistance will result in a shift of the curve to a more upright and vertical position. Decreases in nasal airway resistance shift the curve downward toward a more horizontal position. Secondary to the curvilinear configuration of the flow-pressure relationship, nasal resistance is different at distinct points along this curve, making determination of the overall resistance somewhat more complex. To help standardize rhinomanometry measurements, an international committee that met in Brussels, Belgium, in 1983 determined that resistance should be calculated using airflow measurements obtained at a pressure of 150 Pascals(Pa) during

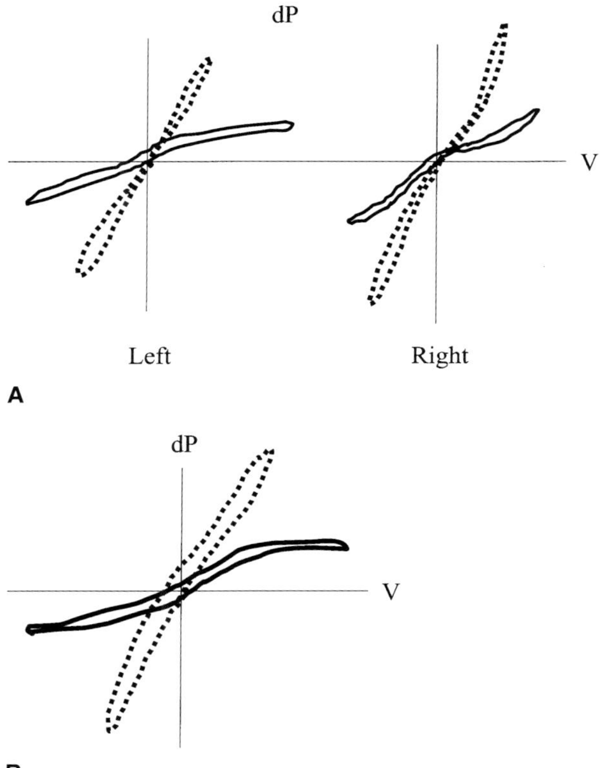

Figure 3 (A) Flow-pressure curves done by anterior rhinomanometry for the left and right nasal passages. The solid curves are normal, nonobstructive nasal passages, whereas the dotted curves represent obstructive or congested nasal passages. (B) Flow-pressure curve done by posterior rhinomanometry. The solid curve shows minimal obstruction, whereas the dotted curve demonstrates a more obstructive total nasal passage.

unilateral active anterior rhinomanometry (31). If bilateral nasal resistance is determined, the flow measurements should be obtained at a pressure of 75 Pa. Patients of Asian descent are unable to generate pressures of 150 Pa during quiet breathing maneuvers; subsequently, flow rates should be measured at 100 Pa or 50 Pa during unilateral or bilateral rhinomanometry, respectively (32). Other ethnic groups are not known to have difficulty in generating 150 Pa.

Despite a relative constancy in total nasal airway resistance, nasal airflow is unequally divided between the right and left nares. Unilateral resistance, controlled by sympathetic nerves supplying venous capacitance vessels, fluctuates

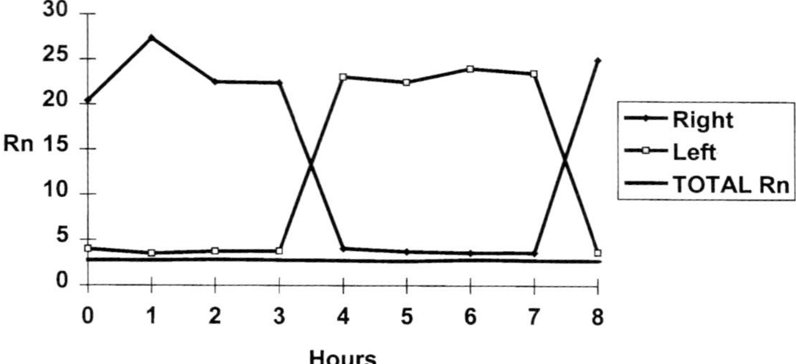

Figure 4 Nasal cycle. Timed plot of airway resistance for the left and right nasal passages and the entire nose (total nasal resistance, Rn). Note that the right nasal passage initially is more congested than the left but decongests over time. Note also that total nasal resistance remains relatively constant, whereas both nasal passages display alternating cycles of resistance.

every 2 to 4 h due to reciprocal oscillation in sympathetic activity, and is known as the nasal cycle (Fig. 4) (33). Due to such fluctuations in resistance, it is recommended that rhinomanometry be measured in each nostril simultaneously and total resistance calculated using the following formula:

$$\frac{1}{R_T} = \frac{1}{R_R} + \frac{1}{R_L}$$

R_T = Resistance total

R_R = Resistance right naris

R_L = Resistance left naris

Measuring nasal resistance with rhinomanometric procedures is classically divided into passive or active, and into anterior or posterior rhinomanometry. Active rhinomanometry requires the patient to generate airflow through the nose by his or her own effort. Passive rhinomanometry is accomplished by external generation of a constant flow of air at a given pressure. The patient requires no respiratory effort for this test. Active rhinomanometry is quick, patients tend to perform it easily, and the International Committee on Standardization of Rhinomanometry recommends it.

All rhinomanometric devices require several common pieces of equipment, including a pneumotachometer with pressure transducer attached for the detection of nasal airflow and a differential pressure transducer attached for determination of transnasal pressure changes. Each is attached to an amplifier for intensification of signal and the data are either displayed by an oscilloscope or processed by a computer for interpretation. Anterior and posterior rhinomanometry primarily differ in the location of the transducer used to measure posterior pharyngeal pressure.

C. Anterior Rhinomanometry

Active anterior rhinomanometry should always be performed with the patient in a comfortable sitting position. A clear, tight-fitting, anesthesia-type face mask with attached pneumotachograph is placed over the mouth and nose and is used to measure nasal airflow (Fig. 5). The anterior pressure is equal to the pressure within the face mask. The posterior pressure is measured by placing a small pressure transducer through a tape-sealed nostril. Posterior pressures measured by this technique closely correlate with true posterior pharyngeal pressure. Airflow is measured through the nonoccluded nostril during several closed-mouth tidal volume breaths. It is imperative that the nostrils are not deformed in any way by the application of the sealing tape or the facemask, because such irregularities will generate abnormal data. Anterior rhinomanometry cannot be used in patients with septal perforation or in those with complete nasal passage occlusion. The pressure volume curves are recorded over several inspiratory and expiratory maneuvers to document consistency and to exclude air leak. The results are expressed in standard SI units (pressure: Pa; flow: cm^3/s) and resistance is calcu-

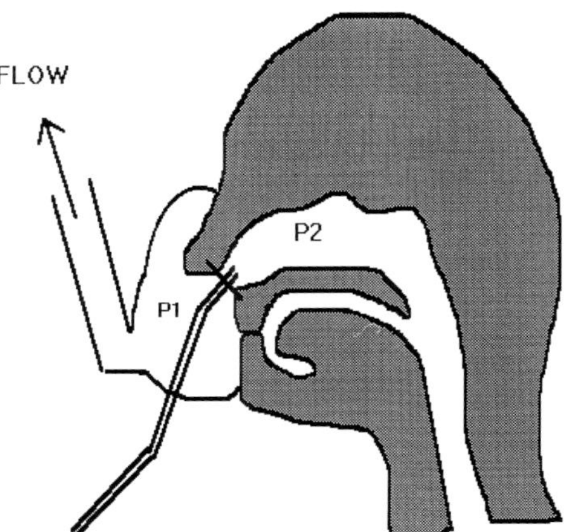

Figure 5 Graphic presentation of anterior rhinomanometry with flow transducer connected to one nasal passage and the pressure transducer directly in contact with the other nasal passage.

lated at a standardized pressure of 150 Pa. Total resistance is calculated by adding the inverses of the resistance of each naris as described previously.

D. Posterior Rhinomanometry

Passive posterior rhinomanometry is similar in technique to that of anterior rhinometry except for the position of the posterior pressure-monitoring device. Unlike the anterior method, the transducer during posterior rhinomanometry is attached to a small tube, which is passed through the oropharynx with the tube's opening located between the tongue and the palate (Fig. 6). The opening is horizontal and should not be occluded at any time during the procedure. The lips are sealed around the tube during the maneuver and nasal airflow is measured through the nares individually or simultaneously. When airflow measurements are obtained through both nares, resistance is calculated at a standardized pressure of 75 Pa. Posterior rhinomanometry has the advantage that total nasal resistance can be determined during one testing maneuver, but it tends to be less well tolerated by the patient being tested. In contrast, total nasal resistance in anterior rhinomanometry is a calculated number. There is a small percentage of patients who are unable to keep a tight seal around the posterior pharyngeal pressure-measuring device or who cannot control their posterior pharyngeal muscles, which occlude the posterior tube opening. Both problems will invalidate test results.

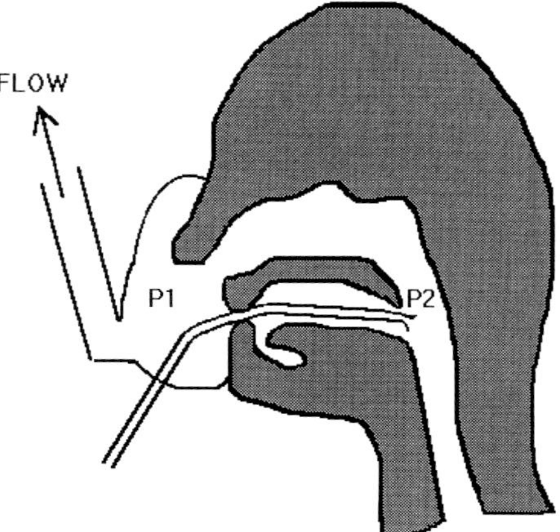

Figure 6 Graphic presentation of posterior rhinomanometry with the flow transducer measuring total nasal airflow and the pressure transducer inside the mouth.

E. Applications of Rhinomanometry

Table 6 lists the clinical and research-related applications of rhinomanometry (34–36). Rhinomanometry is an excellent tool for determining the degree of airflow obstruction before and after surgical procedures and medical interventions. For example, improvement in airflow can be objectively measured after adenoidectomy, rhinoplasty, polypectomy, and septoplasty. In the patient with chronic allergic or nonallergic rhinitis, rhinomanometry can be used to document changes in mucosal edema before and after medical interventions such as topical corticosteroids, antihistamines, immunotherapy, or use of mast cell stabilizers. Rhinomanometry becomes an even more valuable tool when serial measurements are obtained over long periods for a given patient. These measurements permit determination of true baseline values, even with mild individual fluctuations, and provide objective data to complement subjective symptoms both before and after specific therapeutic interventions. Rhinomanometry may also help to distinguish functional causes of upper airway obstruction from structural causes. For example, exercise or decongestants will improve airflow secondary to inflammation and vascular engorgement, whereas fixed abnormalities such as septal deviation

Table 6 Indications and Clinical Uses for Rhinomanometry

Objective measurement of subjective symptoms
Allergic rhinitis
Nonallergic rhinitis
Measure therapeutic benefits to specific therapy
Medical
Anti-inflammatory therapy
Antihistamines
Decongestants
Immunotherapy
Surgical
Adenoidectomy
Nasal polypectomy
Rhinoplasty
Septum repair
Assessment of anatomical variation
Determine response to nasal provocation
Evaluate upper airway resistance in obstructive sleep apnea
Legal evaluation and documentation
Evaluate functional or psychosomatic complaints

do not change after exercise or decongestant use (37). In recent years, rhinomanometry has been used increasingly to determine the amount of upper airway obstruction in patients with obstructive sleep apnea (38,39). These measurements become especially valuable when posterior pressure measurements are made just proximal to the epiglottis, providing true measurements of the resistance of the entire upper airway. Rhinomanometry has proven invaluable in laboratory nasal provocation studies. Airway resistance measurements, both preceding and after intranasal challenge with inflammatory mediators (specific or nonspecific) provide further insight into the physiological changes that occur during the early and late phase inflammatory responses.

Rhinomanometry is a useful tool for clinicians and researchers in determining objective measurements of airway resistance. When used in combination with subjective measures of nasal obstruction, rhinomanometry has helped improve our understanding of nasal flow, nasal obstruction, and patient perceptions of each. Despite numerous applications and relatively common use in research, rhinomanometry has failed to become commonplace in clinical practice. The reasons for limited clinical use are multifactorial, but they most likely relate to the time, equipment cost, and personnel required to conduct such testing. As technology improves and the ability to perform rhinomanometry is simplified, the clinical use of rhinomanometry may increase.

V. SALIENT POINTS

1. Nasal smears obtained from patients with allergic rhinitis are characterized by a predominance of eosinophils and basophilic staining cells.
2. Specific pharmacotherapies for allergic rhinitis, such as topical nasal corticosteroids, significantly reduce the number of eosinophils, basophils, and neutrophils seen in the nasal smears of patients with allergic rhinitis who are treated with these agents.
3. The induction of an in vivo allergic response by the introduction of allergenic stimuli into the nares is known as nasal provocation. This procedure provides a means by which to study the acute and late phase response in patients with allergic rhinitis, as well as any subsequent therapeutic modification of this response.
4. In allergic rhinitis, symptoms of nasal congestion vary greatly among different individuals and correlate poorly with objective measurements of nasal obstruction. Rhinomanometry measures nasal air flow and pressure differences between the anterior nares and posterior pharynx to calculate nasal resistance.
5. Nasal airway resistance contributes to two thirds of the total airway resistance. The primary sites of nasal obstruction to airflow include the nasal vestibule, the nasal valves, and the nasal turbinates.

6. Unilateral nasal airway resistance, which is controlled by sympathetic veins supplying venous capacitance vessels, fluctuates every 2 to 4 h due to oscillations in sympathetic tone. It is referred to as the nasal cycle.

APPENDIX 1

Hansel Stain

1. Allow smear to air dry.
2. Cover the slide with methyl alcohol and allow to dry.
3. Flood the slide with Hansel stain (methanol 95%, eosin, methylene blue, and glycerin 5%) and allow the stain to incubate for 30 seconds.
4. Add a small volume of distilled water for 30 seconds and gently mix with stain to dilute mixture.
5. Pour off the stain and wash with distilled water.
6. Flood with methyl alcohol to de-color until specimen has a pale green color.
7. Air dry.

APPENDIX 2

Wright's Stain

1. Allow smear to air dry.
2. Flood the slide with Wright's stain (eosin and sodium bicarbonate diluted in methyl alcohol and added to methylene blue) and incubate for 2–3 minutes.
3. Layer on phosphate buffer (pH 6.4) and blow gently to mix. Allow to stand 2–3 minutes.
4. Wash with distilled water.
5. Air dry.

REFERENCES

1. Hansel FK. Clinical Allergy. St. Louis: C.V. Mosby Company, 1953.
2. Pipkorn U, Karlsson G. Methods for obtaining specimens from the nasal mucosa for morphological and biochemical analysis. Eur Respir J 1988;1:856–862.
3. Sasaki Y, Araki A, Koga K. The mast cell and eosinophil in nasal secretions. Ann Allergy 1977;39:106–109.

4. Meltzer EO, Orgel HA, Jalowayski AA. Cytology. In: Mygind N, Naclerio RM, eds. Allergic and Non-Allergic Rhinitis: Clinical Aspects. Philadelphia: W.B. Saunders Company, 1993:66–81.
5. Jalowayski AA, Zeiger RS. Examination of nasal or conjunctival epithelium specimens. In: Manual of Allergy and Immunology. Los Angeles: Little, Brown and Company, 1995:432–434.
6. Davies R. Seasonal rhinitis. In: Mackay I, ed. Rhinitis: Mechanism and Management. London: Royal Society of Medicine Services Limited, 1989:97–116.
7. Franklin W. Perennial rhinitis. In: Mackay I, ed. Rhinitis: Mechanism and Management. London: Royal Society of Medicine Services Limited, 1989:117–140.
8. Pipkorn U, Karlsson G, Enerback L. Nasal mucosal response to repeated challenges with pollen allergen. Am Rev Respir Dis 1989;140:729–736.
9. Lee HS, Majima Y, Sakakura Y, Shinogi J, Kawaguchi S, Kim BW. Quantitative cytology of nasal secretions under various conditions. Laryngoscope 1993;103:533–537.
10. Bryan MP, Bryan WTK. Cytologic diagnosis in allergic disorders. Otolaryngol Clin North Am 1974;7:637–666.
11. Orgel HA, Meltzer EO, Kemp JP, Ostrom NK, Welch MJ. Comparison of intranasal cromolyn sodium, 4%, and oral terfenadine for allergic rhinitis: symptoms, nasal cytology, nasal clearance, and rhinomanometry. Ann Allergy 1991;66:237–244.
12. Bascom R, Pipkorn U, Lichtenstein LM, Naclerio RM. The influx of inflammatory cells into nasal washings during the late response to antigen challenge: effects of systemic steroid pretreatment. Am Rev Respir Dis 1988;138:406–412.
13. Simons FER. Antihistamines. In: Middleton E Jr, Reed CE, Ellis EF, Adkinson NF Jr, Yunginger JW, Busse WW, eds. Allergy: Principles and Practice. 5th ed. St. Louis: CV Mosby Co., 1998:612–637.
14. Furin MJ, Norman PS, Creticos PS, Proud D, Kagey-Sobotka A, Lichtenstein LM, Naclerio RM. Immunotherapy decreases antigen-induced eosinophil cell migration into the nasal cavity. J Allergy Clin Immunol 1991;88:27–32.
15. Otsuka H, Mezawa A, Ohnishi M, Okubo K, Seki H, Okuda M. Changes in nasal metachromatic cells during allergen immunotherapy. Clin Exp Allergy 1991;21:115–119.
16. Andersson M, Greiff L, Svensson C, Persson C. Various methods for testing nasal responses in vivo: a critical review. Acta Otolaryngol 1995;115:705–713.
17. Druce HM. Nasal provocation challenge: strategies for experimental design. Ann Allergy 1988;60:191–195.
18. Blackley CH. Experimental researches on the course and nature of catarrhus aestivus (hay-fever and hay-asthma). London: Bailliere, Tindal and Cox, 1873.
19. Schumacher MJ, Pain MCF. Nasal challenge testing in grass pollen hay fever. J Allergy Clin Immunol 1979;64:202–208.
20. Naclerio RM, Meier HL, Kagey-Sobotka A, Adkinson NF, Meyers DA, Norman PS, Lichtenstein LM. Mediator release after nasal airway challenge with allergen. Am Rev Respir Dis 1983;128:597–602.
21. Togias A, Naclerio RM, Proud D, Pipkorn U, Bascom R, Iliopoulos O, Kagey-Sobotka A, Norman PS, Lichtenstein LM. Studies on the allergic and nonallergic nasal inflammation. J Allergy Clin Immunol 1988;81:782–790.

22. Walden SM, Proud D, Bascom R, Lichtenstein LM, Kagey-Sobotka A, Adkinson NF, Naclerio RM. Experimental induced nasal allergic responses. J Allergy Clin Immunol 1988;81:940–949.
23. Lim MC, Taylor RM, Naclerio RM. The histology of allergic rhinitis and its comparison to cellular changes in nasal lavage. Am J Respir Crit Care Med 1995;151:136–144.
24. Georgitis JW, Stone BD, Gottschlich G. Nasal inflammatory mediators release in ragweed allergic rhinitis: correlation with cellular influx in nasal secretions. Int Arch Allergy Appl Immunol 1991;96:231–237.
25. Sipila J, Suonpaa J, Silvoniemi P, Laippala P. Correlation between subjective sensation of nasal patency and rhinomanometry in both unilateral and total nasal assessment. J Otorhinolaryngol Relat Spec 1995;57:260–263.
26. Yaniv E, Hadar T, Shvero J, Raveh E. Objective and subjective nasal airflow. Am J Otolaryngol 1997;18:29–32.
27. Aschan G, Drettner B, Ronge AE. A new technique for measuring nasal airflow resistance to breathing illustrated by the effect of histamine and physical effort. Ann Acad Reg Sci Appsala 1958;2:111–126.
28. Ferris BG, Mead J, Opie LH. Partitioning of respiratory flow resistance in man. J Appl Physiol 1964;19:653–658.
29. Eccles R. Neurological and pharmacological considerations. In: Proctor DF, Anderson I, eds. The nose, upper airways physiology and the atmospheric environment. Amersterdam: Elsevier, 1982:191–214.
30. Polgar G, King GP. The nasal resistance of newborn infants. J Pediatr 1965;67:557–567.
31. Clement PAR. Committee report on standardization of rhinomanometry. Rhinology 1984;22:151–155.
32. Eccles R. Rhinomanometry and nasal challenge. In: Mackay IS, Bull TR, eds. Scott-Brown's Otolaryngology: Rhinology. London: Butterworths, 1987:40–53.
33. Eccles R. The central rhythm of the nasal cycle. Acta Otolaryngol 1978;86:464–468.
34. Maran AGD, Lund VJ. Investigative test. In: Clinical Rhinology. New York: Thieme Medical Publishers, 1990:44–58.
35. Zamansky MJ. The role of rhinomanometry and nasal-pulmonary function tests. In: Goldman JL, ed. The principles and practice of rhinology, New York: John Wiley and Sons, 1987:213–222.
36. Schumacher MJ. Rhinomanometry. J Allergy Clin Immunol 1989;83:711–718.
37. Broms P. Rhinomanometry: procedures and criteria for distinction between skeletal stenosis and mucosal swelling. Acta Otolaryngol 1982;94:361–370.
38. McNicholas WT, Tarlo S, Cole P, Zamel N, Rutherford R, Griffin D, Phillipson EA. Obstructive apneas during sleep in patients with seasonal allergic rhinitis. Am Rev Respir Dis 1982;126:625–628.
39. Anch AM, Remmers JE, Bunce H. Supraglottic airway resistance in normal subjects and patients with occlusive sleep apnea. J Appl Physiol 1982;53:1158–1163.

7

Lung Disease

Ricardo A. Tan
California Allergy and Asthma Medical Group, Los Angeles, California

Sheldon L. Spector
University of California Medical Center and California Allergy and Asthma Medical Group, Los Angeles, California

I. SPIROMETRY AND LUNG FUNCTION

Spirometry is currently the most important diagnostic tool that clinicians have in the assessment of asthmatic patients. It is inexpensive, convenient, and easy to perform in almost any physician's office. The spirometer can measure volume over time, or both flow and volume in a procedure during which the patient takes a full, deep breath, exhales as forcefully and for as long as possible, followed by another full inspiration. The most useful values derived from spirometry include the vital capacity (VC), the forced vital capacity (FVC), the forced expiratory volume in 1 second (FEV_1), peak expiratory flow rate (PEFR), and the forced expiratory flow at 25–75% of the volume expired ($FEF_{25-75\%}$). The maximal voluntary ventilation (MVV) is another useful measure. The pattern of expiration and inspiration can also be recorded as a flow-volume curve to visualize characteristic patterns of obstruction. The information obtained from spirometry provides reproducible information on the presence or severity of airflow obstruction in both large and smaller airways. Characteristic patterns also can differentiate between obstructive and restrictive lung disease. It can confirm the diagnosis of asthma and help in monitoring response to treatment. Numerous studies have shown that symptoms and physical examination frequently underestimate or miss the presence of significant airway narrowing, making spirometry essential for good patient management.

The American Thoracic Society (ATS) provides comprehensive recommendations on spirometric equipment, techniques, and quality control (1). Daily instrument calibration is necessary to ensure accuracy of readings. Precautions against transmission of infection should also be observed (e.g., hand washing, disposable mouthpieces).

A. Indications for Spirometry

Spirometry may be used for: (1) diagnosis of lung disease; (2) monitoring; (3) evaluation of disability; or (4) public health surveys. Spirometry is important for diagnosis of respiratory conditions such as asthma and emphysema. It is also essential in evaluating severity, monitoring the progress, and assessing the response to therapy in these conditions. Spirometry also can help identify individuals at high risk for pulmonary disease, such as smokers and those exposed to toxic occupational agents. Assessment of health status before exercise programs, surgery requiring general anesthesia, and prognosis for procedures such as lung transplant are important indications for spirometry. Effects of environmental factors on large populations can be studied with spirometry (2).

B. VC and FVC

Vital capacity is the maximum amount of air that can be exhaled after maximal inspiration. It also commonly is referred to as the ''slow'' vital capacity to distinguish it from the FVC, which is the maximal amount of air exhaled during a forceful expiration. The FVC is considered to be more reflective of airflow limitation. Both VC and FVC are expressed in liters. The FEV_1, $FEF_{25-75\%}$, and PEFR are all derived from the FVC. Proper technique is crucial for obtaining reliable results. A skilled technician should be able to demonstrate that technique and guide the subject through a full inspiration and a forceful, prolonged exhalation. The subject should exhale for at least 6 s. The FVC maneuver should always be performed at least three times and the highest value used for clinical correlation. Spirometry may be performed in the sitting or standing position (1).

C. FEV_1 and FVC

The FEV_1 (expressed in liters) reflects the volume expired in the first second of the FVC and is the most widely used measure of airflow for diagnosis of asthma. The FEV_1 is largely effort dependent and requires a full, forceful effort from the subject to reflect airflow limitation truly. The effort-dependent portion of the FVC reflects the state of the large airways, the contraction of the expiratory muscles, and the elastic recoil of the lungs (3). Reversible airway obstruction characteristic of asthma can be demonstrated by measuring FEV_1 before and after bronchodilator treatment. The ATS designates a 12% increase from baseline FEV_1 and an absolute change of 200 mL as a positive bronchodilator response (4). The American College of Chest Physicians considers at least a 15% increase from baseline FEV_1 after bronchodilator treatment to be significant (5). After the initial evaluation, the FEV_1 should be used at least every 1 to 2 years to monitor a patient's progress (6). It is highly reproducible if there is good patient effort and technique. The ratio of FEV_1 to FVC can assist in classifying lung disease as obstructive or restrictive. In obstructive disease, airflow limitation causes a diminished FEV_1, whereas FVC may remain normal, causing a lowered FEV_1/FVC ratio. In restrictive disease, the FVC is diminished due to poor lung expansion. The FEV_1 is usually proportionally decreased leading to a normal or elevated FEV_1/FVC ratio. Although this ratio is helpful, the most reliable indicator of restrictive problems is the total lung capacity (TLC). Care must be taken in interpreting ratios when there is a poor expiratory effort. The ratio of a truly low FEV_1 and a low FVC from a suboptimal effort could be falsely normal in an obstructed patient. The FEV_1/FVC ratio should also be interpreted in light of the individual FEV_1 and FVC results. Healthy athletes can sometimes have normal or elevated FEV_1 and a low FEV_1/FVC ratio (4).

D. $FEF_{25-75\%}$

The $FEF_{25-75\%}$, also known as the maximum midexpiratory flow rate, reflects the average flow rate (liters per second) in the middle portion or 25–75% of the volume expired. It is mostly effort independent and has been widely used to reflect the state of the smaller airways. It is not as reproducible and sensitive as the FEV_1. Because the $FEF_{25-75\%}$ is calculated from the slope of the midportion of the volume-time curve of the FVC, a shortened expiration in severe airway obstruction may actually cause the $FEF_{25-75\%}$ to be falsely elevated (3). The

$FEF_{200-1200}$, which is no longer widely used, is a measure of the average flow rate between the first 200 and 1200 mL of volume. It is also known as the maximum expiratory flow rate (MEFR) and roughly correlates with the peak expiratory flow rate. At present, the $FEF_{200-1200}$ does not appear to provide more clinically useful information than the FEV_1 and $FEF_{25-75\%}$ (3).

E. MVV

Maximal voluntary ventilation is the maximum amount of air that a subject can move voluntarily in 1 minute. It is very effort dependent and is measured by having the subject breathe rapidly and fully for about 30 seconds. The maximum volume moved in any 15 seconds is expressed as liters per minute. The MVV is useful for evaluating preoperative lung function, lung function while weaning from mechanical ventilation, respiratory muscle function, and exercise tolerance.

F. Flow-Volume Curves

The flow-volume curve or loop is a recording of the relationship between flow and volume during maximum expiration followed by maximum inspiration (Fig. 1). It is very helpful in diagnosing or evaluating conditions such as asthma or upper airway obstruction that display characteristic patterns in the flow-volume loop. Expiration results as the pressure gradient between the alveolus and the mouth causes air to move outward. The initial upsurge on the graph followed by a gradual downward curve during expiration reflects the forces that affect flow at certain volumes. The first part of the expiratory curve is effort dependent and depends largely on the pressure exerted by the expiratory muscles and the elastic recoil of the lung. The downward sloping part of the curve is largely effort independent and is determined mainly by the elastic recoil of the lung and upstream resistance such as bronchoconstriction, making it a more significant reflection of airflow limitation. The inspiratory part of the loop is more sensitive to central airway obstruction. For every given volume on the horizontal axis, there is a point beyond which flow cannot increase further. This limitation is determined by the equal pressure point, which is the point at which the airway collapses as the pressures inside and outside the airway equalize.

The characteristic pattern of asthma is an increased concavity in the downward curve of the expiratory part of the flow-volume loop. This is also seen in emphysema. Extrathoracic airway obstruction produces a recognizable pattern that helps to identify patients with conditions such as vocal cord dysfunction, which is often misdiagnosed as asthma. The inspiratory loop in extrathoracic obstruction characteristically has a flattened appearance that is due to the collapse of the upper airway from negative pressure generated inside the airway during inhalation (Fig. 2).

Partial flow-volume loops have been used occasionally to eliminate the smooth muscle relaxation that is thought to occur during the deep inhalation

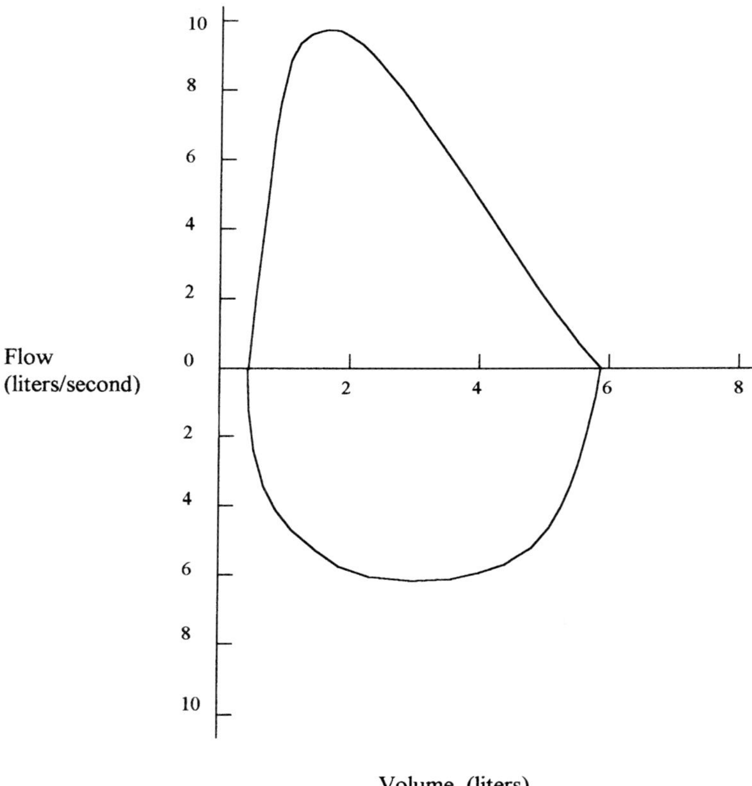

Figure 1 Flow-volume loop in normal subject.

maneuver used to generate full volume loops. This muscle relaxation may result in falsely elevated spirometry values. When obtaining partial flow-volume loops, the subject expires forcefully at the end of regular inspiration. Although not as reproducible as full volume loops, partial flow volume loops are useful in certain situations.

G. Lung Volumes

Measurement of lung volumes provides important information for evaluating lung function in patients with complicated conditions such as mixed obstructive and restrictive disease. Tidal volume (TV), VC, expiratory reserve volume (ERV), and inspiratory capacity (IC) can be measured directly by spirometry. Residual volume and functional residual capacity (FRC) can only be measured

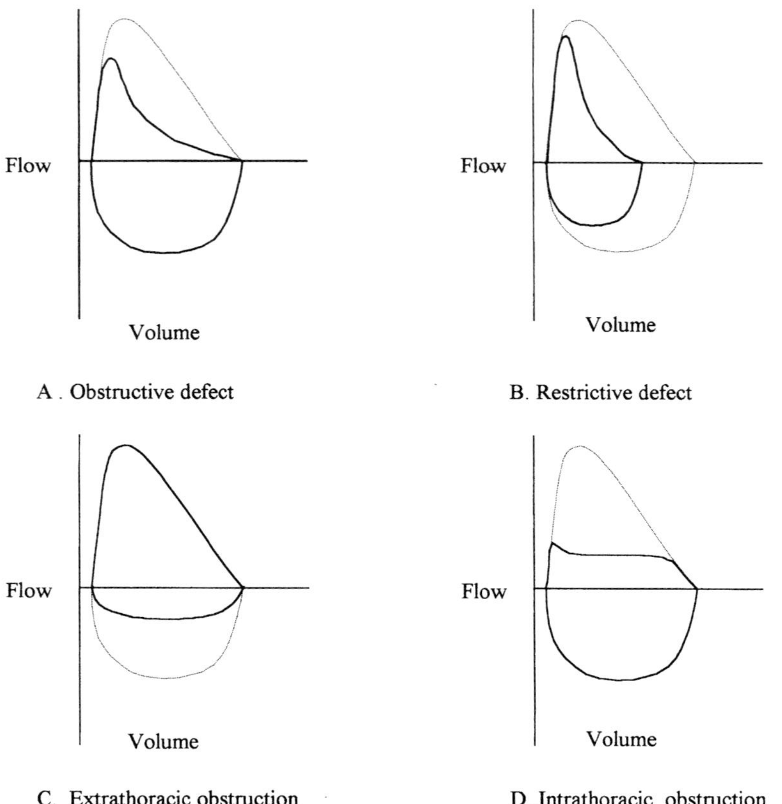

Figure 2 Typical flow volume loop patterns for various pulmonary conditions. (A) Concavity in downward curve in obstructive disease. (B) Diminished flow and volume in restrictive disease. (C) Flattening of inspiratory loop in extrathoracic upper airway obstruction. (D) Flattening of expiratory loop in intrathoracic upper airway obstruction.

indirectly by means of more complicated procedures (for example, body plethysmography or gas dilution techniques, such as helium dilution and nitrogen washout). These procedures are usually available only in research and hospital-based facilities.

As mentioned previously, VC is the maximal amount of air that can be exhaled after maximal inspiration. Tidal volume is the amount inhaled and exhaled during quiet (normal) breathing. Residual volume is the amount of air remaining in the lung after the end of maximum expiration, whereas FRC is the amount of air remaining after normal expiration. Both FRC and RV are increased in asthma. Expiratory reserve volume is the additional amount that can be expelled after a normal expiration. Inspiratory capacity is the maximum amount of air that can be inspired after normal expiration. Total lung capacity is the sum of RV and VC. Vital capacity can also be computed as the sum of IC and ERV. Several sets of predicted values for total lung capacity and residual volume have been derived from different studies, but only the Crapo study, which is based on measurements obtained from nonsmoking adults, conforms to the ATS standards for spirometry (7).

H. Reference Values

Numerous studies have been conducted to determine reference values for spirometry and pulmonary function testing. However, no single set of values can be universally applied to all populations. The ATS has extensively reviewed and listed these studies, along with their strengths and limitations. Because of variability among individuals and populations, the ATS recommends that practitioners should be familiar with the applicability and limitations of different sets of published reference values. If a computerized spirometer is being used, physicians should know which set of reference values has been programmed to designate results as normal, elevated, or decreased. Most reference tables list age and height as variables and have separate tables for men and women. Racial ancestry and past and present health are also important variables (4). Among the studies often used for predicted values are those done by Crapo (8) and Dockery (9), both of which were done on nonsmoking Caucasian men and women. Racial background is an important variable that may not be taken into account by most practitioners. In general, non-Caucasian populations show lower values for lung volumes. Rossiter et al. suggested a correction factor of 0.88 when reference values for Caucasians are used for Americans of African descent (10).

The varying ranges for predicted ''normal'' values make it imperative for the practitioner to correlate all pulmonary function test results with individual patients. The patient's age, size, sex, and racial background should be considered. The ATS recommends against using 80% of predicted as the lower limit of normal for pulmonary function test results because it applies only to individuals with average characteristics and may arbitrarily classify healthy persons as abnormal (4). Monitoring changes in a patient's spirometry values over time provides the best way of evaluating his or her respiratory status at any point in time.

II. PEAK FLOW

The PEFR is the highest expiratory flow produced with forceful expiration after maximal inspiration. It is expressed in liters per minute. The peak flow meter is a popular, portable, easy, and relatively inexpensive way to monitor lung function outside of the physician's office. The PEFR measures only the most effort-dependent part of the FVC and is similar to the MEFR. It is most useful in moderate-to-severe asthma because it may miss subtle airflow limitation in mild episodes. Peak flow meters can be used to monitor asthma status and assess response to bronchodilator therapy during acute asthma attacks at home. The PEFR may also help confirm the presence of asthma in patients with normal spirometry by demonstrating a difference of 20% or more between morning and afternoon peak flow readings over 1 to 2 weeks.

There are numerous peak flow devices now available, which vary from simple tubes to computerized models. Only those that conform to the criteria set by the ATS should be used (1). The ATS recommends that devices should permit readings from 60 to 400 L/min for children and 100 to 850 L/min for adults. It is very important that patients are taught the proper technique for using the peak flow meter. The patient should be standing and should inhale fully, place the flow meter in his or her mouth, close the lips around it to form a tight seal, and exhale through the meter with maximal force. Unlike the FVC, the PEFR can be obtained properly with an exhalation time limited to 1 to 2 seconds. Three peak flow readings should be obtained and recorded each time the device is used (1,6).

Studies have shown that many patients underestimate the severity of asthma attacks when subjective symptoms are their only guide (11,12). These findings make the relatively objective peak flow meter more important in home monitoring. A patient's personal best peak flow should be established during an asymptomatic period and should form the basis of comparison for subsequent readings. During acute attacks, peak flow readings should be used to guide therapy. Patients using peak flow meters should be given written action plans, including when to take their medications or adjust the dosages and when to call the physician or go to the emergency department. The 1997 National Institutes of Health (NIH) asthma guidelines (6) recommend the use of peak flow meters at least once daily to monitor chronic asthma and its response to therapy. Daily peak flow readings are best taken in the morning prior to bronchodilator use. If the reading is less than 80% of the patient's personal best, the peak flow should be checked again throughout the day according to the patient's action plan.

Although results of studies directly comparing usual care and addition of peak flow monitoring have been inconclusive (13,14), it is generally agreed that long-term peak flow monitoring will more likely benefit moderate-to-severe asthmatics.

III. BRONCHOSCOPY

Bronchoscopy provides for direct visualization of the tracheobronchial tree and collection of specimens with an endoscopic device. The rigid bronchoscope was introduced in the 1900s and is still used today for certain procedures such as dilatation of bronchial strictures and laser therapy. With the introduction of the flexible fiberoptic bronchoscope, the procedure became more efficient, easier to perform, and more comfortable for patients.

Indications for bronchoscopy may be diagnostic, therapeutic or investigative. Bronchoscopy is indicated in the diagnosis and evaluation of lung masses, pulmonary infiltrates, hemoptysis, abnormal sputum cytology, recurrent laryngeal nerve paralysis, stridor or wheezing, unexplained cough, lung abscess, acute pulmonary injury and trauma, bronchiectasis, bronchopleural fistulas, and other conditions. It is required in staging lung cancer. It is helpful therapeutically for removing foreign bodies, applying laser therapy, and assisting in endotracheal tube and tracheostomy placement. In asthma, it has been used primarily for research purposes. It has allowed research to confirm the inflammatory nature of asthma by facilitating bronchial biopsies and bronchoalveolar lavage (BAL). Although it is rarely needed in clinical practice to diagnose or monitor asthma, it is useful in ruling out conditions that may mimic asthma such as foreign body obstruction or endobronchial tumors. Bronchoscopy should not be done without informed consent from the patient and without a skilled bronchoscopist or adequate facilities for resuscitation or oxygenation. Relative contraindications include uncontrolled asthma, bleeding disorders, pregnancy, pulmonary hypertension, superior vena cava obstruction, unstable cardiac disease, hypoxemia, and hypercapnia (15).

A full history, physical examination, and screening laboratory tests must be obtained prior to bronchoscopy to ensure that no contraindications to the procedure are present. Preoperative medications include morphine or meperidine, as well as the anticholinergic agent, atropine. Benzodiazepines, such as diazepam, may be added to help the anxious patient relax. Certain patients are intubated prior to bronchoscopy if necessary. The bronchoscope may be inserted through the nose or the mouth while 2% lidocaine is administered at intervals as the scope enters the trachea and bronchi. The nasal passages, larynx, and vocal cords are all inspected fully before the scope progresses into the bronchi. Equipment for obtaining specimens may be passed through the scope, including brushes and forceps for biopsies, and needles for aspiration and biopsies. Fluid is instilled through the scope and suctioned to obtain BAL fluid.

A. Safety of Bronchoscopy

With the increased use of bronchoscopy, bronchial biopsy, and bronchoalveolar lavage for research rather than diagnostic or therapeutic indications, the safety of asthmatic research subjects has been a concern. The NIH released guidelines in 1991 regarding the investigative use of bronchoscopy, lavage, and bronchial biopsies in asthma and other airway diseases (16). The NIH recommends that patients with asthma should undergo a full evaluation of baseline pulmonary function in addition to the usual precautions. Severe asthmatics that are to be studied should have arterial blood gases monitored. Asthmatics with a history of acute severe respiratory failure should not be selected. In general, the NIH believes that the safety of investigative bronchoscopy in asthma has been well studied and documented. When peak flow monitoring was done for 2 weeks after bronchoscopy and biopsy in asthmatic subjects, no delayed adverse effects in pulmonary function were seen (17).

B. Bronchial Biopsies

The same precautions exercised before bronchoscopy are important in performing bronchial biopsies. In asthmatic patients, a spirometry is essential to make sure the patient is stable prior to the procedure. Arterial blood gas monitoring may be needed in some instances. If patient evaluation and preparation are carefully followed, bronchial biopsies appear to be safe and well tolerated by patients with asthma (16).

Brush and forceps biopsy of airway mucosa as well as transbronchial lung biopsy can be performed through the bronchoscope. In the brush biopsy, cells and pieces of tissue are collected in the bristles of the biopsy brush as it is moved across the mucosa, and the specimen is smeared on a slide for study. Forceps biopsies obtain larger pieces of mucosa and deeper tissue than brush specimens. Transbronchial lung biopsies are ideally performed under fluoroscopic guidance. Bleeding is the most common complication of bronchial biopsies and may be avoided by instilling epinephrine into the area to be biopsied. The NIH recommends that brushings be limited to two to four areas and that only three to six 2-mm biopsies be obtained in a single procedure from a combination of the main carina and one or more segmental or subsegmental carinae (16).

Bronchial biopsies and BAL have made possible major advances in the concept and understanding of the pathophysiology of asthma as a chronic inflammatory condition. Research using these techniques continues to provide new information on the mechanisms of inflammation and the cells, mediators, and cytokines involved.

C. Findings in Asthma

Studies using endobronchial biopsies have established asthma as a disorder characterized by chronic inflammation. Damaged airway epithelium characterized by shedding of epithelial cells and widened intercellular spaces are seen in most biopsies obtained from the lungs of asthmatic subjects. Whereas normal epithelium consists mostly of pseudostratified ciliated epithelium, there is an increased proportion of goblet cells to ciliated cells in the bronchi of asthmatics. Lymphocytes comprise 60–90%, whereas mast cells account for less than 20% of the inflammatory cells found in normal airway mucosal biopsy specimens. Most pathological studies report a general increase in numbers of lymphocytes and mast cells as well as eosinophils and macrophages in the airways of asthmatics compared to control subjects. The increase in eosinophil number appears to correlate directly with the severity of asthma. Biopsy studies of the pulmonary epithelium have noted basement membrane thickening in asthmatic subjects that may play a role in airway remodeling. The contributions of collagen, fibronectin, tenascin, and laminins to this process are under investigation (18).

IV. BRONCHOALVEOLAR LAVAGE

Bronchoalveolar lavage and bronchial biopsy usually are performed via flexible bronchoscopy. In BAL, fluid is introduced through the bronchoscope into the bronchi and alveoli and then aspirated to obtain fluid containing cellular and protein material. Bronchoalveolar lavage has both diagnostic and therapeutic indications. It is used most commonly to obtain bronchoalveolar fluid and identify cellular and protein profiles characteristic of specific pulmonary diseases such as sarcoidosis, hypersensitivity pneumonitis, idiopathic pulmonary fibrosis, alveolar proteinosis, and eosinophilic granuloma. For example, BAL fluid has a preponderance of CD4 (helper) compared to the CD8 (suppressor) type of T lymphocytes in sarcoidosis patients, whereas the reverse is true in patients with hypersensitivity pneumonitis. Lavage fluid facilitates identification of *Pneumocystis carinii*, an opportunistic pathogen that causes pneumonia in immunocompromised patients. Therapeutic lavage is occasionally used in subjects with alveolar proteinosis or cystic fibrosis to remove impacted secretions. Bronchoalveolar lavage and bronchial biopsies are research tools that have enhanced understanding of asthmatic inflammation at both cellular and molecular levels.

Bronchoalveolar lavage, however, also has technical limitations. The invasive nature of the procedure itself can mechanically disrupt the integrity of the cells and proteins being studied. The BAL specimens are obtained from mucosal surfaces and may not reflect any cellular changes in submucosal airway tissue. The main limitation of BAL fluid examination is the variable dilution of specimens. Because the amount of fluid infused and returned cannot be exactly the same with each procedure, the values for cell numbers and protein concentrations are not accurate or consistent. There is no standard dye or marker that helps to determine the dilution of a given specimen.

The methods and protocols used for BAL vary and are not standardized. The bronchoscope is usually wedged into a bronchus in the lung segment to be studied. The right middle lobe, lingula, and lower lobes are preferred sites because they provide a larger return of lavage fluid than the upper lobes (16). Sterile saline is infused through the bronchoscope in 20- to 50-mL increments. The NIH recommends the instillation of not more than 400 mL of fluid during a single procedure. Larger amounts have been associated with hypoxemia and atelectasis. After each instillation, fluid is withdrawn by aspiration into a syringe or by the force of gravity. Aspiration should be gentle to prevent trauma to the cells and mucosa. Approximately 50–60% of the instilled fluid is recovered by both gravity and low suction (50–70 mm Hg). The recovered fluid is centrifuged and the cells are separated for study. The protein-laden supernatant fluid can remain viable at room temperature for a few hours but it also may be frozen for storage. A workshop on bronchoscopy concluded that two lavage procedures within 24 hours, if necessary, are safe and well tolerated (16).

A. Findings in Asthma

Bronchoalveolar lavage fluid has been used in asthma to elucidate the pathophysiology of airway inflammation and to study the effects of various pharmacological and nonpharmacological interventions. Most of the inflammatory cells, cytokines, and chemical mediators involved in asthma are increased in BAL fluid. Macrophages comprise up to 90% of BAL fluid cells. Eosinophils account for less than 1% of BAL fluid cells in nonasthmatics, but they account for 2–11% of cells in BAL fluid obtained from asthmatic individuals (19). This increase in eosinophils is a prominent characteristic of BAL fluid in asthmatics. Eosinophils in asthma usually exist in an activated state with elevated levels of major basic protein, eosinophil cationic protein, and eosinophil-derived neurotoxin (20,21). Bronchoalveolar lavage fluid contains mucosal type (MC_T) mast cells, which activate and degranulate in symptomatic asthma (22). Although mast cells constitute less than 0.5% of BAL fluid cells in nonasthmatics, they can account for up to 3% of BAL fluid cells obtained from asthmatics. Lymphocytes are the predominant cells observed in lung biopsy specimens, but they account for only 10–20% of BAL fluid cells, and the BAL lymphocyte concentration appears to be the same in both asthmatic and nonasthmatic individuals. However, BAL fluid obtained from asthmatics has increased levels of interleukin (IL)-2 receptors, which provides evidence of T-lymphocyte activation (23). Basophils may be increased in BAL fluid obtained from asthmatics, but this usually occurs only during the late-phase response to allergen challenge. Numerous cytokines interact in a complex network to influence inflammation in asthma. A characteristic set of cytokines produced by the T-helper 2 (TH2) subset of T-lymphocytes has been established as crucial in humorally mediated immunity and in allergic inflammation, including asthma. The TH2 cytokines include IL-4, which promotes isotype switching of B-lymphocytes during IgE synthesis, and IL-5, which promotes eosinophil production and survival. Both of these cytokines are increased in the BAL fluid of asthmatic subjects. Other cytokines that are increased in asthmatic BAL fluid include IL-1, IL-2, IL-6, IL-8, IL-13, IL-16, interferon-γ, transforming growth factor-α (TGF-α), macrophage-inflammatory protein-1α (MIP-1α), tumor necrosis factor-α (TNF-α), granulocyte-macrophage colony stimulating factor (GM-CSF), and regulated upon activation, normal T-cell expressed and secreted (RANTES). The complex interactions between these cytokines and their target cells in asthma are under investigation.

Inflammatory mediators such as the cysteinyl leukotrienes, prostaglandins, kinins, histamine, and tryptase, all of which play a role in asthma, are elevated in BAL obtained from asthmatics. Increased levels of adhesion molecules, including ICAM-1 (CD54), VCAM-1 (CD106), and E-selectin (CD62E) have also been found. Increased numbers of epithelial cells shed into BAL fluid also characterize asthma, and their presence indicates damaged airway epithelium (21).

V. BRONCHOPROVOCATION

Bronchoprovocation, or bronchial challenge testing, is used to assess subjects for nonspecific or specific bronchial hyperresponsiveness by exposing them to inhaled stimuli in a controlled setting and measuring their response by spirometry. Bronchoprovocation testing with methacholine or histamine is widely used to confirm the presence of asthma in patients with atypical symptoms, such as chronic cough without wheezing or dyspnea. Bronchial challenge with specific stimuli, such as allergens and occupational agents, can identify or confirm the correlation between exposure and symptoms. In many cases, skin testing of allergens does not correlate accurately with airway reactivity to the same substances. Inhaled challenge with exercise, cold air and non-ionic aerosols can also detect airway hyperresponsiveness. Leukotrienes, prostaglandins, and adenosine have also been used for bronchoprovocation in research studies. Bronchoprovocation also is used to study the efficacy of therapeutic agents in decreasing the bronchial challenge responses expected from known triggers of symptoms (24).

General considerations regarding precautions, procedures, and methods are applicable to most bronchial challenge tests. Any modifications of these principles will be mentioned in the sections that follow. In general, challenge testing should be done when the degree of a subject's airway responsiveness is as close to baseline as possible. The subject's baseline FEV_1 should be at least 70% of the value predicted for the reference group. Symptomatic pulmonary disease is a contraindication for the procedure. Because anxiety or anticipation may influence the bronchial response, it is important that the subject be informed that the result of the test may indicate an increase, decrease, or no change in lung function. Circadian rhythms also may play a role in the response to challenge, but no specific recommendations on the best time of day for testing are available. Challenges should not be performed after recent allergen exposure, exercise, exposure to pollutants, or during ongoing or recent viral infections, all of which can increase bronchial hyperresponsiveness and affect test results. Coffee, chocolate, cola drinks, and smoking should be avoided at least 6 hours prior to challenge. β-Adrenergic agents, short-acting theophylline preparations, α-adrenergic agents, and anticholinergic agents should be stopped at least 8 hours before testing. Sustained-release β-agonists and theophylline preparations should be stopped at least 12 hours prior to testing. Antihistamines should be avoided for 48 hours or longer, depending on the half-life of the drug. Mast-cell stabilizers, such as cromolyn and nedocromil, may be continued prior to inhaled bronchoconstrictor (histamine or methacholine) but should be avoided 24 hours before allergen, occupational agent, or exercise challenge (24).

The FEV_1 is the pulmonary function value used most widely to assess bronchial responsiveness because it is convenient and very easy to perform. It is less variable than other values such as $FEF_{25-75\%}$. Other tests used to evaluate bronchial response are VC, PEFR, MMFR or $FEF_{25-75\%}$, FRC, specific airway resistance (SRaw), and specific airway conductance (SGaw). At least a 20% fall from baseline FEV_1 is generally considered a significant response to bronchial challenge. The minimal changes considered positive for other parameters include VC (−10%), PEFR (−25%), MMFR (−25%), FRC (+25%), SRaw (+35%) and SGaw airway conductance (−35%).

A. Inhaled Bronchoconstrictor Agents

Methacholine and histamine are the bronchoconstrictor agents used most widely to assess airway responsiveness, a key feature of asthma. The responses elicited are usually short-lived and therefore ideal for testing. A challenge is especially appropriate for persons with dyspnea or cough of unclear etiology. Methacholine is generally preferred because histamine may cause side effects, such as headache and tachycardia, and histamine has a tendency to cause tachyphylaxis after repeated challenges. Airway responsiveness to these bronchoconstrictor agents correlates well with asthma severity.

Several standardized protocols for bronchoprovocation are available. Among the methods most widely used are those described by Cockcroft (25), Chai (26), and Yan (27). Most protocols start with five breaths of a saline solution control, and a drop of 15% or more in the FEV_1 is a contraindication to the bronchial challenge. The subject is next given five breaths at a time of progressively increasing concentrations of methacholine or histamine. For safety, the initial concentration used for both agents is usually less than 0.1 mg/mL. Spirometry is performed after each set of five breaths. The concentration ($PC_{20}FEV_1$) or cumulative dose ($PD_{20}FEV_1$) of methacholine or histamine measures the response to provocation required to decrease the subject's baseline FEV_1 by 20%. The concentration is expressed as mg/mL, whereas the cumulative dose is expressed as cumulative micromoles or cumulative breath units. Each breath unit is equivalent to one breath of a

1 mg/mL concentration (28). After five inhalations of the usual maximal concentration of 10 mg/mL (histamine) or 25 mg/mL (methacholine), fewer than 5% of normal patients will have a 20% fall in FEV_1 (26). Approximately 85–100% of asthmatics will have a $PC_{20}FEV_1$ of 8 mg/mL or less of methacholine or histamine (25,29). Cockcroft has classified asthmatics with $PC_{20}FEV_1$ of 2–8 mg/mL to methacholine as mild; 0.25 to less than 2 mg/mL as moderate; and less than 0.25 mg/mL as severe (25). Persons with allergic rhinitis but no history of asthma symptoms may have $PC_{20}FEV_1$ values of 8 mg/mL or less, but may exhibit a plateau in the dose-response curve, whereas asthmatics continue to show a decline in FEV_1 as the dose of methacholine or histamine is increased (30).

B. Nonisotonic Aerosols

Osmolar changes in the airway mucosa, whether positive or negative, have long been believed to lead to airflow limitation. In recent years, bronchoprovocation has increasingly used nonisotonic aerosols, such as water, and hypotonic and hypertonic solutions. These aerosols are especially helpful for physicians who prefer to use nonpharmacological alternatives for evaluating airway hyperresponsiveness. Bronchoprovocation with nonisotonic aerosols is inexpensive, easy to perform, and relatively free of side effects (31). Bronchodilators and mast cell stabilizers, such as cromolyn and nedocromil, may diminish the bronchial response to nonisotonic aerosols and should be stopped at least 6–8 hours before the provocation procedure.

All challenge methods use the ultrasonic nebulizer, which delivers more aerosol than regular nebulizers. Water, which is hypotonic, and hypertonic saline solutions of 2.7%, 3.6%, and 4.5% sodium chloride are commonly used. A mouthpiece or facemask enables delivery of the aerosol, with a single exposure or several exposures at increasing lengths of time or concentration. Exposure time usually starts at 30 seconds and is doubled with each subsequent exposure to a maximum of 8 minutes. More than 80% of asthmatics will have a fall in FEV_1 of 20% or more after 15–20 mL of aerosol is delivered. It appears that nonisotonic aerosols are less sensitive than methacholine or histamine in detecting airway hyperresponsiveness. Because normal subjects only have a 7% or less decrease in FEV_1 after an exposure of up to 50 mL of nonisotonic aerosols, some experts have proposed that establishing clinical significance at a 12% or greater decrease in FEV_1 may enhance the sensitivity of this challenge method (31). Specific airways resistance also can be used to measure the bronchial response to nonisotonic aerosols, with an increase of 100% or 6 cm H_2O/L/sec denoting a positive response (32).

Nonisotonic aerosols appear to cause changes in osmolarity rather than producing bronchoconstriction directly. These changes cause mast cells to release inflammatory mediators such as histamine, prostaglandins, and cysteinyl leukotrienes. These mediators produce airway obstruction through bronchoconstriction, edema, increased mucus production, and influx of inflammatory cells. This osmolar mechanism also has been proposed as the basis for exercise-induced asthma. Due to their indirect mechanism, nonisotonic aerosols are felt to be less sensitive but more specific for moderate to severe asthma than methacholine or histamine (31).

C. Allergen Bronchoprovocation

A good clinical history and skin testing remain the primary diagnostic tools for identifying allergenic triggers of asthma. The necessity of bronchial challenge with specific allergens remains controversial. However, bronchial challenge testing with allergens may clarify the role of specific allergens when skin testing cannot be performed because of severe eczema or other skin disorders or when RAST testing is considered inadequate. It may also reinforce for the patient the presence or absence of a clinical correlation between allergen exposure and pulmonary symptoms. Bronchoprovocation with allergens is another important research tool for the investigation of mechanisms and mediators of inflammation, identification of new allergens, evaluation of the response to immunotherapy, and assessment of the efficacy of new therapeutic agents, among other uses (24).

Mast-cell heterogeneity may account for the disparity sometimes seen between skin test and bronchial challenge results. The production of immunoglobulin (Ig)E may also vary in different sites. In animal studies, mast cells in the respiratory tract react differently than skin mast cells (33). Although at least one study concludes that bronchoprovocation offers no advantage over skin or in vitro testing (34), many practitioners feel that bronchoprovocation provides important additional information in certain clinical situations.

The accuracy of the bronchial challenge results depends in large part on the potency of the allergen vaccine used. Over the last decade, standardization of commonly used vaccines based on their biological potency has been ongoing. Although relatively few in number, standardized allergen vaccines are superior and produce more reproducible findings than vaccines that are graded according to older criteria, such as weight or protein content. (Standardized allergen vaccines are discussed in Chapter 1.)

There is no single protocol for determining the safest initial concentration for an allergen provocative challenge. In general, the lowest concentration producing an erythema-surrounded wheal larger than 5 mm (2+) by intradermal skin testing would be a safe, initial challenge concentration. Fish (28) suggests that subjects with 2+ skin test responses to concentrations less than 0.05 μg/mL can be started safely at inhalation doses of 0.025 to 0.05 μg/mL to avoid prolonged testing.

The allergen challenge is delivered in aerosol form with a nebulizer. A control diluent substance, usually saline, is delivered first. The decrease in FEV_1, if any occurs after diluent challenge, should be less than 10% from the baseline. A greater decrease would indicate nonspecific reactivity, which would adversely affect test results. The allergen to be tested is prepared in multiple dilutions and given in a graded dose protocol (Table 1). Five successive breaths of the most dilute preparation are given first. The FEV_1 is checked after delivery of each allergen concentration. A sustained decrease in FEV_1 of 20% or more for at least 3 minutes is considered a positive result. If the response is negative, successively higher concentrations are given in the same manner at 12–15 minute intervals. If the result is borderline or equivocal, the patient should take fewer than five breaths with the next inhalation. The challenge is continued until the patient has a positive response, or a concentration approximating 1:500 wt/vol is reached. The significance of testing with a 1:100 wt/vol concentration or its equivalent is unclear because of possible irritant effects (24).

The FEV_1 is plotted against the cumulative inhalation units, each of which is equivalent to one breath of 1:500 wt/vol dilution, to produce a dose-response curve. The dose in cumulative inhalation units that is needed to decrease the FEV_1 by 20% from the baseline is referred to as the provocative dose ($PD_{20}FEV_1$). The lower the $PD_{20}FEV_1$, the more allergic the patient is to the test substance (24).

Unlike inhaled methacholine and histamine, for which the effects are short lived, allergen challenges can produce both immediate and late-phase responses. Therefore, it is important for a patient's respiratory status to be monitored and

Table 1 Cumulative Doses for Bronchial Inhalation Challenge with Allergen at Five Breaths per Dilution

Allergen concentration (w/v)*	Inhalation units/ five breaths[†]	Cumulative units/ five breaths
1:1,000,000	0.025	0.025
1:500,000	0.05	0.075
1:100,000	0.25	0.325
1:50,000	0.5	0.825
1:10,000	2.5	3.32
1:5,000	5.0	8.32
1:1,000	25.0	33.3
1:500	50.0	83.3
1:100	250.0	300.3

* At concentrations of antigens of 1:100 and above, the clinical meaning is unclear.
[†] One inhalation unit = one breath 1:500 w/v dilution.
Abbreviation: w/v = weight per volume.

checked up to 24 hours after challenge. Late-phase responses usually appear 6–8 hours after the challenge, last longer than immediate responses, and may persist for several weeks (28). *Alternaria* and *Dermatophagoides* appear to cause late-phase reactions in up to 90% of patients (35). Due to the risk of severe reactions, allergen bronchoprovocation should only be performed in facilities with emergency medications and resuscitation equipment available.

D. Exercise and Hyperventilation

Exercise and hyperventilation have long been observed to be significant triggers of bronchospasm. Some asthmatics only exhibit symptoms after exercise. Bronchial challenge with exercise or hyperventilation is useful for assessing bronchial hyperreactivity, as well as diagnosing exercise-induced asthma (EIA).

Exercise-induced asthma is characterized by transient airway obstruction, which occurs after strenuous exertion. Inhalation of large volumes of dry, cold air during exercise leads to loss of heat and water from the bronchial mucosa. Proposed mechanisms for bronchoconstriction in EIA include: (1) mucosal drying and increased osmolarity, which stimulate mast cell degranulation (36) and (2) rapid airway rewarming after exercise, which causes vascular congestion, increased permeability, and airway edema (37). In contrast to methacholine and histamine, which produce direct constriction of bronchial smooth muscle, exercise and hyperventilation appear to be more reflective of the actual inflammatory process in the bronchi.

Typically, EIA symptoms start after exercise, peak 8–15 minutes after exercise, and spontaneously resolve in about 60 minutes. A decline in the FEV_1 after exercise of 10% or more is usually considered diagnostic. A refractory period, during which repeat exercise causes less bronchospasm, has been observed to last up to 3 hours after recovery. Enhanced ventilation and cold, dry, inspired air increase the risk for EIA.

Exercise challenge testing is usually accomplished by using a treadmill or cycle ergometer. The subject exercises for approximately 6–8 minutes with the goal of reaching about 80% of the predicted maximal heart rate or 50–60% of the predicted maximum oxygen consumption or VO_{2max} (37). A fall of more than 10% in the FEV_1 after exercise is diagnostic of EIA (38). Some authors, however, believe that a 15% drop is needed for diagnosis (37). Some accomplished athletes may not show EIA during laboratory testing. Athletes in sports with variable exertion, such as boxing or hockey, can be tested both before and after their usual sports activities. The diagnosis is established when a fall in FEV_1 of more than 10–15% after exercise is observed.

Because the rate of ventilation influences EIA, isocapneic hyperventilation can also be used to test for EIA. Isocapneic hyperventilation requires more equipment, but it is easier to perform for patients who are unable to exercise. The subject breathes through a valve box with a pump set to a specific minute ventilation. A reservoir balloon is attached to the valve box and the patient breathes with enough force to prevent deflation of the balloon. A low concentration of carbon dioxide is delivered to the patient to prevent hypocapnia. The usual aim is to achieve approximately 60–70% of maximum voluntary ventilation. A fall of 10% in the FEV_1 after hyperventilation suggests asthma. Other authors recommend a 15% decline for diagnosis (39).

E. Occupational Asthma

Occupational causes of asthma are suspected in patients who appear to have worsening of symptoms in the workplace. These symptoms may appear immediately after starting work or after years of exposure. Both IgE- and non–IgE-mediated mechanisms have been proposed for bronchospasm caused by occupational agents. Use of a peak flow meter or spirometry, if available, to compare lung function at and away from the workplace may be adequate for a diagnosis of occupational asthma. However, bronchial challenge testing in a laboratory may be necessary in some cases to document definitively the presence or absence of a correlation between occupational exposure and asthma. This documentation may be essential for the physician to make recommendations to preserve the patient's health, and for the patient who may be faced with the difficult decision of leaving a job.

Occupational agents that can cause asthma include high-molecular-weight agents, such as natural proteins, and low-molecular-weight chemicals, such as diisocyanates. Occupational chemicals implicated in workplace asthma include anhydrides (e.g., trimellitic anhydride in epoxy resins), antibiotics (e.g., penicillin), diisocyanates (e.g., hexamethylene diisocyanate used for spray painting), precious metals (e.g., platinum salts), wood dusts (e.g., plicatic acid in western red cedar), and dyes. Diisocyanates and plicatic acid appear to cause asthma by non–IgE-mediated mechanisms (40).

High-molecular-weight allergens are usually derived from plant and animal proteins. There are numerous proteins implicated in occupational asthma. Among those most commonly encountered are vegetable gums (e.g., acacia), enzymes (e.g., *Bacillus subtilis* in detergent workers), animal proteins (e.g., laboratory animals), insects (e.g., storage mites in farm and granary workers), plant proteins (e.g., latex in health workers or wheat flour in bakers), and legumes (e.g., soybeans, castor beans) (40).

Specific inhalation challenges are currently performed only in hospital or research facilities with appropriate equipment. Challenge testing uses specialized inhalation chambers where exposure to test substances can be rigorously controlled. If possible, the level of the suspected agent is measured in the workplace and this level is then used to guide the dose used in testing. The challenge process may require several days of testing. Patients usually undergo a methacholine challenge to determine baseline airway hyperreactivity prior to testing with the suspected agent. On the first day, the subject is exposed only to room air, and control values for FEV_1 are obtained at regular intervals during and after exposure. On subsequent days, the patient is exposed to the test agent inside the chamber and the FEV_1 is assessed in the same manner. The initial exposure time is usually 30 minutes but the exposure time is increased gradually over successive days up to 4 hours. A sustained decrease in FEV_1 of 20% or more at any time is considered a positive response and the testing is stopped (41).

F. Segmental Bronchoprovocation

Segmental bronchial challenge is used increasingly in research studies to obtain a precise picture of physiological changes in specific segments of the lungs. In this technique, allergen is instilled through a bronchoscope into a lung segment and BAL fluid is obtained immediately after the challenge. The BAL fluid is then studied for changes in cell and protein content. This procedure is obviously more invasive than the regular allergen challenge, but it has helped to provide important data on the allergic response in asthma (42).

VI. SALIENT POINTS

1. Spirometry is the most important diagnostic tool in the evaluation and monitoring of asthma and is essential in the initial evaluation of other pulmonary diseases.
2. The most useful values derived from spirometry are FEV_1, FVC, $FEF_{25-75\%}$, and PEFR. Age, sex, height, and race are all variables that affect predicted reference values.
3. Improvement of FEV_1 after bronchodilator treatment can confirm the diagnosis of asthma.
4. The peak flow meter is an easy and convenient way to monitor lung function outside the physician's office. Patients with chronic asthma, especially moderate to severe, should monitor their PEFR regularly because studies have shown that symptoms alone are not reliable indicators of airflow limitation.
5. Bronchoscopy is primarily used in asthma for investigative or research purposes. It enables visualization of the bronchial tree and collection of bronchial biopsies and BAL fluid. With proper precautions, it is safe to perform in asthma.
6. Bronchoalveolar lavage remains an invaluable tool in the study of asthma pathophysiology. The study of BAL fluid from asthmatics has

increased our knowledge of the chemical processes and mediators involved in acute and chronic asthma.

7. Bronchoprovocation with inhaled bronchoconstrictor substances (methacholine and histamine) and nonisotonic aerosols can be used to determine the presence of nonspecific airway hyperresponsiveness.
8. Exercise and hyperventilation challenges are useful in the diagnosis of exercise-induced asthma.
9. Bronchoprovocation with allergens is occasionally necessary to establish the correlation between exposure and symptoms if the patient history and allergen-specific skin or serum antibody testing are inadequate. It is also used in the research setting to investigate asthma pathophysiology and the efficacy of therapeutic interventions.
10. Bronchoprovocation with occupational agents may be useful is diagnosing occupational asthma.

REFERENCES

1. American Thoracic Society. Standardization of spirometry: 1994 update. Am J Respir Crit Care Med 1995; 152:1107–1136.
2. Crapo RO. Pulmonary function testing. N Engl J Med 1994; 331:25–30.
3. McFadden ER Jr. Pulmonary structure, physiology, and clinical correlates in asthma. In: Middleton E Jr, Reed CE, Ellis EF, Adkinson NF Jr, Yunginger JW, Busse WW, eds. Allergy: Principles and Practice. 4th ed. St. Louis: Mosby, 1993:672–693.
4. American Thoracic Society. Lung function testing: selection of reference values and interpretive strategies. Am Rev Resp Dis 1991; 144:1202–1218.
5. Committee report. Criteria for the assessment of reversibility in airways obstruction: report of the committee on emphysema. American College of Chest Physicians. Chest 1974; 65:552–553.
6. National Institutes of Health. Expert Panel Report 2: Guidelines for the diagnosis and management of asthma. Bethesda, MD: National Institutes of Health, 1997.
7. Crapo RO, Morris AH, Clayton PD, Nixon CR. Lung volumes in healthy nonsmoking adults. Bull Eur Physiopathol Respir 1982; 18:419–425.
8. Crapo RO, Morris AH, Gardner RM. Reference spirometric values using techniques and equipment that meet ATS recommendations. Am Rev Respir Dis 1981; 123: 659–664.
9. Dockery DW, Ware JH, Ferris BG Jr, Glicksberg DS, Fay ME, Spiro A 3rd, Speizer FE. Distribution of forced expiratory volume in one second and forced vital capacity in healthy, white, adult never-smokers in six US cities. Am Rev Respir Dis 1985; 131:511–520.
10. Rossiter CE, Weill H. Ethnic differences in lung function: evidence for proportional differences. Int J Epidemiol 1974; 3:55–61.
11. Kendrick AH, Higgs CM, Whitfield MJ, Laszlo G. Accuracy of perception of severity of asthma: patients treated in general practice. BMJ 1993; 307:422–424.

12. Kikuchi Y, Okabe S, Tamura G, Hida W, Homma M, Shirato K, Takishima T. Chemosensitivity and perception of dyspnea in patients with a history of near-fatal asthma. N Engl J Med 1994; 330:1329–1334.
13. Charlton I, Charlton G, Broomfield J, Mullee MA. Evaluation of peak flow and symptoms only self-management plans for control of asthma in general practice. BMJ 1990; 301:1355–1359.
14. Grampian Asthma Study of Integrated Care. Effectiveness of routine self monitoring of peak flow in patients with asthma. BMJ 1994; 308:564–567.
15. American Thoracic Society. Guidelines for fiberoptic bronchoscopy. Am Rev Respir Dis 1987; 136:1066.
16. National Institutes of Health. Workshop summary and guidelines: investigative use of bronchoscopy, lavage and bronchial biopsies in asthma and other airway diseases. J Allergy Clin Immunol 1991; 38:808–814.
17. Jarjour NN, Peters SP, Djukanovic R, Calhoun WJ. Investigative use of bronchoscopy in asthma. Am J Respir Crit Care Med 1998; 157:692–697.
18. Laitinen A, Laitinen LA, Virtanen IT. Bronchial biopsies. In: Barnes PJ, Grunstein MM, Leff AR, Woolcock AJ, eds. Asthma. Philadelphia: Lippincott-Raven Publishers, 1997:225–239.
19. Wenzel SE. Abnormalities of cell and mediator levels in bronchoalveolar lavage fluid of patients with mild asthma. J Allergy Clin Immunol 1996; 98:S17–21.
20. Bousquet J, Chanez P, Lacoste JY, Barneon G, Ghavanian N, Enander I, Venge P, Ahlstedt S, Simony-Lafontaine J, Godard P. Eosinophilic inflammation in asthma. N Engl J Med 1990; 323:1033–1039.
21. Liu MC. Bronchoalveolar lavage in studies. In: Barnes PJ, Grunstein MM, Leff AR, Woolcock AJ, eds. Asthma. Philadelphia: Lippincott-Raven Publishers, 1997:225–239.
22. Broide DH, Gleich GJ, Cuomo AJ, Coburn DA, Federman EC, Schwartz LB, Wasserman SI. Evidence of ongoing mast cell and eosinophil degranulation in symptomatic asthma airway. J Allergy Clin Immunol 1991; 88:637–648.
23. Wilson JW, Djukanovic R, Howard PH, Holgate ST. Lymphocyte activation in bronchoalveolar lavage and peripheral blood in atopic asthma. Am Rev Respir Dis 1992; 145:958–960.
24. Spector SL. Allergen inhalation challenges. In: Spector SL, ed. Provocative Testing in Clinical Practice. New York: Marcel Dekker, Inc, 1995:325–368.
25. Cockcroft DW, Killian DN, Mellon JJ, Hargreave FE. Bronchial reactivity to inhaled histamine: a method and clinical survey. Clin Allergy 1977; 7:235.
26. Chai H, Farr RS, Froehlich LA, Mathison DA, McLean JA, Rosenthal RR, Sheffer AL, Spector SL, Townley RG. Standardization of bronchial inhalation challenge procedures. J Allergy Clin Immunology 1975; 56:323–327.
27. Yan K, Salome CM, Woolcock AJ. Rapid method for measurement of bronchial responsiveness. Thorax 1983; 38:760–765.
28. Fish JE. Bronchial challenge testing. In: Middleton E Jr, et al, eds. Allergy: Principles and Practice. 4th ed. St. Louis: Mosby, 1993:613–627.
29. Hopp RJ, Bewtra AK, Nair NM, Townley RG. Specificity and sensitivity of methacholine inhalation challenge in normal and asthmatic children. J Allergy Clin Immunol 1984; 74:154–158.

30. Sterk PJ, Daniel EE, Zamel N, Hargreave FE. Limited maximal airway narrowing in nonasthmatic subjects. Am Rev Respir Dis 1985; 132:865–870.
31. Anderson SD, Smith CM, Rodwell LT, du Toit JI, Riedler J, Robertson CF. The use of nonisotonic aerosols for evaluating bronchial hyperresponsiveness. In: Spector SL, ed. Provocative Testing in Clinical Practice. New York: Marcel Dekker Inc, 1995:249–278.
32. Shepard D, Rizk NW, Boushey HA, Bethel RA. Mechanism of cough and bronchoconstriction induced by distilled water aerosol. Am Rev Respir Dis 1983; 127:691–694.
33. Patterson R, Suszko IM, Zeiss CR Jr. Reactions of primate respiratory mast cells. J Allergy Clin Immunol 1972; 50:7.
34. Bruce CA, Rosenthal RR, Lichtenstein LM, Norman PS. Quantitative inhalation bronchial challenge in ragweed hay fever patients: a comparison with ragweed-allergic asthmatics. J Allergy Clin Immunol 1975; 56:331–337.
35. Metzger WJ, Hunninghake GW, Richerson HB: Late asthmatic responses: inquiry into mechanisms and significance. Clin Rev Allergy 1985; 3:145.
36. Sheppard D, Eschenbacher WL. Respiratory water loss as a stimulus to exercise-induced bronchoconstriction in asthma. J Allergy Clin Immunol 1984; 73:640–642.
37. McFadden ER Jr. Exercise-induced airway obstruction. Clin Chest Med 1995; 16: 671–682.
38. Spector SL. Update on exercise-induced asthma. Ann Allergy 1993; 71:571–577.
39. Godfrey S. Bronchial challenge by exercise or hyperventilation. In: Spector SL, ed. Provocative challenge procedures: background and methodology. Mount Kisco, NY. Futura Publishing Company, 1989:365–394.
40. Bernstein DI. Allergic reactions to workplace allergens. JAMA 1997; 278:1907–1913.
41. Hendrick DJ, Salvaggio JE. The use of inhalation bronchial challenge for occupational diseases. In: Spector SL, ed. Provocative Testing in Clinical Practice. New York: Marcel Dekker, Inc, 1995:479–511.
42. Jarjour NN, Calhoun WJ, Kelly EAB, Gleich GJ, Schwartz LB, Busse WW. The immediate and late allergic response to segmental bronchopulmonary provocation in asthma. Am J Respir Crit Care Med 1997; 155:1515–1521.

8

Food Allergy: Current Diagnostic Methods and Interpretation of Results

John M. James
Colorado Allergy and Asthma Centers, P.C., Ft. Collins, Colorado

A. Wesley Burks, Jr.
University of Arkansas for Medical Sciences and Arkansas Children's Hospital, Little Rock, Arkansas

I. INTRODUCTION

As many as 30% of surveyed households in the United States report at least one individual who is thought to be allergic to a food or food ingredient (1). Epidemiological studies using well-controlled food challenges to confirm suspected food allergy, however, have demonstrated a much lower prevalence, 2–5% of children and less than 2% of adults (2–4). This discrepancy in public

Table 1 Confirmation of Food Allergy Using Double-Blind, Placebo-Controlled Food Challenges

Reference	Population	Food Challenges	Positive DBPCFC	% Positive DBPCFC
Bock 1990	Children	1014	245	24%
Sampson 1985	Children with atopic dermatitis	370	101	27%
Jansen 1994	General adult Dutch population	19	9	47%
Host 1990	Danish infants	117	39	33%
Bernhisel-Broadbent 1989	Children	130	43	33%
Bernhisel-Broadbent 1992	Children Young adults	50	15	30%

opinion underscores the importance of understanding the diagnostic methods used in the clinical evaluation and confirmation of adverse reactions to foods.

In vivo and in vitro diagnostic tests, as well as oral provocative food challenges, are extremely useful methods for evaluating patients with histories of adverse food reactions. Of these, a properly performed oral food challenge is the most reliable method by which to confirm or refute adverse food reactions, especially food allergy, because the patient ingests the food suspected of causing symptoms. Oral provocative food challenges have established that approximately 30–50% of patients with clinical histories of an adverse food reaction and a positive puncture skin test to the incriminated food have positive, confirmatory oral food challenges (5–13) (Table 1). Although the majority of the published data has focused on clinical research investigations, the importance of oral food challenges should not be underestimated in outpatient clinical practice settings.

This chapter will discuss the appropriate uses and limitations of in vivo and in vitro diagnostic testing in the evaluation of adverse food reactions. Special emphasis will be placed on oral provocative food challenges in terms of their current design and application, as well as the interpretation of their results. This chapter will provide the clinician with a reliable diagnostic approach to patients with histories of adverse reactions after the ingestion of foods and food additives.

II. EVALUATION OF THE PATIENT WITH A SUSPECTED ADVERSE FOOD REACTION

A. Medical History

The diagnostic approach to the patient with a suspected adverse food reaction should begin with a comprehensive medical history and physical examination

(3,4). The overall usefulness of the medical history, however, may vary. For example, in cases in which a patient has a history of acute anaphylaxis after ingestion of a food (e.g., peanuts or shellfish), the clinical history may be instrumental in diagnosing food allergy. Convincing histories of cause and effect might even preclude the need for further diagnostic testing. In contrast, less convincing histories of food allergy often require further testing, in as much as less than 50% of patients with both a history suggestive of allergic reactions to food and a positive skin test to the food are substantiated by double-blind, placebo-controlled food challenge (DBPCFC) (6–14). Moreover, the clinical history may fail to suggest an underlying pathogenic role of food allergens in some chronic disorders, such as atopic dermatitis (15,16). Finally, the value of the history also depends on the patient's recollection of the actual signs and symptoms and the clinician's ability to differentiate between immunological and nonimmunological disorders.

Several pieces of information are important to establish when an allergic reaction to a food or food additive is being considered:

1. The food suspected to have provoked the reaction (Fig. 1)
2. The quantity of the food ingested
3. The length of time between ingestion and development of symptoms
4. A description of the clinical signs and symptoms provoked
5. If similar symptoms developed on other occasions when the food was ingested
6. If other factors (e.g., exercise) were necessary to provoke the reaction
7. The length of time since the last reaction

Although many foods and food additives have the potential to cause an allergic reaction, a few select foods account for approximately 90% of these allergic reactions. In children, these foods are eggs, milk, peanuts, soybeans, wheat, tree nuts, and fish (especially in Scandinavian countries). In adults, these foods are typically peanuts, tree nuts, fish, and shellfish (Fig. 1).

A diet diary is frequently used as an adjunct to the medical history. Patients are asked to keep a chronological record of all foods ingested over a specified period and to record any symptoms they experience during this time. The diary can then be reviewed at a subsequent office visit to determine if there is any relation between the foods ingested and the symptoms experienced. It is uncommon for this method to detect an unrecognized association between a food and a patient's symptoms.

A dietary history should include all ingredients of the suspected meal. The food provoking the reaction may be a contaminant (intentional or inadvertent) in the meal. For example, peanuts or peanut butter are frequently added to cookies, candies, pastries, or sauces such as chili, spaghetti, and barbecue sauces. Peanut butter is often used to hold together the overlapping ends of egg rolls

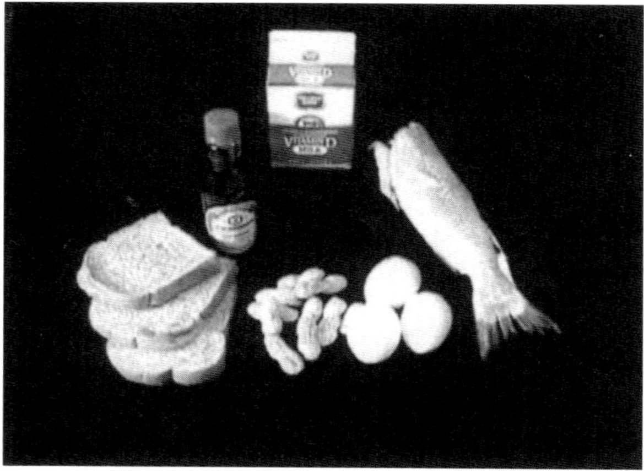

a

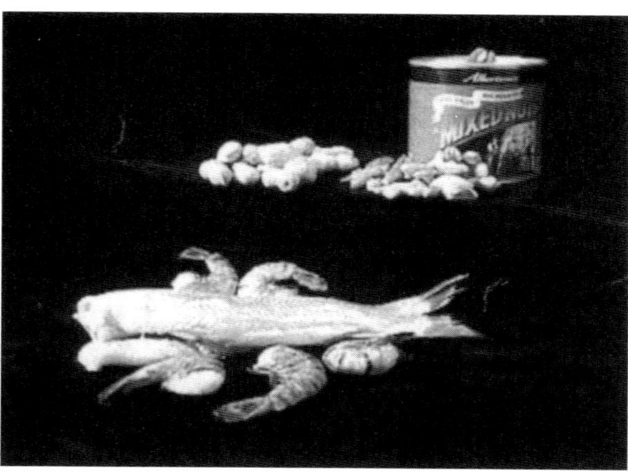

b

Figure 1 Major food allergens. (a) The major food allergens in children are eggs, milk, peanuts, soybeans, wheat, fish, and tree nuts (not shown). (b) The major food allergens in adults are peanuts, tree nuts, fish, and shellfish.

(17). In addition, Chinese restaurants often use "cold pressed" peanut oil in their cooking or reuse the same wok to cook a variety of different meals, resulting in the transfer of residual peanut protein (18). Another infrequent cause of food contamination occurs during the manufacturing process, when scraps of candy are "reworked" into the next batch of similar candy or when the line of production switches from one product to another at the processing plant.

Elimination diets are mainly used in the treatment of food allergy once the diagnosis has been confirmed, but they also may aid in the diagnosis of adverse food reactions. If a certain food or group of foods is suspected of provoking the adverse reaction, they are completely eliminated from the diet, typically for 7–14 days. The success of an elimination diet depends on several factors, including: (1) the correct identification of the food allergen or allergens involved; (2) the ability of the patient to maintain a diet completely free of all forms of the possible offending allergen, and (3) the assumption that other factors will not provoke similar symptoms during the study period.

Satisfying all of these requirements may be very difficult, which limits the usefulness of an elimination diet. For example, resolution of symptoms after substitution with a soy formula or casein hydrolysate formula (e.g., Alimentum®, Nutramigen®, Pregestamil®) is highly suggestive of cow's milk allergy in a young infant who reacts to cow's milk formula, but it also could reflect lactose intolerance. Unfortunately, elimination diets are rarely diagnostic of food allergy, particularly in chronic disorders such as atopic dermatitis or asthma. Finally, one investigation demonstrated that strong parental beliefs about food allergy can, in some cases, lead to unnecessary dietary restrictions severe enough to produce malnourishment in children (19).

B. In Vivo Diagnostic Testing

Based on the information derived from these initial steps, various laboratory studies may be helpful. Allergy prick skin tests are highly reproducible and often are used to screen patients with suspected immunoglobulin (Ig)E-mediated food allergies (3,4). The criteria established by Bock and others have proven useful to many investigators and clinicians (20). The glycerinated food vaccines (1 : 10 or 1 : 20 w/v) and appropriate positive (histamine) and negative (saline) controls are applied percutaneously by either the prick or puncture technique. If appropriate and high quality food vaccines are used, a food allergen eliciting a wheal at least 3 mm or greater than the negative control is considered positive; anything else is considered negative. A negative skin test confirms the absence of an IgE-mediated reaction (overall negative predictive accuracy is greater than 95% (21–23). A positive skin test to a food indicates only the possibility that the patient has symptomatic reactivity to that specific food (overall the positive predictive accuracy is less than 50%). Moreover, the presence of IgE cross-reactivity (in vivo and in vitro) among different constituents of a particular botanical food allergen group is typically much greater than the confirmed rate of clinical cross-reactivity when oral food challenges are performed (Table 2).

The percutaneous (puncture or prick) skin test is an excellent means for excluding IgE-mediated food allergies (21–23). There are some minor exceptions to this general statement. First, IgE-mediated sensitivity to several fruits and veg-

Table 2 Food Allergen Cross-Reactivity

	Specific IgE to Multiple Members of the Same Taxonomic Family	Clinical Reactivity
Milk (different species)	Common	Common
Legumes	Common	Uncommon
Cereal grains	Common	Uncommon
Fish	Common	Uncommon
Crustaceans	Common	Data unavailable
Mollusks	Common	Data unavailable
Tree nuts	Common	Uncommon
Egg and chicken	Occasional	Rare
Milk and beef	Occasional	Uncommon

etables (apples, oranges, bananas, pears, melons, potatoes, carrots, and celery) is frequently not detected with commercially prepared vaccines or reagents; this is thought to result from the lability and denaturation of the responsible food allergen during commercial preparation of the vaccine. Skin-prick testing with fresh preparations of these fruits and vegetables (i.e., prick and prick technique) has been shown to be a simple, reproducible, and reliable method of detecting IgE antibodies to these foods (24). Second, children younger than 1 year of age may have an IgE-mediated food allergy without a positive skin test or have smaller skin test wheal sizes, possibly due to the relative lack of skin reactivity.

An intradermal skin test is a more sensitive method when compared to the skin-prick test, but it is much less specific than a blinded oral food challenge. In other words, intradermal positive skin tests for foods have not been demonstrated to have a high degree of clinical correlation and reliability (20,22). In addition, intradermal skin testing has a greater risk of inducing a systemic reaction than does skin-prick testing. Therefore, intradermal skin testing with food allergens is not recommended.

Intragastric provocation under endoscopic control (IPEC) has been evaluated as a potential diagnostic method for food allergy (25). In this investigational procedure, small quantities of the suspected food vaccine (1 : 10 solution of food in normal saline) are applied to the gastric mucosa as the site is observed endoscopically and the mucosal reaction is scored. Intragastric provocation under endoscopic control provoked reactions on the gastric mucosa in all patients with food allergy previously documented by DBPCFC. The tissue histamine levels and stainable mast cells in biopsies of the site were decreased compared to prechallenge samples. Other tests used during this investigation included skin-prick tests and radioallergosorbent tests (RAST), which were positive in only one-half these patients. Applicability of this technique is limited because its specificity has not been evaluated in skin test-positive, nonreactive patients and many patients experience systemic symptoms during the procedure making it no safer than oral challenges.

C. In Vitro Diagnostic Testing

Radioallergosorbent tests and similar in vitro assays [including enzyme-linked immunosorbent assays (ELISAs)] have been used for the identification of food-specific IgE antibodies. These tests are often used to screen for IgE-mediated food allergies. Whereas RAST is slightly less sensitive than skin testing, one study comparing RAST with DBPCFCs found skin-prick tests and RASTs to have similar sensitivity and specificity when a RAST score of three or greater was considered positive (21). In this study, if a two was considered positive, there was a slight improvement in sensitivity whereas the specificity decreased significantly. In general, in vitro measurement of serum food-specific IgE performed in high-quality laboratories provides information similar to skin-prick tests (21).

The recent development of the CAP system fluoroenzyme immunoassay (FEIA) (Pharmacia & Upjohn Diagnostics AB, Uppsala, Sweden) has provided a more quantitative method of determining allergen-specific IgE to inhalant and food allergens. A recent investigation of patients with food allergy compared food-specific IgE concentrations determined by this system to the results obtained from skin-prick testing and DBPCFCs (26). When compared to the outcome of the food challenges, the predictive value of CAP system FEIA is generally comparable to those of skin-prick tests in predicting symptomatic food allergy. Moreover, by quantitating food-specific IgE antibodies with this automated system, the investigators were able to identify a subset of patients who are highly likely ($> 95\%$) to have allergic reactions to egg, milk, peanut, or fish. For example, a level of greater than 15 kU_A/L (kilounits of allergen-specific IgE per liter) of specific IgE to peanut has greater than 95% accuracy in predicting a positive food challenge. The authors published positive and negative predictive values using the CAP system FEIA, which will aid in the diagnosis of patients with possible food-allergic reactions. The predictive values of CAP system FEIA results are currently limited to several major food allergens (egg, milk, peanut, or fish). This type of testing potentially may eliminate the need to perform DBPCFCs in a significant number of patients suspected of having IgE-mediated food allergy.

Basophil histamine release assays (BHRs) are in vitro assays of IgE-mediated reactions that typically have been restricted to research and academic settings. The use of whole blood in the newer, semiautomated assays circumvents the problem of high spontaneous basophil histamine release seen in food-allergic individuals continuing to ingest the responsible allergen (27). Results from BHR were compared to similar results obtained by skin-prick tests, RAST, food antigen-induced intestinal mast cell histamine release, and food challenges in suspected food-allergic children (28). The food allergen-induced BHR correlated most closely with RAST results and was not more predictive of clinical allergic sensitivity than either the skin-prick test or RAST.

The intestinal mast cell histamine release (IMCHR) assay is a method performed primarily in research settings. It uses dispersed intestinal mast cells obtained from biopsy specimens (29). In this assay, the representative food antigen is added to the mast-cell preparation, and the resulting percentage of histamine release is measured. Compared to skin-prick tests, RAST, and BHR, IMCHR correlated most closely to the outcome of oral food challenge in which gastrointestinal tract symptoms were confirmed. This investigation suggests that local inflammatory mediator release may explain some gastrointestinal symptoms not generally thought to be mediated by an IgE mechanism.

Other diagnostic tests that have no demonstrable clinical value include food-specific IgG or IgG4 antibody levels, food antigen-antibody complexes, evidence of lymphocyte activation (^{3}H-thymidine uptake, interleukin [IL]-2 production, leukocyte inhibitory factor, etc.), and sublingual or intracutaneous provocation (30).

III. HISTORICAL PERSPECTIVE OF ORAL PROVOCATIVE FOOD CHALLENGES

Although adverse reactions after food ingestion have been recognized and discussed for centuries, a basic understanding of the pathogenesis of these reactions was absent until the 20th century. The past 20 years in particular have witnessed a significant advancement in our basic understanding of adverse reactions to foods, including food allergy and food intolerance (31). One of the most significant developments has been the use of oral food challenges to evaluate the role of food allergy in a variety of atopic and nonatopic diseases. Based on the clinical history and the results of in vivo or in vitro diagnostic studies, well-designed oral provocative food challenges are critical for confirming or refuting the role of a specific food or food additive as the cause of the symptoms observed in an adverse food reaction. Anecdotal reports are unreliable, because many are refuted by provocative challenge. This does not suggest that all adverse food reactions have to be evaluated by oral provocative food challenge. However, appropriate oral provocative food challenges need to be included in the overall study design in basic and clinical research involving food allergy. The next section of this chapter will highlight the various types of oral food challenges used to evaluate adverse reactions to foods and food additives.

IV. ORAL FOOD CHALLENGES: GENERAL INTRODUCTORY COMMENTS

A. Advance Preparation for Oral Food Challenges

Bock and others have written a manual that outlines practical guidelines and methods for performing oral food challenges in the office setting (5). Before performing any oral food challenge procedure, the physician must discuss it thoroughly with the patient and parent or guardian, if necessary. The physician must explain the overall purpose of the procedure, the benefits, and the possible adverse reactions, especially if an anaphylactic reaction may occur during the challenge. In addition, the patient and the parent/guardian should be assured that any adverse reaction would be treated appropriately and rapidly. The person obtaining consent for the challenge procedure should allow sufficient time to answer all questions before the procedure is scheduled. The setting of the food challenge (office or hospital) depends on the reported severity of the patient's previous adverse reaction to the incriminated food, the timing of the symptoms after ingestion, and the availability of medications, equipment, and trained personnel to manage a severe allergic reaction, if one occurs.

B. Medical Conditions Precluding an Oral Food Challenge

There are selected medical conditions and prior medical histories that preclude an oral food challenge procedure. First, patients with an unstable medical condition, such as uncontrolled hypertension, should be scheduled for an oral food challenge only when the condition is controlled. Second, patients with an acute illness with or without fever that would confound the overall evaluation and interpretation of adverse symptoms (e.g., rhinorrhea, emesis, diarrhea, coughing, or wheezing) should not be scheduled for a food challenge until the illness has completely resolved. Third, any patient with unstable asthma, especially with a forced expiratory volume in 1 second (FEV_1) less than 70% of predicted for the reference group, should not undertake an oral food challenge because of the increased risk of exacerbating adverse respiratory symptoms and, possibly, anaphylaxis. Finally, patients with a convincing history of a severe anaphylactic reaction after the isolated ingestion of a specific food (e.g., peanuts, tree nuts, shellfish) do not need to have their history confirmed by an oral food challenge.

C. Medication Avoidance Prior to Performing an Oral Food Challenge

All patient medications must be carefully reviewed before the food challenge procedure is performed. Certain modifications in medication administration schedules may be needed to prevent the masking of important clinical symptoms that could be observed during the food challenge. For example, antihistamines can ameliorate urticaria, sneezing, and rhinorrhea, and bronchodilators can reduce laryngeal edema, coughing, and wheezing. Specific medications should be stopped for a designated time before a challenge procedure. These include antihistamines (96 hours), β-agonists (12 hours), theophylline (12 hours), and cromolyn (12 hours). Unfortunately, withholding these medications could cause confusion between adverse symptoms provoked by the food challenge and those symptoms caused by changes in the patient's medical regimen. Therefore, some modification of these restrictions may be needed, especially in the patients with underlying moderate-to-severe asthma.

D. Preparation of Challenge Constituents

Selection of foods for challenge is based upon historical information or results of appropriate laboratory studies, such as percutaneous skin tests or in vitro measurements of specific IgE antibodies to food. For open food challenges, the food is prepared in the usual fashion and served in typical proportions. Therefore, no special preparation of the suspect food is needed (see below). For single-blind and double-blind, placebo-controlled oral food challenges, dehydrated forms of the specific challenge food may be purchased from commercial bakeries, local grocery stores, health food stores, or camping outlets and disguised in an appropriate vehicle. Multiple vehicles used to hide or disguise foods in these challenges include opaque capsules, elemental formulas, tapioca-fruit mixture, applesauce, tuna fish, and hamburger. The selection of the vehicle will depend on the individual patient and the specific clinical history of the adverse food reaction. To remove all bias from interpretation of a challenge, a disinterested third party (medical assistant, nurse, or dietitian) should prepare the challenge foods and determine the random order of the challenges by which all double-blind, placebo-controlled oral food challenges will be administered.

E. Oral Food Challenge Procedures: Description of Different Methods

1. Open Food Challenges

Description. In open food challenges, the patient ingests the suspect food after it has been prepared in its customary fashion. Both the patient and the observer (usually a physician or nurse) are aware of the food contents.

When to consider. The open food challenge is best used in clinical practice when patient and physician bias is minimal and the skin test to the suspect food is negative. If a specific food reaction is unlikely, the food may be replaced in the diet at home with confidence that the food will be tolerated. Open challenges may be more appropriate in an office setting if the skin test to a specific food allergen is positive. Whenever the results of the open challenge are equivocal, a blinded challenge should be performed to confirm the clinical reaction. Finally, open food challenges are used after negative DBPCFC to exclude the rare possibility of a false negative DBPCFC.

Precautions/treatment of reactions. An open food challenge should never be performed at home if there is even a remote chance of the patient developing severe symptoms.

Interpretation of results. Open food challenges are especially useful when the symptoms are not reproduced, thus eliminating the incriminated food as a culprit. Patients holding strong beliefs about an adverse subjective reaction to a particular food are highly likely to react to that food during an open food challenge.

Pitfalls. Failure to anticipate the possibility of the remote chance that a patient will experience a severe reaction when the open food challenge is performed at home could result in serious adverse reactions after the challenge. Patients or observers holding strong beliefs about the outcome of the challenge may influence the interpretation of the actual results. Therefore, results of open food challenges are too imprecise for clinical research protocols investigating food allergy.

2. Single-Blind Food Challenges

Description. In single-blind food challenges, the patient ingests the suspected food in a disguised form, but the observer is aware of the contents of the food challenge. These challenges are designed to reduce patient bias. This challenge method, however, cannot completely eliminate subjective attitudes regarding the outcome of the challenge.

When to consider. These food challenges are suitable for clinical practice and may be useful in screening patients for entry into clinical research studies in which the history will be unequivocally confirmed by DBPCFC. Negative challenges are useful in eliminating the diagnosis of food allergy suggested by patient history.

Performing the challenge. The challenge can be performed in the manner described above for an open challenge or in a more rigorous manner, as discussed below for DBPCFC.

Interpretation of results. A single-blind food challenge is generally sufficient to establish a diagnosis by objective criteria. When strictly subjective symptoms are being investigated, at least two sets of challenges or a well-designed DBPCFC (see below) are necessary to confirm the diagnosis. The main objection to single-blind food challenges is the potential for bias, which the observer can communicate nonverbally to the patient.

Pitfalls. Potential pitfalls are identical to those discussed previously for open food challenges.

3. Double-Blind Placebo-Controlled Food Challenges

Description: In DBPCFCs, the patient ingests a suspected food that has been disguised so that both patient and observer are unaware of the contents of the challenge (5). This type of challenge is designed to reduce subjective attitudes of both patient and observer during the procedure. These challenges should always be conducted in an office or hospital setting.

When to consider. For research purposes, the DBPCFC is considered the "gold standard" for diagnosing food allergy. The DBPCFC is currently the only completely objective method for determining the validity of a reported adverse reaction to a food. It may be necessary in clinical practice to confirm results of a positive open or single-blind food challenge and the DBPCFC is an essential component of clinical research studies of food allergy.

Performing the challenge. Ideally, an equal number of challenges should be performed for both the test food and the placebo. Eight to 10 g of dehydrated, powdered food in opaque capsules or in 100 mL of juice should be administered over 60 to 90 minutes. The initial dose is generally less than 500 mg (Table 3). Each challenge should be evaluated and scored (Table 4). All patients should be observed for a minimum of 2 hours before discharge.

Interpretation of results. Several published investigations have used the DBPCFC to confirm the diagnosis of food allergy (Table 1). In a 16-year period, Bock and Atkins used DBPCFC to investigate patterns of food hypersensitivity in children (6). Of the 480 children monitored during this investigation, 185 (39%) had positive DBPCFC; some of the patients had more than one positive challenge. In all, 245 (24%) of 1014 DBPCFC showed positive results and confirmed the presence of food allergy in children with histories of adverse food reactions. Eggs, cow's milk, peanuts, and tree nuts were responsible for the overwhelming majority of these positive food challenges. A comprehensive, prospec-

Table 3 Sample Schedule for Double-Blind, Placebo-Controlled Food Challenge

Time	Food Dosage	Time	Placebo Dosage
8:00 AM	0.5 g	11:00 AM	0.5 g
8:15 AM	1.0 g	11:15 AM	1.0 g
8:30 AM	2.0 g	11:30 AM	2.0 g
8:45 AM	3.0 g	11:45 AM	3.0 g
9:00 AM	3.5 g	12:00 PM	3.5 g

Table 4 Sample Recording Sheet for Double-Blind, Placebo-Controlled Food Challenge

Food Challenge Information Form

Previous reaction suspected of being due to food.
Date:__________
Sx:__________

Time for ingestion of suspected agent to first sx.__________
Time from appearance of first sx. to peak of rx.__________
Treatment received__________

Skin test results: Food__________ Skin test: Positive Negative

Other relevant illnesses (HBP, CAD, ASTHMA, etc.)__________

Medications taken on day of challenge:__________

CHALLENGE SUBSTANCE:__________
Carrier Food:__________
BASELINE BP_____ BASELINE FEV_1_____ (L):_____ (% predicted)

Time Given	Dose	Time Evaluated	BP	CHALLENGE FEV_1 (L)	Reaction

I understand that this food challenge procedure may cause an allergic reaction in me, including, but not limited to swelling, itching, hives, asthma, wheezing or anaphylaxis (severe allergic reaction). I agree that this test is indicated and necessary.

Patient:__________

Parent or Guardian:__________

Witness:__________

Source: Ref. 5.

tive study of cow's milk allergy in 1749 Danish children found that only 39 (33%) of the 117 infants with a clinical history suggestive of this allergy had their histories confirmed with a positive DBPCFC (7). Jansen and others investigated the prevalence of food allergy and intolerance in a random sample of 1483 Dutch adults and observed a gap between self-reported food allergy/intolerance and objective symptoms confirmed by DBPCFC. Less than 50% of the challenges confirmed the clinical history (8). When DBPCFC is used in children with atopic dermatitis, approximately 30% and 60% of the challenges confirmed the presence of food allergy in those patients with mild-to-moderate and severe atopic dermatitis, respectively (9,10). Bernhisel-Broadbent and colleagues used DBPCFC to evaluate the clinical relevance of positive skin tests to multiple legumes (11). The percentage of patients with a positive skin test and a corresponding positive confirmatory DBPCFC to that legume was as follows: peanut 52%, soybean 33%, pea 11%, green bean 0%, and lima bean 0%. Similarly, the same investigators have demonstrated that patients with fish allergy may have positive skin tests to multiple fish species, but DBPCFC typically confirms symptomatic fish allergy to one or two individual fish species (12). Finally, the prevalence of intolerance to food additives has been evaluated with DBPCFC, and 50% of these challenges confirmed the clinical histories (13).

Pitfalls. There are no major pitfalls, but all negative challenges must be confirmed by an open challenge. Rarely, false negative DBPCFCs have been reported and likely are the result of the preparation of the food substance for the challenge (e.g., lyophilization of fish) (12).

V. CONCLUSIONS

This chapter has provided an overview of the appropriate use and limitations of in vitro and in vivo diagnostic testing (including oral provocative food challenges) in the evaluation of adverse food reactions. More time, energy, and preparation are needed for the successful completion of DBPCFC, but this type of food challenge is still considered the ''gold standard'' for the diagnosis of food allergy. After the diagnosis of food allergy is established, the only proven therapy is strict elimination of the offending allergen (3,4). This is important to emphasize because prescribing an elimination diet is like prescribing a medication: it can have positive effects, but it also can have side effects. Elimination diets may lead to malnutrition or eating disorders, especially if they encompass a large number of foods or are used for extended periods (19). Patients and their families should be taught to read food labels carefully and should be provided with educational material to help them detect potential sources of hidden food allergens (32). Patient and family education is vital to the success of the elimination diet. Families should receive instructional material that will help them to remember which foods contain the allergen they should avoid. The major food allergens are listed in Figure 1; however, it can be difficult to determine what food will contain a hidden allergen without carefully reading a product label or checking with the food manufacturer. At present, there is no evidence to support the use of oral or parenteral immunotherapy for the treatment of food allergy.

Immunologic responsiveness to food allergens is generally very specific. Patients rarely react to more than one member of a botanical or animal family. Importantly, initiation of an elimination diet totally excluding only those foods identified to provoke food allergic reactions will result in symptomatic improvement. Clinical studies of both children and adults indicate that symptomatic reactivity to food allergens is often lost over time, except for peanuts, tree nuts, fish, and shellfish. Avoidance of the implicated food generally will lead to resolution of the food allergy within a few years and is unlikely to induce malnutrition or other eating disorders.

VI. SALIENT POINTS

1. Adverse food reactions may result from food allergy (hypersensitivity) or food intolerance. Food allergy results from an abnormal immunologic response after the ingestion of a food, whereas food intolerance is the result of nonimmunologic mechanisms.
2. Although the medical history, physical examination, and selected diagnostic laboratory studies are useful in the diagnosis of food allergy, well-designed oral provocative food challenges are the best method for confirming an adverse reaction to a food or food additive.
3. The major foods causing allergic reactions in different age groups:

Children	*Adults*
milk	peanuts
egg	tree nuts
peanuts	fish
soybeans	shellfish
wheat	
fish	
tree nuts	

4. Studies of possible clinical cross-reactivity among various members of a given botanical or animal family have shown that it is uncommon for patients to react in oral challenge to several members of a given family. Patients should be evaluated on an individual basis before recommending total dietary restriction of a particular family.

5. A positive skin test to a food indicates that the patient may have symptomatic reactivity to that specific food (overall the positive predictive accuracy is less than 50%). A negative skin test confirms the absence of an IgE-mediated reaction (overall negative predictive accuracy is greater than 95%).
6. A presumptive diagnosis of food allergy based on a patient's history and skin-prick tests or RAST results should be confirmed clinically, unless the patient has experienced severe anaphylaxis after the isolated ingestion of a specific food.

REFERENCES

1. Altman DR, Chiaramonte LT. Public perception of food allergy. J Allergy Clin Immunol 1996;97:1247–1251.
2. Bock SA. Prospective appraisal of complaints of adverse reactions to foods during the first three years of life. Pediatrics 1987;79:683–688.
3. James JM. Adverse reactions to foods. In: Ziegler EE, Filer LJ, eds. Present Knowledge in Nutrition. Washington: ISLI Press, 1996:604–611.
4. Sampson HA. Food allergy. JAMA 1997;278:1888–1894.
5. Bock SA, Sampson HA, Atkins FM, Zeiger RS, Lehrer S, Sachs M, Bush RK, Metcalfe DD. Double-blind placebo-controlled food challenge as an office procedure: A manual. J Allergy Clin Immunol 1988;82:986–997.
6. Bock SA, Atkins FM. Patterns of food hypersensitivity during sixteen years of double-blind, placebo-controlled food challenges. J Pediatr 1990;117:561–567.
7. Host A, Halken S. A prospective study of cow milk allergy in Danish infants during the first 3 years of life. Allergy 1990;45:587–596.
8. Jansen JJN, Kardinaal AFM, Huijbers G, Vlieg-Boerstra BJ, Martens BPM, Ockhuizen T. Prevalence of food allergy and intolerance in the adult Dutch population. J Allergy Clin Immunol 1994;93:446–456.
9. Burks AW, Mallory SB, Williams LW, Shirrell MA. Atopic dermatitis: Clinical relevance of food hypersensitivity reactions. J Pediatr 1988;113:447–451.
10. Sampson HA, McCaskill CM. Food hypersensitivity and atopic dermatitis: Evaluation of 113 patients. J Pediatr 1985;107:669–675.
11. Bernhisel-Broadbent J, Sampson HA. Cross-allergenicity in the legume botanical family in children with food hypersensitivity. J Allergy Clin Immunol 1989;83:435–440.
12. Bernhisel-Broadbent J, Scanlon SM, Sampson HA. Fish hypersensitivity: in vitro and oral challenge results in fish-allergic patients. J Allergy Clin Immunol 1992;89:730–737.
13. Fuglsnag G, Madsen C, Saval P, Osterballe O. Prevalence of intolerance to food additives among Danish school children. Pediatr Allergy Immunol 1993;4:123–129.
14. Burks AW, James JM, Hiegel A, Wilson G, Wheeler JG, Jones SM, Zuerlein N. Atopic dermatitis and food hypersensitivity reactions. J Pediatr 1988;132:132–136.
15. Sampson HA, Scanlon SM. Natural history of food hypersensitivity in children with atopic dermatitis. J Pediatr 1989;115:23–27.

16. Sampson HA. Role of immediate food hypersensitivity in the pathogenesis of atopic dermatitis. J Allergy Clin Immunol 1983;71:473–480.
17. Loza C, Brostoff J. Peanut allergy. Clin Exp Allergy 1995;25:493–502.
18. Hoffman DR, Collins-Williams C. Cold-pressed peanut oils may contain peanut allergen. J Allergy Clin Immunol 1994;93:801–802.
19. Roesler TA, Barry PC, Bock SA. Factitious food allergy and failure to thrive. Arch Pediatr Adolesc Med 1994;148:1150–1155.
20. Bock SA, Buckley J, Houst A, May CD. Proper use of skin tests with food extracts in diagnosis of food hypersensitivity. Clin Allergy 1978;8:559–564.
21. Sampson HA, Albergo R. Comparison of results of skin tests, RAST, and double-blind placebo-controlled food challenges in children with atopic dermatitis. J Allergy Clin Immunol 1984;74:26–33.
22. Atkins FM, Steinberg SS, Metcalfe DD. Evaluation of immediate adverse reactions to foods in adult patients. I. Correlation of demographic, laboratory, and prick skin test data with response to controlled oral food challenges. J Allergy Clin Immunol 1985;75:348–355.
23. Sampson HA. Comparative study of commercial food antigen extracts for the diagnosis of food hypersensitivity. J Allergy Clin Immunol 1988;82:718–726.
24. Ortolani C, Ispano M, Pastorello EA, Ispano M, Pastorello EA, Ansaloni R, Magri GC. Comparison of results of skin prick tests (with fresh foods and commercial extracts) and RAST in 100 patients with oral allergy syndrome. J Allergy Clin Immunol 1989;83:683–690.
25. Reimann HJ, Ring J, Ultsch B, Wendt P. Intragastric provocation under endoscopic control (IPEC) in food allergy: Mast cell and histamine changes in gastric mucosa. Clin Allergy 1985;15:195–202.
26. Sampson HA, Ho D. Relationship between food-specific IgE concentrations and the risk of positive food challenges in children and adolescents. J Allergy Clin Immunol 1997;100:444–451.
27. Sampson HA, Broadbent KR, Bernhisel-Broadbent J. Spontaneous release of histamine from basophils and histamine-releasing factor in patients with atopic dermatitis and food hypersensitivity. N Engl J Med 1989;321:228–232.
28. Nolte H, Schiotz PO, Kruse A, Skov S. Comparison of intestinal mast cell and basophil histamine release in children with food allergic reactions. Allergy 1989;44:554–565.
29. Selkekk BH. A comparison between in vitro jejunal mast cell degranulation and intragastric challenge in patients with suspected food intolerance. Scand J Gastroenterol 1985;20:299–303.
30. Condemi JJ. Unproved diagnostic and therapeutic techniques. In: Metcalfe DD, Sampson HA, Simon RA, eds. Food Allergy: Adverse reactions to foods and food additives. 2d ed. Cambridge: Blackwell Science, 1997:541–550.
31. Anderson JA. Milestones marking the knowledge of adverse reactions to food in the decade of the 1980's. Ann Allergy 1994;72:143–154.
32. Barnes-Koerner C, Sampson HA. Diets and nutrition in food allergy. In: Metcalfe DD, Sampson HA, Simon RA. Food Allergy: Adverse Reactions to Foods and Food Additives. 2d ed. Cambridge: Blackwell Science, 1997:461–484.

9

Determining Allergic Versus Nonallergic Drug Reactions

Gailen D. Marshall, Jr.
University of Texas Medical School, Houston, Texas

Phillip L. Lieberman
University of Tennessee College of Medicine, Memphis, Tennessee

I. INTRODUCTION

With the biochemical diversity and steadily increasing the number of commercially available pharmaceutical agents, the incidence of adverse drug reactions is also increasing. Even though allergists are most commonly consulted after a significant adverse drug reaction, due to type I [immunoglobulin (IgE)] hypersensitivity, other distinct immune reactions are possible (1). Additionally, many adverse drug reactions are nonimmunologic in origin. Such reactions may be categorized as predictable because they are dose-dependent, they derive from physiologic action of the drug and, under appropriate circumstances, they can occur in most people who take the drug. Predictable adverse drug reactions include toxic effects due to excess drug exposure (e.g., somnolence in opiate analgesics), drug interactions, or psychological effects prompted by anxiety over known or previously experienced side effects (such as mucosal irritation, gastrointestinal upset, skin rash, malaise, fatigue, etc.). Conversely, administration of a drug may produce unpredictable reactions, which are typically not dose-dependent and may be seen only in particularly susceptible patients. Unexpected adverse reactions may include idiosyncratic reactions or drug intolerance in which a standard dose produces extreme side effects not experienced at a reduced dose. Finally, initial immune-based drug reactions are unpredictable, but subsequent reactions may be predictable under appropriate conditions. Allergic and other immune-based drug reactions cause 6–10% of all observed adverse drug reactions, and the risk of an allergic reaction for most drugs is 1–3% (2).

II. MECHANISMS OF IMMUNE-BASED DRUG REACTIONS

An immune-based reaction requires that a drug must either elicit a new immune response or provoke a response based on immunologic sensitization due to prior antigenic exposure. Immune-based adverse drug reactions require certain chemical characteristics. Generally, the lower the molecular weight of a compound, the less antigenic it is. Likewise, molecular complexity increases antigenicity as does electrical charge (because of increased protein-binding affinity). Finally, the nature of the biological molecule dictates its relative antigenicity: protein > polysaccharide > lipid.

Exposure is another major component of immune-based drug reactions. Adverse reactions to first-time exposure are rarely due to immune-mediated mechanisms. Clinical sensitization takes days or even weeks to develop and become clinically apparent. An exception to this is cross-reactivity. Adverse drug reactions frequently occur on initial exposure to a drug that has significant cross-reactivity with a drug to which the patient had previously developed an immune-based sensitivity.

There are four major mechanisms by which a drug can cause an immune-based adverse reaction. These are based upon the Gell and Coombs classification for hypersensitivity states and include (1) type I or *immediate* (IgE-mediated) *hypersensitivity*; (2) type II or *cytotoxic antibody*; (3) type III or *immune complex reactions*; and (4) type IV or *delayed* (T-cell-mediated) *hypersensitivity*. The term *drug allergy* ideally should be restricted to those reactions mediated by Type I mechanisms since, as will be discussed, desensitization is clinically possible only for mast cell reactions. Dermatologists for many years have called cutaneous, T cell–mediated drug reactions, allergic contact dermatitis, and many textbooks categorize all immune-based drug reactions as drug allergy.

Type I. Immunoglobulin E is the antibody isotype designed to afford antigen-specific host protection against parasites in conjunction with mast cells and eosinophils (3). A first exposure (sensitization) is necessary to cause specific IgE formation. This antigen-specific IgE subsequently binds to mast cells found in multiple organs, including respiratory, gastrointestinal, and cardiovascular sites. Subsequent allergen exposure causes mast-cell-bound IgE cross-linkage, which results in mast cell degranulation and activation. Histamine is the major preformed product released by human mast cells. It results in many of the signs and symptoms of immediate hypersensitivity, such as pruritus, urticaria, angioedema, sneezing, wheezing, abdominal cramping, diarrhea, cardiac dysrhythmias, and hypotension/shock that typically begin minutes after drug exposure in sensitive patients (4). Mast cells also have the ability to synthesize many mediators, which can provoke more delayed reactions occurring 6–24 hours later.

Type II. In these reactions a series of plasma proteins collectively termed *complements* bind to the cell-bound antibodies to initiate a biochemical cascade resulting in target cell lysis (cytolysis). Specific antibodies can develop after repeated drug administration. If the drug binds to one of these antibodies on a cell membrane site in the skin or on an erythrocyte, subsequent cytotoxicity can occur. The drug may also result in loss of self-tolerance for erythrocyte antigens, forming autoantibodies that ultimately leads to an autoimmune hemolytic anemia (5).

Type III. These reactions result from the deposition of soluble antigen-antibody complexes on various organ surfaces (such as the kidney, lung, synovium, etc.) where they activate complement. These activated complement components, among other actions, attract inflammatory cells to the site of the immune complex depositions. The inflammatory cells attempt tissue phagocytosis and release proteolytic enzymes that damage the tissues. This type III mechanism is responsible for the serum sickness reactions that occur with some drugs, particularly antimicrobials (6).

Type IV. These are the only drug reactions that do not involve antibodies. Rather, sensitized T cells secrete small peptides called *cytokines* that activate macrophages to form *granulomas*, apparently to contain an actual or perceived infectious agent. Diseases such as tuberculosis, leprosy, and sarcoidosis all occur as a result of this mechanism. The most common manifestation of Type IV drug reactions is contact hypersensitivity to various topical medications, particularly antimicrobials (7).

This chapter will review the principles for diagnosing allergic versus other immune-mediated drug reactions. It will focus on the description and reliability of various in vivo and in vitro tests available to the allergy specialist.

III. HOW TO EVALUATE SUSPECTED ALLERGIC REACTIONS TO SPECIFIC DRUGS

A. General Principles for Assessment

The specific procedures for evaluating drug allergy are limited to relatively few drugs. This is due in part to the limited resources available for the basic and clinical research necessary to document the validity and utility of a specific testing procedure. A representative summary of drug reaction mechanisms, diagnostic capabilities, and therapeutic principles is presented in Table 1.

Several steps should be taken routinely when an individual suspected of having a drug allergy is about to undergo any sort of diagnostic or therapeutic procedure involving the suspected drug. First, the need for the specific drug because no antigenically distinct alternatives are available should be established and documented in the medical record. In the case of antimicrobials contemplated in a patient with previously life-threatening reactions, for example, an infectious disease specialist typically would establish this need. Second, a careful prechallenge physical assessment should be performed to look for underlying signs and symptoms (e.g., rashes, mucosal edema, wheezing, orthostatic hypotension, etc.) that might be misinterpreted as an early allergic reaction. Additionally, careful documentation should be done for each test or challenge protocol, including doses administered and reactions observed. Finally, informed consent, including a dis-

Table 1 Diagnostic and Therapeutic Principles in Drug-Induced Immune Reactions

Drug	IgE/mast cell[a]	Skin testing[b]	Prophylaxis[c]	Test dosing[d]	Desensitization[e]
Penicillin	+/+	+[f]	−[g]	−	+
Insulin	+/+	+	−	+	+
Lidocaine	−/?[h]	+	−	+	−
Radiocontrast	−/+	−	+	+	−
NSAIDs	−/+	−	+[i]	+	−
Sulfonamides	−/?	−	−	+	−

[a] Mast cells and their mediators triggered by IgE or non–IgE-mediated mechanisms.
[b] Accepted skin test protocols are available to look for immediate hypersensitivity reactions.
[c] Pretreatment with various combinations of antihistamines and corticosteroids.
[d] Gradually increasing doses of drug with careful monitoring to detect adverse reactions. The intervals are based upon the suspected mechanisms (immediate versus late).
[e] Specifically designed to treat IgE-mediated reactions.
[f] Involved or useful.
[g] Not involved or not useful.
[h] Involvement or usefulness not established.
[i] Prophylaxis with antileukotriene drugs may be useful.

cussion of the procedure and its potential complications, including death, should be obtained from the patient and documented.

B. β-Lactam Antibiotics

Penicillin drug allergy is one of the most commonly reported, particularly in older individuals. Early preparations of penicillin contained impurities, rather than the penicillin molecule itself, to which the patient may have been reactive (8). Furthermore, many so-called penicillin allergies [such as the microvasculitis associated with ampicillin (9)] are actually inflammatory rashes that are not IgE-mediated. Thus, many patients have presumed that a penicillin allergy existed and have used alternative drugs for many years.

Immunoglobulin-E-mediated reactions to the penicillin molecule do occur. Penicillin is a β-lactam ring-containing molecule (molecular weight approximately 300 Da) that must bind to skin or serum protein in order to be immunogenic. Estimates of true penicillin allergy range from less than 1% to more than 10% of patients who have previously received the drug. There is no increased risk for developing penicillin allergy in patients who are sensitive to the *Penicillium spp.* molds, nor is atopy in general a risk factor for developing penicillin-specific allergic reactions (10). There is cross-reactivity between penicillin-specific IgE and other β-lactam drugs including cephalosporins and the newer β-lactams (11). In general, the true cross-reactivity for cephalosporins appears to decrease progressively from first to third generations (12). Among the newer β-lactams, imipenem, a carbapenem, appears to be highly cross-reactive in penicillin-allergic patients, whereas aztreonam, a true monobactam, has very low cross-reactivity and thus should be safe to use in all but the most highly sensitive patients (13). The potential importance of a reaction due to cross-reactivity should be based upon the specific history of an individual patient. If the purported allergy was a transient morbilliform or maculopapular rash, for example, it is unlikely that the patient is at significant risk for an IgE-mediated reaction after the administration of either a cephalosporin or a monobactam. However, if the patient reports a history of penicillin-induced anaphylaxis, careful monitoring of the administration of these potentially cross-reactive drugs is appropriate. As discussed below, penicillin testing may also be useful.

Penicillin skin testing helps, in the context of the clinical history, to identify a patient at increased risk for a significant IgE-mediated adverse reaction to penicillin. It is estimated that the risk of immune-based reactions to penicillin in skin test-negative patients is 1.5 per million doses administered (14) and, in a previously sensitive patient whose skin test is negative, the risk is not greater than that of the population at large (3–7%) (15). Thus, proper skin testing for penicillin will enable an accurate assessment of risk for individual patients.

Penicillin Skin Testing Procedure. For proper assessment of immediate hypersensitivity the reagents used must be able to test for both major and minor determinants of penicillin. The terms *major* and *minor* do not pertain to importance but rather to abundance where penicillin metabolism is concerned. Minor determinants account for up to 16% of all penicillin allergy reactions. Reagents include histamine sulfate (as a positive control), diluent (usually phosphate-buffered saline as a negative control), benzyl-penicilloyl-polylysine (Pre-Pen, the major determinant), minor determinant mixture (MDM), not commercially available in the United States, but prepared from benzyl penicillin powder (Table 2) and, when MDM is not available, aqueous penicillin G. The dilutions tested and resulting reactions, along with positive and negative controls, are logged on a skin testing sheet, which is filed in the patient's medical record. Many allergists include a signed, informed consent form along with the skin testing sheet. Clearly labeled vials containing the MDM (and/or penicillin G) are prepared in log dilutions from 1,000,000 units/mL to at least 100 units/mL (up to 1 unit/mL for patients suspected of extreme hypersensitivity).

At any point a positive reaction is gained, penicillin testing is stopped and the patient is readied for desensitization. The procedure begins by testing the patient with histamine, saline diluent, and Pre-Pen (full strength) with the percutaneous (prick) method. Twenty minutes later, the reactions are read and recorded.

Table 2 Penicillin Minor Determinant Mixture (MDM) Skin Test Reagent[a]

Materials
1 vial benzyl penicillin (32 g)
50% sodium hydroxide (NaOH) solution
Concentrated sulfuric acid (H_2SO_4)

Procedure
1. Benzylpenicillin is slowly dissolved in approx. 125 mL distilled water (10 mM solution).
2. Add NaOH solution (usually about 8 mL) to bring pH to 12 over 90 minutes.
3. After 2 hours, return the pH to 5.0 with dropwise H_2SO_4 (usually about 5 mL).
4. This mixture (benzylpenicilloate) is frozen and lyophylized to powder.
5. Take 12.5 g of benzylpenicilloate and heat to 76 °C for 24 hours. This yields benzylpenilloic acid.
6. Combine, in equimolar concentrations (10 mM each), benzylypenicillin, benzylpenicilloate, and benzylpenilloic acid in phosphate-buffered saline (pH 7.4).
7. Aliquot and freeze at −20 °C. The material remains stable for 1 year.

[a] *Source*: Courtesy of Adkinson NF. Tests for immunological reactions to drugs and occupational agents. In: Rose, NR, Conway de Macario E, Folds JD, Lane HC, Nakamura RM, eds. Manual of Laboratory Immunology, 5th ed. Washington D.C.: ASM Press, 1997:896–987.

A wheal-and-flare response with a wheal of 3 mm above that of saline is considered a positive reaction. If the percutaneous Pre-Pen is negative, 0.03 mL is injected intradermally along with a saline control. Twenty minutes later, any reactivity is noted. Next are the 1000, 10,000, and 100,000 units/mL dilutions of minor determinant mix (or Pen G) are tested percutaneously (higher dilutions should be used in patients with a high suspicion of sensitivity). Finally, intradermal testing should be done with 100, 1000, and 10,000 units/mL dilutions, each at 20-minute intervals. If all testing is negative in a patient who has a positive wheal and flare from the histamine control, that patient only has a 1% chance of having a serious immediate hypersensitivity reaction. However, accelerated (e.g., serum sickness) or late (e.g., dermatitis) reactions may still occur, and patients should be warned to look for these possibilities.

C. Insulin

The use of bovine, porcine, or recombinant human insulin in patients with diabetes mellitus is commonly associated with the production of serum anti-insulin antibodies, usually of the IgG isotype (16). However, IgE formation specific for insulin molecules (bovine > porcine > recombinant human) is also common. Fully 50% of patients who receive chronic insulin injections develop positive immediate skin tests (17). Most have only mild, local urticarial reactions. Anaphylactic reactions to insulin are uncommon. In patients who experience insulin-induced anaphylaxis, the classic history is a hiatus from bovine insulin injections followed by restarting injections. Because up to half the patients receiving insulin may have a positive immediate skin test, only a negative skin test is valuable, inasmuch as the sensitivity of the test appears high. In patients with clinical histories consistent with an insulin injection–associated systemic reaction, other components of the insulin preparation should be considered. Indeed, sensitivity to excipients such as protamine has been confused with insulin allergy. This is particularly important when it is considered that standard skin testing for insulin sensitivity uses *regular* insulin, which contains no protamine.

Skin Testing. Using regular insulin preparations of bovine, porcine, and recombinant human insulin, saline dilutions of 1:10, 1:100 and, depending upon severity of the reported reaction, 1:1000 of each preparation are made. (Bovine insulin is no longer commercially available in the United States.) The individual is tested percutaneously with each dilution at 20-min intervals, along with baseline positive and negative controls (Table 3). Ideally, a negative reaction is sought but, because a positive reaction is commonly observed, the least positive reaction (i.e., the reaction showing a positive only at the lowest dilution) is used for subsequent desensitization.

Table 3 Insulin Allergy Skin Test Protocol[a]

		Reaction (mm)[b]		
Dilution[c]	Route	Bovine	Porcine	Human
1:100	PC[d]			
1:10	PC			
Full strength	PC			
1:1000	ID[e]			
1:100	ID			
1:10	ID			
Histamine	PC			
Saline	PC			
	ID			

[a] Each of the three species of regular insulin tested together.
[b] Wheal measured in millimeters. Positive reaction is at least 3 mm greater than saline control.
[c] Diluted in normal saline.
[d] Percutaneous prick through a drop of the test reagent.
[e] Intradermal injection of .03 cc of the test reagent.
Source: Ref. 16.

D. Lidocaine

It is commonly reported by patients and their dentists that they are ''allergic'' to one or more of the caine drugs. Yet actual caine sensitivity is exceedingly rare. Usually, the most frequently reported side effects of caine injections for local anesthesia are due to vasovagal reactions (fainting), overdose toxicity (perhaps from injecting into highly vascular areas), or toxicity from epinephrine (i.e., cardiovascular) anxiety reactions (18).

It is imperative that the local anesthetic to which the patient reportedly reacted be identified. Local anesthetic agents are of two biochemical categories: esters and amides. Typically, the category other than the one to which the patient had the reaction is utilized for testing. The preparation must not contain epinephrine as its vasoconstrictive properties could cause a false negative reaction.

One method of skin testing for local anesthetic allergy is outlined in Table 4. The anesthetic is diluted 1:10 and 1:100 in normal saline. Percutaneous testing is done with the full strength anesthetic preparation, followed at 15-minute intervals by subcutaneous injections of 0.1-mL aliquots of 1:100, 1:10, and full strength anesthetic. Finally, undiluted aliquots of 1 mL and then 2 mL are injected subcutaneously. A local reaction that is 3 mm larger than the saline diluent is considered a positive reaction. If this test procedure is negative, the referring physician or dentist can be informed that the patient does not have a greater risk

Table 4 Skin Testing Protocol for Local Anesthetic Sensitivity[a]

Dilution[b]	Volume(cc)	Route	Reaction[c]
F.S.[d]	0.03	PC	
1:100	0.1	SC	
1:10	0.1	SC	
F.S.	0.1	SC	
F.S.	1.0	SC	
F.S.	2.0	SC	

[a] Test injections given at 15-minute intervals.
[b] Diluted in normal saline.
[c] Positive reaction is a wheal at least 3 mm larger than the saline control.
[d] Full strength, 2–4%, without epinephrine.
Source: Ref. 19.

of experiencing an immediate-type reaction to the specific local anesthetic tested than does a member of the general population (19).

E. Radiocontrast Media

Because the incidence of radiocontrast media (RCM) reactions is so low in the general population, many underestimate the importance of identifying patients at high risk for potentially life-threatening reactions so that appropriate preventative and therapeutic measures can be taken. Indeed, although only 1% of all RCM-based procedures result in a clinically significant reaction, up to 33% of previous reactors will have subsequent reactions of equal or greater severity. Many if not most patients undergoing RCM-based imaging procedures have underlying illnesses that could be exacerbated by a severe RCM reaction. Thus, prospective identification of specific risk factors has clinical utility in the cost-effective care of patients undergoing these procedures.

Test dosing. Identification of the patient at high risk for major reactions is important in weighing the risk/benefit of a radiocontrast procedure. There is no skin-testing procedure that can accurately predict responders. However, a specific graded challenge procedure may be of benefit to predict those at highest risk of repeat reactions. In a study reported by Yocum and colleagues (20), 204 previous RCM reactors categorized according to their history of reaction (vague versus specific), their challenge result (positive versus negative) and pretreatment (diphenhydramine versus none) demonstrated a clear utility of the procedure to identify high-risk patients likely to have repeat reactions with subsequent RCM exposure. Such patients would require the highest pretreatment and monitoring possible.

In the pretest procedure, increasing doses of the proposed radiocontrast agent (usually iso-osmolar when available) are given intravenously at 15-minute intervals until a total of 6 mL of full-strength RCM is reached (Table 5). The patient is monitored carefully for definite signs of an anaphylactoid reaction (such as wheezing, hypotension, urticaria, angioedema, etc.). Based on this, the pretest is recorded as positive or negative.

Yocum and colleagues showed that positive pretest reactors had a 66.7% (12/18) probability of repeat reaction without prophylaxis. Vague history with negative pretest had only a 4.9% (2/41) reaction rate with subsequent RCM administration. Only 4.2% (3/71) of patients with a high probability history, negative pretest, and prophylaxis with diphenhydramine reacted to their repeat RCM procedure while a comparable group with no prophylaxis had a reaction rate of 20.7% (11/53).

F. Sulfonamides

With increased use of trimethoprim-sulfamethoxazole (TMP-SMX) for prophylaxis against *Pneumocystis carinii* (PCP) in patients infected with the human immunodeficiency virus (HIV), increased adverse reactions to sulfonamides have become a progressively alarming problem. The most common immune-based reaction is a generalized maculopapular rash. This usually occurs several days

Table 5 Pretest for Radiocontrast Sensitivity[a]

Dilution[b]	Volume(cc)	Reaction[c]
−1:10,000	0.1	
1:1,000	0.1	
1:100	0.1	
1:10	0.1	
F.S.	0.1	
F.S.	1.0	
F.S.	5.0	

Abbreviation: F.S., full strength.

[a] Sensitivity determined after intravenous administration of the radiocontrast material at 15-minute intervals.

[b] Dilution made in normal saline.

[c] Reaction is an indication of systemic mast-cell activity.

Source: Ref. 20.

Table 6 Trimethoprim-Sulfamethoxazole (TMP-SMX) Test Dosing Protocols

A. Oral[a]	
Day 1	0.1 cc
Day 2	1 cc
Day 3	3 cc
Day 4	10 cc (or full-strength tablet)
B. Intravenous Rush (Emergency)[b]	
Dose (mg)[c]	
0.8	
7.2	
40	
80	
400	
680	

[a] TMP-SMX elixir used where 10 cc represents full adult dose.
[b] Given I.V. at 20-minute intervals.
[c] Dose based on SMX component.
Source: Ref. 23.

after beginning therapy. Immunoglobulin E is not a major immunologic mediator in most TMP-SMX rashes (21). Such skin reactions should be distinguished from those involving mucous membranes (Stevens-Johnson syndrome) or exfoliation (toxic epidermal necrolysis). In these cases, further use of sulfonamides is contraindicated.

Unfortunately, there is no currently accepted in vivo or in vitro test for determining immune-mediated sensitivity to sulfonamides. Recent efforts have been made to develop skin test reagents but these are developmental and not available for general use. To date, only test dosing is an acceptable method in patients with history of TMP-SMX sensitivity for whom this drug is a medical necessity. This would primarily involve the HIV-infected group who needed TMP-SMX for prophylaxis against or treatment of *P. carinii* pneumonia (22). Many different methods are reported, some taking days and others a few hours (23). Obviously, caution is paramount and, due to the risk of a late (48–72 hours after dosing) reaction, great caution should be exercised whenever possible. Generally, a slow procedure (oral or intravenous) can be given over 4 days (Table 6A) (24). When critical, the drug can be administered in a test-dosing procedure in as little as 2 to 4 hours (Table 6B) (25). If a significant reaction occurs during test dosing, patients should be treated with high-dose corticosteroids with or without antihistamines, depending upon the nature of the symptoms. Although Stevens–Johnson syndrome also may be treated with corticosteroids, the success rate is much poorer than for a maculopapular rash. Test doses of sulfonamides are contraindicated in patients who have experienced Stevens–Johnson syndrome or toxic epidermal necrolysis following sulfonamide administration.

G. Aspirin

The prototypic nonsteroidal anti-inflammatory agent (NSAID) is aspirin. It is still common to elicit a history of aspirin ''allergy,'' yet usually what is meant is gastrointestinal upset. But a defined population of individuals will have what appears to be mast-cell-mediated reactions of either respiratory or cutaneous origin (26). The triad of asthma, nasal polyposis, and aspirin sensitivity is well described as Samter's syndrome (27). Although the precise mechanism is unknown, it is thought to involve the cyclo-oxygenase inhibition by the NSAIDS with possible increase in 5-lipoxygenase activity resulting in increased leukotriene synthesis (28) and the resulting systemic symptoms. A defined sensitivity to one NSAID should be considered to apply to all other NSAIDs (including aspirin), with the exception of the nonacetylated salicylates, such as salsalate, which weakly inhibit the cyclo-oxygenase pathway, or acetaminophen.

When an NSAID is considered clinically essential for a chronic inflammatory state, desensitization can be attempted. Generally, after desensitization, respiratory symptoms can be successfully eliminated virtually completely (29), whereas cutaneous symptoms (such as urticaria) are successfully eliminated less than 40% of the time (30). Due to availability of different strengths and preparation, successful test dosing with aspirin can be used even when another NSAID will be used therapeutically (31). There is a refractory period after test dosing that lasts from 2–5 days. However, as in other drug desensitization protocols, the general rule to prevent recurrent sensitivity is to permit dose intervals of no greater than four half-lives. Otherwise, the entire test-dose protocol must be repeated (32). The standard test dosing is done over 2 days at 8:00 AM, 11:00 AM, and 2:00 PM (Table 7). If the individual history is significant for severe reactions, the procedure can be accomplished over 3 days. The desensitized state can be maintained indefinitely, as long as NSAID administration continues daily or every other day.

H. Multiple Drug Allergy (Pseudoallergy)

One of the most commonly abused medical terms is ''allergy'' as it pertains to drug sensitivity. As discussed above, an allergic reaction should, as a rule, only be suspected when certain clinical signs and symptoms present within a defined time frame after taking the drug. An often puzzling clinical situation for allergists

Table 7 Aspirin Desensitization Protocol[a]

Day[b]	Time	Dose
1	8:00 AM	3 mg
	11:00 AM	6 mg
	2:00 PM	10 mg
2	8:00 AM	15 mg
	11:00 AM	32 mg
	2:00 PM	65 mg
3	8:00 AM	150 mg
	11:00 AM	325 mg
	2:00 PM	650 mg

[a] Aspirin elixir is used for dosing purposes. At 325 mg, one can switch to tablets.
[b] With low suspicion of aspirin/NSAID sensitivity, protocol can begin on day 2.
Source: Refs. 29, 30.

is a patient who presents with a history of multiple sensitivities to a variety of antigenically unrelated drugs (usually antibiotics). Because the only antibiotic that can reliably be skin tested is penicillin, this can create a dilemma for the allergist to establish which drugs can be taken safely. The answer is a double-blind, placebo-controlled provocative challenge (33).

To properly and safely perform a double-blind challenge, a careful history must be taken. The time between drug administration and appearance of symptoms must be documented, and the nature of the symptoms also must be noted. The patient's need for the specific medication should also be carefully documented. A careful prechallenge physical assessment should be performed to look for signs and symptoms that might otherwise be misinterpreted as an early allergic reaction. Each administered dose and observed reaction should be documented carefully and thoroughly. Finally, informed consent should be obtained from the patient and documented following a discussion of the procedure and its potential complications, including death. If the history appears to be consistent with an anaphylactoid reaction, a test dosing (intravenous or oral) procedure can be initiated. The drug in question, along with a placebo, is prepared by the pharmacist and coded. The first challenge is done by administering graded increases in the dose of medication (or placebo) beginning at 1% of the dose and doubling at 15-minute intervals with careful observation. Regardless of the reaction (or lack thereof), the patient returns (usually several days later) for a repeat challenge with the other preparation. After both challenges have been performed, the code is broken. In most instances, the patient is as likely to have a reaction to the placebo as to the drug in question. After a negative double-blind, placebo-controlled challenge, the patient can be reassured that he or she is not sensitive (from an allergic mechanism) to the particular drug in question out of proportion to the population at large.

The major caveat to double-blind, placebo-controlled challenges is the placebo itself. It should be as close to the drug in question in color, consistency, and taste, as possible to keep the patient (and physician) from identifying the solutions. Such differences cna invalidate the entire procedure.

IV. SUMMARY

Drug sensitivity is a major clinical problem that is incompletely understood. Much effort continues in identifying patients at risk for developing drug sensitivities, predicting the various immune mechanisms most likely to be activated by a specific drug, and developing more reliable tests to identify the drug-allergic patient.

V. SALIENT POINTS

1. The incidence of adverse drug reactions (ADR) is estimated at up to 1% of all drug doses given.
2. Immunologic reactions to drugs can be allergic (IgE-mediated), antibody-mediated (IgM or IgG-mediated), or cell-mediated (delayed-type hypersensitivity).
3. An estimated 1% of all administered drug doses cause IgE-mediated AR.
4. If a drug suspected of causing an allergic reaction in a patient is to be used again in that patient, the benefit of using that drug must clearly outweigh the risk of another reaction.
5. Very few skin test reagents reliably confirm the presence of a specific drug allergy. Use of other reagents provides results that are speculative but not definitive.
6. For most suspected drug allergic reactions, confirmation of allergic status demands a double-blind, placebo-controlled challenge. Before such a procedure is done, it is critical to establish that there are no alternative drugs available, that the risk-benefit ratio is sufficient to justify the risk, and that the patient understands the potential risks for morbidity and mortality.

REFERENCES

1. Anderson JA. Allergic and allergic-like reactions to drugs and other therapeutic agents. In: Lieberman P, Anderson J, eds. Allergic Diseases: Diagnosis and Treatment. Totowa, NJ: Humana Press, 1997:275–292.
2. DeSwarte RD, Patterson R. Drug allergy. In: Patterson R, Grammer LC, Greenberger PA, eds. Allergic Diseases: Diagnosis and Management, 5th ed. Philadelphia: Lippincott-Raven, 1997: 317–412.
3. Miller HR. Mucosal mast cells and the allergic response against nematode parasites. Vet Immunol Immunopathol 1996; 54:331–336.
4. Van Cauwenberge P, Van Haver K. Immunological aspects and inflammatory mechanisms of allergic reactions. Acta Otolaryngol 1993; 113:383–386.
5. Girdwood RH. Drug-induced anemias. Drugs 1976; 11:394–404.
6. Uetrecht J. Drug metabolism by leukocytes and its role in drug-induced lupus and other idiosyncratic drug reactions. Crit Rev Toxicol 1990; 20:213–235.
7. Ramsay DL, Parnes RE, Dubin N. Response of mycosis fungoides to topical chemotherapy with mechlorethamine. Arch Dermatol 1984; 120:1585–1590.
8. Blanca M. Allergic reactions to penicillin: A changing world? Allergy 1995; 50: 777–782.
9. Adcock BB, Rodman DP. Ampicillin-specific rashes. Arch Fam Med 1996; 5:301–304.
10. Van Arsdel PP. Classification and risk factors for drug allergy. Immunol Allergy Clin North Am 1991; 11:475–492.
11. Kishiyama JL, Adelman DC. The cross-reactivity and immunology of beta-lactam antibiotics. Drug Saf 1994; 10:318–327.
12. Anne S, Reisman RE. Risk of administering cephalosporin antibiotics to patients with histories of penicillin allergy. Ann Allergy Asthma Immunol 1995; 74:167–170.
13. Hantson P, de Coninck B, Horn JL, Mahieu P. Immediate hypersensitivity to aztreonam and imipenem. BMJ 1991; 302:294–295.
14. Sarti W. Routine use of skin testing for immediate sensitivity for immediate penicillin allergy to 6764 patients in an outpatient clinic. Ann Allergy 1985; 55:157–161.
15. Gruchalla RS. Antibiotic drug allergy: challenges of diagnosis and treatment. Arb Paul Ehrlich Inst Bundesamt Sera Impfstoffe Frankf A M 1997; 91:237–249.
16. Grammer L. Insulin allergy. Clin Rev Allergy 1986; 4:189–200.
17. Patterson R, Roberts M, Grammer LC. Insulin allergy: reevaluation after two decades. Ann Allergy 1990; 64:459–462.
18. Jackson D, Chen AH, Bennett CR. Identifying true lidocaine allergy. J Am Dent Assoc 1994; 125:1362–1366.
19. Chandler MJ, Grammer LC, Patterson R. Provocative challenge with local anesthetics in patients with a prior history of reaction. J Allergy Clin Immunol 1987; 79: 883–886.
20. Yocum MD, Heller AM, Abels RI. Efficacy of intravenous pretesting and antihistamine prophylaxis in radiocontrast media-sensitive patients. J Allergy Clin Immunol 1978; 62:309–313.

21. Hennessy S, Strom BL, Berlin JA, Brennan PJ. Predicting cutaneous hypersensitivity reactions to cotrimoxazole in HIV-infected individuals receiving primary *Pneumocystis carinii* pneumonia prophylaxis. J Gen Intern Med 1995; 10:380–386.
22. Tapper ML. Successful prophylaxis of *Pneumocystis carnii* pneumonia with trimethoprim-sulfamethoxazole in AIDS. J AIDS 1989; 2:389–395.
23. White MV, Haddad ZH, Brunner E, Sainz C. Desensitization to trimethoprim sulfamethoxazole in patients with acquired immune deficiency syndrome and *Pneumocystis carnii* pneumonia. Ann Allergy 1989; 62:177–179.
24. Finegold I. Oral desensitization to trimethoprim-sulfamethoxazole in a patient with acquired immune deficiency syndrome. J Allergy Clin Immunol 1986; 78:905–908.
25. Palusci VJ, Kaul A, Lawrence RM, Haines KA, Kwittken PL. Rapid oral desensitization to trimethoprim-sulfamethoxazole in infants and children. Pediatr Infect Dis J 1996; 15:456–460.
26. Settipane GA. Aspirin sensitivity and allergy. Biomed Pharmacother 1988; 42:493–498.
27. Zeitz HJ. Bronchial asthma, nasal polyps, and aspirin sensitivity: Samter's syndrome. Clin Chest Med 1988; 9:567–576.
28. Cowburn AS, Sladek K, Soja J, Adamek L, Nizankowska E, Szczeklik A, Lam BK, Penrose JF, Austen FK, Holgate ST, Sampson AP. Overexpression of leukotriene C4 synthase in bronchial biopsies from patients with aspirin-intolerant asthma. J Clin Invest 1998; 101:834–846.
29. Stevenson DD, Hankammer MA, Mathison DA, Christiansen SC, Simon RA. Aspirin desensitization treatment of aspirin-sensitive patients with rhinosinusitis-asthma: Long-term outcomes. J Allergy Clin Immunol 1996; 98:751–758.
30. Grzelewska-Rzymowska I, Szmidt M, Rozniecki J. Aspirin-induced urticaria—A clinical study. J Invest Allergol Clin Immunol 1992; 2:39–42.
31. Zhu DX, Zhao JL, Mo L, Li HL. Drug allergy: identification and characterization of IgE-reactivities to aspirin and related compounds. J Invest Allergol Clin Immunol 1997; 7:160–168.
32. Bernstein JA. Allergic drug reactions. How to minimize the risks. Postgrad Med 1995; 98:159–160.
33. Reider MJ. In vivo and in vitro testing for adverse drug reactions. Pediatr Clin North Am 1997; 44:93–111.

10

Fiberoptic Rhinoscopy

Howard M. Druce
UMDNJ–New Jersey Medical School, Newark, New Jersey

Dennis K. Ledford
University of South Florida College of Medicine and the James A. Haley Veterans Hospital, Tampa, Florida

I. INTRODUCTION

Fiberoptic rhinoscopy is the best nonsurgical technique to visualize both the normal anatomy and any pathology of the nose and pharynx. The indications for and techniques used in this procedure are discussed in this chapter.

Only a small proportion of the surface area of the nares can be visualized by a nasal speculum. A head mirror and nasopharyngeal mirrors are required to see more. However, the mirror examination technique cannot usually be mastered during a 2–4 week medical school rotation on an otolaryngology or allergy/immunology elective. Furthermore, many subjects cannot be examined, regardless of the physician's skill, due to a hyperresponsive gag reflex. This is unfortunate, because 25% of physician office visits are made for upper respiratory tract complaints. Fiberoptic rhinoscopy is not difficult to learn. However, recognizing and distinguishing normal findings from those that are abnormal requires considerable time and experience. Rhinoscopy also can be videotaped for patient education, teaching purposes, and consultation with other physicians. The videotape provides a permanent record of the procedure.

The diagnostic utility of rhinoscopy is illustrated in the following case report. A 52-year-old male presented with a 12-year history of obstruction of his left nasal passage. There were no symptoms of allergic rhinitis, nasal polyps, anosmia, bleeding, or previous surgery of the upper airway, although nasal obstruction was worse in the morning. Over-the-counter medications did not help, and he had not previously sought medical care.

Rhinomanometry, which measures nasal airway resistance, indicated that there was increased resistance to airflow in the right nares but not in the left. Anterior rhinoscopy revealed no septal deviation or polyp, and the nasal mucosal membranes were normal. Videotaped fiberoptic rhinoscopy revealed a mass on the nasal floor attached to the septum. A consulting otolaryngologist examined the videotape before the patient left the clinic and felt that the mass was a squamous cell carcinoma. Computerized tomography of the sinuses and nasal and oral pharynx was normal. A surgical biopsy showed an epithelialized inflammatory polyp and not carcinoma.

This case illustrates the importance of rhinoscopy, because it enables the physician to visualize various portions of the upper airway, from the nasal vestibule to the larynx. The part above the level of the soft palate is the nasopharynx, communicating posteriorly with the nasal choanae and the eustachian tube, also called the tubus tubarium. The lower portion of the upper airway consists of two sections: the oropharynx, which lies between the soft palate and the upper edge of the epiglottis, and the laryngopharynx, which lies below the upper edge of the epiglottis and opens into the larynx and esophagus. In most cases of rhinitis, fiberoptic rhinoscopy is not necessary to make a diagnosis. However, this safe technique visually confirms suspected findings in typical cases of rhinitis and is a cost-effective diagnostic tool in atypical or complicated cases.

II. WHO SHOULD DO RHINOSCOPY AND ITS INDICATIONS

Fiberoptic rhinoscopy is a technique used to visualize the anatomy of the nares and the pharynx and is considered by most physicians to be a difficult procedure.

Table 1 Possible Indications for Flexible Rhinoscopy

General
Any upper airway symptom for which the diagnosis cannot be ascertained by a complete history and physical
Nose and Nasopharynx
Anosmia
Assess result of surgical intervention
Earache, recurrent or chronic otitis media
Epistaxis
Facial pain
Headache
Nasal obstruction (especially unilateral)
Rhinorrhea
Sinusitis
Snoring, mouth breathing
Regional adenopathy (head and neck)
Oropharynx and Laryngopharynx
Chronic cough
Dysphagia or globus
Hoarseness
Other change in voice quality
Vocal cord dysfunction

Source: Ref. 4.

However, in reality, the simple technique of the fiberoptic rhinoscopic examination can be used to great advantage by generalists, who examine 25% of all patients with upper respiratory tract complaints (1,2).

Rhinoscopy is indicated whenever direct visualization of the nares and pharynx would facilitate making a correct diagnosis, for example, to identify the presence of chronic sinusitis, nasal polyps, tumor, or vocal cord abnormalities (Table 1). Fiberoptic rhinoscopy is not a technique that permits biopsy or sampling of secretions.

III. HOW TO DO RHINOSCOPY

A narrow-bore instrument designed for fiberoptic rhinoscopy is required. There are several manufacturers and models, and ideally a physician should try several different instruments before purchasing one, especially if the physician is left-handed. A pediatric 3-mm diameter rhinoscope without an aspiration channel is the instrument most physicians use. Most manufacturers also offer several light sources with variable intensities, and it is useful to test each scope with its respective light source or sources. As with any instrument, the accessibility for service when the scope is broken is equally important in choosing the device, because it is easy to damage a fiberoptic rhinoscope.

Rigid rhinoscopes with fixed angulation are also available. These instruments permit visualization of areas of the airway that may not be accessible with the fiberoptic, flexible rhinoscope. The optics in rigid scopes are superior to the fiberoptic scopes. However, the examination is more uncomfortable for the patient, requires more preparation with topical anesthesia and decongestion of the airway, and is more time-consuming. Examination with rigid rhinoscopes is generally performed by otolaryngologic surgeons. The information provided in this chapter applies to fiberoptic rhinoscopy.

A. Setup

A special area or room for rhinoscopy is ideal; however, in most offices, this is not possible and the equipment is kept on a cart and moved into position whenever it is used. There are no ports or orifices to collect secretions and contaminate the rhinoscope. Therefore, cleaning with soap and water reduces the risk of contamination after the instrument is used. To eliminate the possibility of transmitting infection, sterilization of the rhinoscope with ethylene oxide or soaking in 2–3% glutaraldehyde solution is necessary. Higher concentrations of glutaraldehyde or other solutions may damage the fiberoptic coating. Manufacturers provide details for the preferred method of sterilization for their respective instruments.

If the rhinoscope is used without a video camera, the physician should face the patient and look directly into the eyepiece of the rhinoscope as it is inserted into the nares. When the rhinoscope is used with a television monitor, the monitor should be placed next to the patient at the physician's eye level so he or she can view the monitor comfortably as the rhinoscope is inserted into the nares.

Ideally, the patient should sit in an otolarnygologic chair so that its height can be adjusted and the patient's head immobilized against the headrest. A concave or ''donut'' shaped headrest is best suited for this purpose; however, a small pillow can also be used. If a special chair is not available, a regular office chair will suffice, with the patient's head immobilized against a wall. With reassurance and foreknowledge of the procedure, most patients can be examined even when leaning forward in a regular chair without head immobilization.

B. Patient Preparation

The procedure should be explained to the patient and written informed consent may be helpful to document preparation. Because the procedure is very safe, some institutions and physicians do not require a signed consent form prior to rhinoscopy.

The patient is instructed to sit upright and place his or her head firmly against the back of the chair or wall. It is unnecessary to use a topical decongestant or local anesthetic if the patient is cooperative, with patent nares. However, usually the nares are decongested with topical agents such as 1% ephinephrine or 1% ephedrine, one spray in each nostril through a self-administered squeeze bottle. The spray bottle is discarded after use, or the application tip is replaced or sterilized. Long-acting topical decongestants, such as oxymetazoline, are also effective. Topical anesthesia is preferred by some physicians or patients. Lidocaine solution, 1–4%, topically applied by spray is a useful preparation if anesthesia is desired. Another alternative is to apply 4% viscous lidocaine on a sterile swab between the nasal septum and middle and inferior turbinates for 5 minutes before the procedure. The fiberoptic portion of the rhinoscope also can be lubricated with viscous lidocaine before its insertion into the nares as an alternative or additional anesthetic.

Singh and others (3) conducted a double-blind study of 60 subjects investigating whether the use of topical anesthesia improved patient tolerance of the procedure. Each subject had 5% cocaine solution sprayed into one nostril and normal saline into the other. The pain/discomfort and gag scores associated with rhinoscopy were not statistically different with cocaine versus normal saline. Subjects with septal deviations, which can make the examination more uncomfortable, reported no significant difference in discomfort with or without the use of topical anesthesia. Forty-two (70%) of the patients had a moderate to marked septal deviation. Thirty-three percent (14 subjects) of these individuals reported pain with rhinoscopy after cocaine application to the nares with the septal deviation compared to 37% (15 subjects) with saline pretreatment of the nares with the septal deviation. Ease-of-procedure scores for both sides (with and without septal deviation) were comparable, irrespective of the use of anesthetic.

If the patient is not cooperative, rhinoscopy should not be performed. If the nares are too narrow to accommodate the scope, the patient should be referred to an otolaryngologist for evaluation, either by rhinoscopy with anesthesia or an indirect nasopharyngeal examination.

To avoid confusion, the physician may prefer to select the same side of the nose for initial examination. Other physicians prefer to visualize the most patent naris first to minimize potential discomfort during the initial phase of the examination. The rhinoscope is introduced into the naris and gradually inserted, and the entire pharynx examined in a systematic fashion (Fig. 1). Special attention should be paid to the ostiomeatal complex in patients with suspected sinusitis (see Fig. 10.2, color insert). Pressure in this area from the tip of the rhinoscope can be particularly painful. A rigid rhinoscope, with appropriate anesthesia, often is necessary to visualize the ostia in the middle meatus. The sphenoethmoid recess

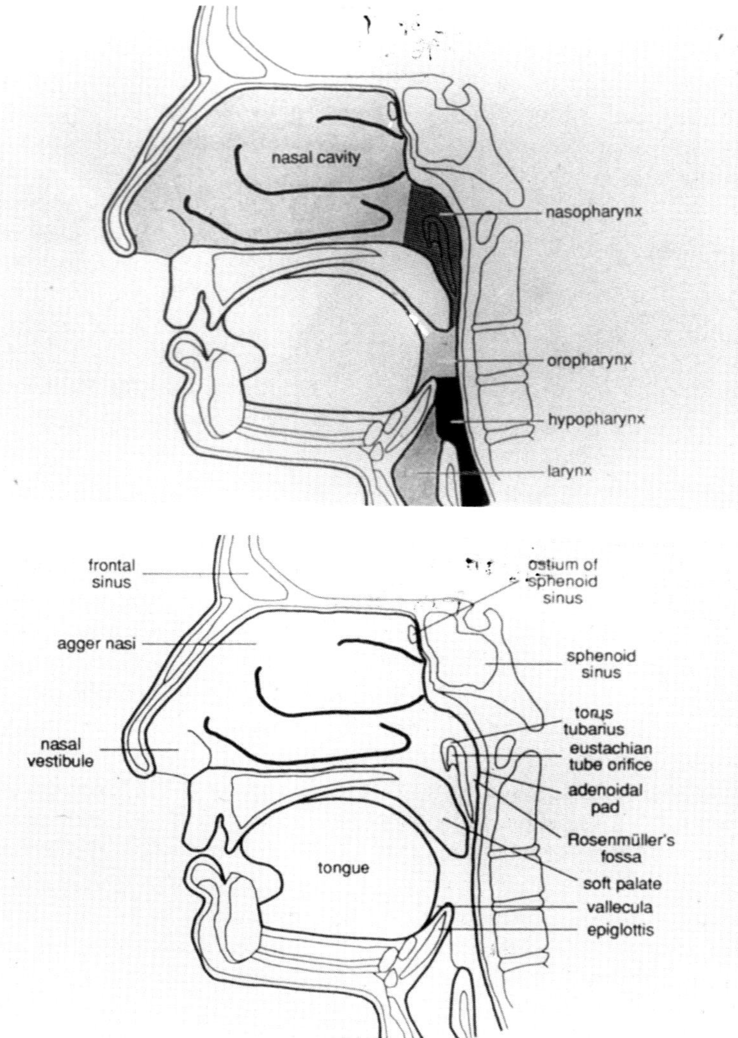

Figure 1 Lateral views of structures seen with fiberoptic rhinoscopy.

is examined by maximally dorsally flexing the scope. This permits observation of the superior turbinate, the sphenoid ostium, and the posterior ethmoid ostium. Active infection in these sinuses is usually identified by the presence of purulent drainage traversing the posterior nasopharyngeal wall or by recognizing purulence in the ostia. The adenoid tissue is visualized immediately posterior to the nasal choanae. Adenoiditis, adenoid hyperplasia, or a Tornwaldt's bursa (an embryonic remnant of Rathke's pouch that can be responsible for halitosis or a sensation of thick postnasal drainage) can be identified. The opening of the eustachian tube, or the torus tubarium, is just lateral to the adenoid. The intervening cleft is the fossa of Rossenmüller, a site of origin for nasopharyngeal carcinoma that is difficult to visualize without rhinoscopy.

Detailed accounts of the anatomy of the upper airway and methods used to perform rhinoscopy are presented elsewhere (4,5).

C. How to Record Results

Details of patient preparation and rhinoscopic findings should be incorporated into the patient's record (Table 2). Standardized reporting forms ensure that the same procedure is followed for all patients examined and the findings are appropriately recorded. An example of these forms can be obtained at the annual meetings of the American Academy of Allergy, Asthma and Immunology, Milwaukee, Wisconsin, and the American College of Allergy, Asthma and Immunology, Chicago, Illinois. A video recording of the procedure is useful to document the examination and permit review at a later time.

D. Typical Findings: Tips and Pitfalls

Considerable practice is necessary to recognize the normal anatomical variations that occur in the nares and pharynx. For example, the color of the nasal mucosa can vary from pale gray to deep red. Mild-to-moderate septal deviation is almost always present, and the degree of deviation can appear magnified by the convex optics of the rhinoscopic lens. A frequent error on routine anterior nasal examination is to interpret a clear gelatinous accumulation of mucus high in the nasal cavity as a polyp. This error in interpretation of findings is unlikely to occur with fiberoptic rhinoscopy. Sinusitis in the posterior ethmoid or sphenoid sinuses is usually recognized by a stream of purulent mucus on the posterior wall of the nose or by purulence in the sinus ostia. Sinusitis affecting the maxillary, frontal, or anterior ethmoid sinuses results in erythema and mucopurulent discharge in the middle meatus (the space between the inferior and middle turbinates) or by a stream of mucopus draining over the inferior turbinate. Adenoiditis, which may cause symptoms similar to sinusitis, can be identified by direct visualization of the adenoid tissue posterior to the nose.

Table 2 Observations on Flexible Rhinoscopy

- Nasopharynx
  - Mucosa
    - Color, consistency, edema
  - Nasal cavity
    - Antral window
    - After surgery
  - Ostiomeatal complex and sphenoethmoid recess
    - Appearance, secretions, polyps
  - Septum
    - Alignment, spurs, bleeding points, crusts, ulcers
- Laryngopharynx
  - Eustachian tube
    - Patency, inflammation, movement
  - Adenoid tissue
    - Size, exudate, after surgery, Tornwaldt's bursa (present or absent)
  - Lingual tonsil
  - Rosenmüller's fossa
  - Palatine tonsils
  - Secretions
- Larynx
  - Appearance and function—normal or abnormal
  - Arytenoid cartilage mucosa—edema, erythema
  - Epiglottis—color, edema
  - False cords—color, edema
  - Pyriform sinus—foreign bodies
  - True vocal cords—polyps or nodules, motion

Lingual tonsil enlargement is common in subjects with upper airway complaints but frequently is asymptomatic and thus of questionable clinical significance. The laryngeal examination may provide an explanation of hoarseness or cough. Paradoxical closure of the false or true vocal cords (indicative of vocal cord dysfunction), asymmetry of the vocal cords (indicative of vocal cord paralysis or malignancy), vocal cord erythema or nodules (indicative of laryngitis, papillomas, or voice abuse), and inflammatory changes of the mucosa overlying the arytenoid cartilage [suggestive of gastroesophageal reflux (GERD)] are findings of importance. Observing the larynx during phonation, both high and low pitch, during natural respiration and during a forced exhalation maneuver is helpful in assessing the function of the larynx and identifying vocal cord dysfunction. The latter condition emulates asthma with wheezing and cough and often is the cause of asthma-like symptoms that do not respond to appropriate asthma therapy.

E. Use in Diagnosing Diseases of the Nose, Pharynx, and Sinuses

Headaches commonly occur with acute sinusitis. The diagnosis is usually obvious because of the associated nasal and sinus symptoms. However, headache caused by chronic sinusitis or other upper airway pathology can be more difficult to identify. Clerico (6) reported a series of 10 patients in whom rhinoscopy and computerized tomography were useful to ascertain a sinonasal cause of chronic headaches, despite the absence of airway symptoms. All of these subjects had had previous neurology evaluations and various, unsuccessful therapeutic trials for chronic headache. Nine of the 10 subjects had an unexpected diagnosis confirmed by rhinoscopy or computerized tomography of the sinsues, and 8 of these experienced long-term improvement from appropriate treatment. The diagnoses included concha bullosa, enlarged agger nasi cells, septal deviation with inspissation of secretions, narrowed sphenoethmoid recess, septal spur, and sinusitis. The findings of rhinoscopy and the radiographic studies were complementary, and rhinoscopy alone would have made the diagnosis in four or five of these subjects.

The medical literature provides differing opinions as to who should undergo fiberoptic rhinoscopy when presenting with nasal or sinus complaints. Benninger (7) described his experience with 100 consecutive new patient evaluations by an otolaryngologist. Patients were excluded if their only complaint was obstruction and they had a septal deviation as the only clinical finding. The diagnoses with a complete history and physical examination, including anterior nasal examination (without rhinoscopy), was compared to the diagnoses after fiberoptic rhinoscopy. The conclusion was that fiberoptic rhinoscopy need not be a part of the evaluation of all patients with nasal or sinus complaints but is useful in confirming a diagnosis, particularly when anterior rhinoscopy is limited by anatomical obstruction. By contrast, Jorissen (9) advocates that rhinoscopy should be routine to completely examine the airway. Endoscopic and radiographic findings are complementary, each with strengths and weaknesses. The strengths of the fiberoptic rhinoscopic examination include the evaluation and monitoring of efficacy of therapy or the progress of disease, differentiation of soft-tissue abnormalities such as tissue hyperplasia or polyps from mucosal edema, assessment of the color and nature of secretions (for example clear, mucoid, or purulent), and evaluation of the functional significance of septal deviations, choanal narrowing, and synechiae (scar tissue connecting the turbinates and the nasal septum) (8–14) (see Figs. 10.4 and 10.5, color insert).

Fiberoptic rhinoscopy is technically more difficult to perform in children because of their smaller nasal and upper airway anatomy and due to the frequent lack of cooperation of the subject, particularly when younger than 5 years. Clinical series of children, including one comprising 817 subjects, demonstrate that fiberoptic nasopharyngeal examination is feasible in most cases (15). The authors of the 817-subject study conclude that rhinoscopy is tolerated by most children, that adenoid hyperplasia is more accurately assessed by rhinoscopy than by lateral skull radiography, and that rhinoscopy is of significant clinical value in the evaluation of children for adenoidectomy (see Fig. 10.3, color insert). Utility of rhinoscopy has also been demonstrated in cystic fibrosis for the assessment of the common frequent complications of sinusitis and nasal polyposis (16,17). Thus, fiberoptic rhinoscopy is a valuable tool in the management of pediatric upper airway disease.

In summary, rhinoscopy is a useful procedure to diagnose or monitor a variety of problems that occur in the nares and pharynx (18). A list of suggested indications for rhinoscopy is included in a report of the American Academy of Allergy, Asthma and Immunology (19).

IV. COMPARISON OF PROCEDURES FOR DIAGNOSING SINUSITIS

Various imaging techniques are useful to document abnormal nasal and paranasal sinus anatomy and disease. Computerized tomography (CT) has largely replaced conventional radiographs for this purpose. However, overreliance on CT without preoperative rhinoscopy may lead to unnecessary surgery (20).

Katz and others (21) reported on 35 patients who were evaluated by history, physical examination, laboratory tests, and sinus radiographs, magnetic resonance imaging (MRI), and flexible rhinoscopy. Fiberoptic rhinoscopy provided diagnostic findings of sinusitis in 13 of 29 cases, but all of these cases were detected by radiograph. The MRI studies identified two additional cases. A completely normal rhinoscopic examination virtually eliminated the possibility of clinical sinusitis. Castellanos and Axelrod (22) showed in a series of 246 patients that fiberoptic rhinoscopy detected sinusitis in 148 subjects, with radiographs being diagnostic in only 84. Rhinoscopy is superior to sinus radiographs in making a sinusitis diagnosis, although CT or MRI scanning is more sensitive than rhinoscopy (23). However, the clinical importance of most of these rhinoscopically normal cases of sinusitis is insignificant. The cost, delay in getting information, radiation exposure for CT (average of 2.2 to 6.8 rad), and possible need for sedation are additional disadvantages for doing these imaging techniques. Rhinoscopy complements, and may be superior to, other techniques in diagnosing sinusitis and is a useful procedure for monitoring therapeutic response.

V. USE IN AUDITORY DISORDERS

Endoscopy is useful to visualize the eustachian tube orifices and assess an anatomical explanation for eustachian tube dysfunction. Mucopurulent discharge from the eustachian tube may be associated with acute and chronic inflammation

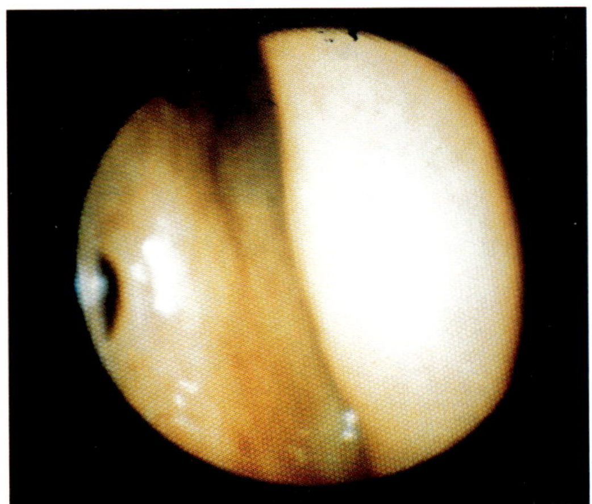

Figure 10.2 Superior meatus with posterior ethmoidal ostium.

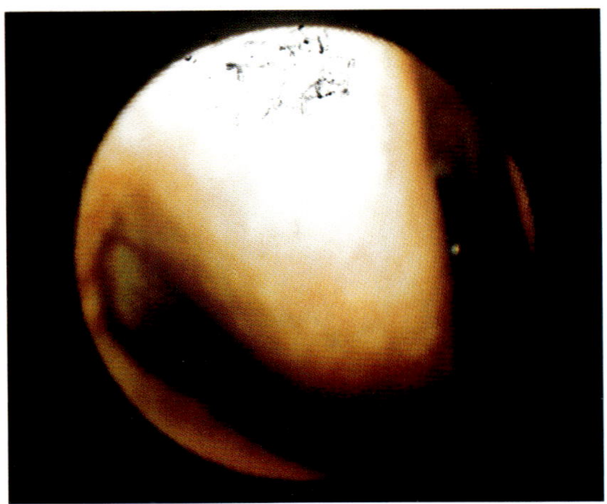

Figure 10.3 Left choana with pus from middle meatus.

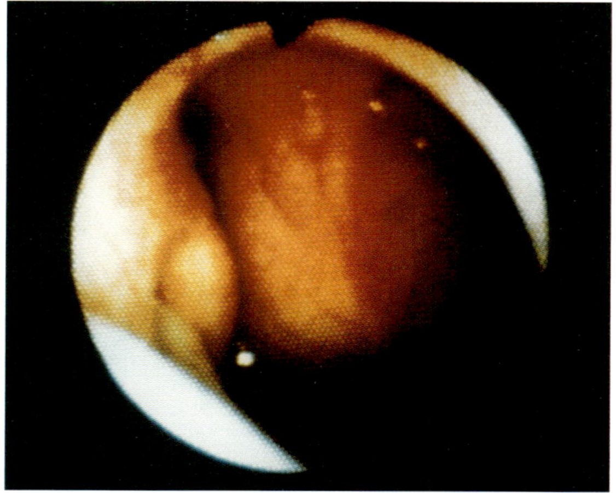

Figure 10.4 Adenoids protruding to nasal cavity.

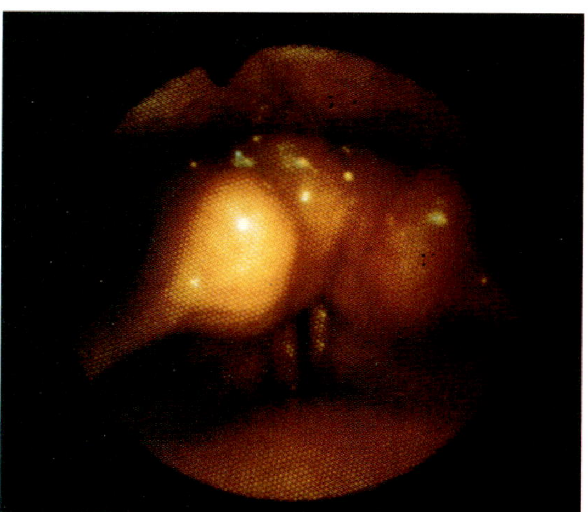

Figure 10.5 Vocal cord polyp.

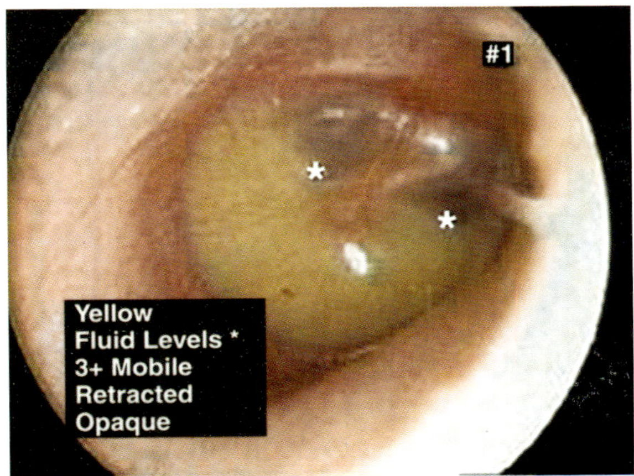

Figure 11.1 Yellow (pus) fluid levels in acute otitis media. (*Source:* Kaleida PH, Hoberman A. Otoendoscopic Examinations, Training Tape #3, Universal Health Communications, Inc: Boynton Beach, FL, 1994.)

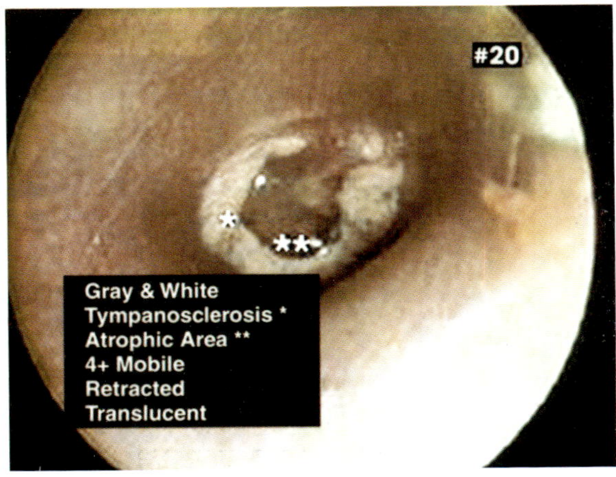

Figure 11.2 Tympanosclerosis and atrophic area of tympanic membrane. (*Source:* Kaleida PH, Hoberman A. Otoendoscopic Examinations, Training Tape #3, Universal Health Communications, Inc: Boynton Beach, FL, 1994.)

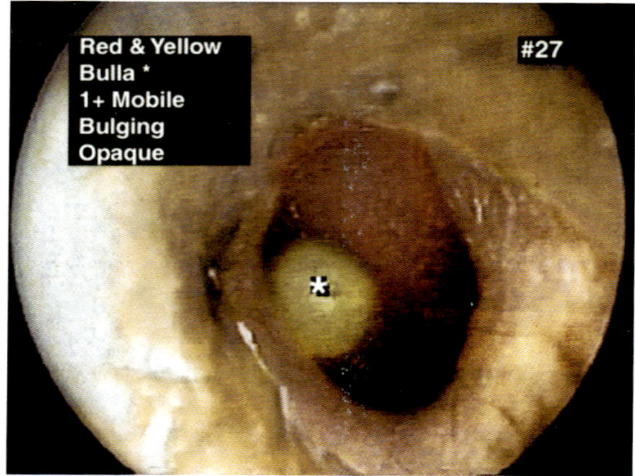

Figure 11.3 Bullous myringitis (acute otitis media). (*Source:* Kaleida PH, Hoberman A. Otoendoscopic Examinations, Training Tape #3, Universal Health Communications, Inc: Boynton Beach, FL, 1994.)

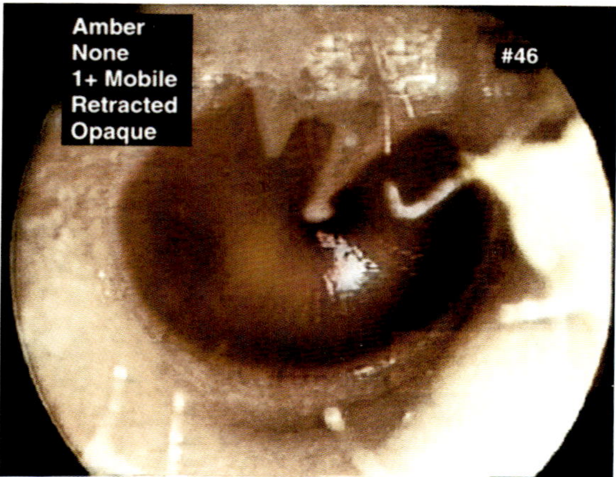

Figure 11.4 Amber, retracted tympanic membrane in otitis media with effusion. (*Source:* Kaleida PH, Hoberman A. Otoendoscopic Examinations, Training Tape #3, Universal Health Communications, Inc: Boynton Beach, FL, 1994.)

or infection of the middle ear. Filiaci and others (24) characterized the nasal anatomy using fiberoptic rhinoscopy in 35 subjects with chronic, purulent middle ear effusion. They also measured allergic sensitivity, rhinomanometry, mucociliary transport, and nasal response to histamine. Thirty-one of the affected individuals exhibited abnormal rhinoscopic findings. The authors concluded that a thorough assessment of the upper airway, particularly by rhinoscopy, is useful in patients with chronic middle-ear disease (24).

VI. USE IN OROPHARYNGEAL DISORDERS: EXAMINATION OF THE VOCAL CORDS

Laryngeal symptoms or signs are common in subjects who consult an allergist/immunologist. These laryngeal abnormalities or complaints may be the result of nasal disease or may emulate upper airway disorders. Examples of these laryngeal symptoms include "postnasal drip" with hoarseness, frequent clearing of the "throat," dryness and burning of the posterior pharynx, sensation of fullness or a foreign body in the throat, or cough. Indications for rhinoscopy to visualize the laryngeal pharynx are listed in Table 1.

Patients with GERD may also present to an allergist/immunologist. Gastroesophageal reflux is a very frequent cause of "throat clearing," hoarseness, sore throat, and chronic cough. Gastric contents regurgitating into the posterior pharynx cause erythema and edema of the mucosa overlying the arytenoid cartilages, which attach to the posterior vocal cords and articulate with the cricoid cartilage. The arytenoid-cricoid articulation provides the freedom for rotation of the vocal cords to open for respiration or to approximate with swallowing or speech. Erythema and edema of this anatomical area is often a physical sign of GERD. These findings are not specific for this disease, and a trial of antireflux therapy is indicated, or a further diagnostic work-up may be necessary to determine whether GERD is responsible for these complaints. A consultation with a gastroenterologist or a 24-h pH probe study may be helpful. The latter monitors and records the presence of acid in the distal and proximal esophagus to confirm reflux esophagitis.

VII. CONCLUSION

More than 25% of all individuals who seek medical care do so because of nasal and pharyngeal complaints. Fiberoptic rhinoscopy is a useful and cost-effective method by which potential diagnoses can be confirmed or eliminated. Most physicians are capable of learning this procedure and using it for better diagnosis to treat their patients with upper respiratory tract complaints.

VIII. SALIENT POINTS

1. Fiberoptic rhinoscopy is the best nonsurgical, nonradiographic technique available to examine the upper airway completely.
2. Twenty-five percent of all outpatient physician visits are for evaluation of upper airway complaints.
3. Fiberoptic rhinoscopy permits visualization of the nares, pharynx, and larynx, but this instrument does not permit biopsy or sampling of secretions.
4. The technique of fiberoptic rhinoscopy examination is relatively straightforward; however, experience and practice are necessary for the examiner to recognize significantly abnormal findings.
5. Diagnoses for which fiberoptic rhinoscopy is particularly useful include sinusitis, nasal polyposis, unilateral nasal obstruction, adenoiditis or adenoid hyperplasia, upper airway malignancy, vocal cord dysfunction, laryngitis, vocal cord nodules, dysphonia, vocal cord paralysis, and airway complications of gastroesophageal reflux.
6. Advantages of rhinoscopy compared to computerized tomography of the upper airway include reduced cost, more rapid availability of diagnostic information, and avoidance of radiation exposure.
7. Minimal topical anesthesia or no anesthesia is usually required for the procedure.
8. Almost every subject who is cooperative can be examined with a fiberoptic rhinoscope, particularly if the 3- or 4-mm diameter rhinoscope is used.
9. The rhinoscope must be cleaned and sterilized between examinations, but this process is simplified because the instrument does not have a port or orifice to retain secretions. Cleaning with soap and water followed by soaking in an appropriate sterilizing solution, such as 2–3% glutaraldehyde, is sufficient.
10. Most physicians, including generalists, are capable of learning and incorporating this useful, diagnostic procedure into their practice.

REFERENCES

1. Hocutt JE, Corey GA, Rodney WM. Nasolaryngoscopy for family physicians. Am Fam Practice 1990; 42: 1257–68.
2. Patton DD. Office procedures. Nasopharyngoscopy. Prim Care 1997; 24:359–374.
3. Singh V, Brockbank MJ, Todd GB. Flexible transnasal endoscopy: is local anesthetic necessary? J Laryngol Otol 1997; 111:616–8.

4. Selner JC, Dolen WK, Spofford B, Koepke JW. Rhinolaryngoscopy. 2d ed. Allergy Respiratory Institute of Colorado, Denver, CO, 1989.
5. Dolen WK, Selner JC. Upper airway endoscopy. In: Gershwin ME, Incaudo GA, eds. Diseases of the Sinuses, 1st ed. Totowa, NJ: Humana Press, 1996: 469–485.
6. Clerico DM. Sinus headaches reconsidered: referred cephalgia of rhinologic origin masquerading as refractory primary headaches. Headache 1995; 35:185–192.
7. Benninger MS. Nasal endoscopy: its role in office diagnosis. Am J Rhinol 1997; 11:177–180.
8. Ferguson BJ. Acute and chronic sinusitis. Postgrad Med 1995; 97:45–57.
9. Jorissen M. Recent trends in the diagnosis and treatment of sinusitis. Eur Radiol 1996; 6:170–176.
10. Blake P. The role of endoscopy and computed tomography in the diagnosis and treatment of sinusitis. N Z Med J 1994; 107:327–328.
11. Chow JM. The diagnosis and management of sinusitis. Compr Ther 1995; 21:74–79.
12. Mabry RL. Allergic and infective rhinosinusitis: differential diagnosis and interrelationship. Otolaryngol Head Neck Surg 1994; 111:335–339.
13. Lockey RF. Management of chronic sinusitis. Hosp Pract 1996; Mar 16:141–151.
14. Gwaltney JM, Jones DW, Kennedy DW. Medical management of sinusitis: educational goals and management guidelines. The international conference on sinus disease. Ann Otol Rhinol Laryngol Suppl 1995; 167:22–30.
15. Wang DY, Bernheim N, Kaufman L, Clement P. Assessment of adenoid size in children by fiberoptic examination. Clin Otolaryngol 1997; 22:172–177.
16. Nishioka GJ, Cook PR. Paranasal sinus disease in patients with cystic fibrosis. Otolaryngol Clin North Am 1996; 29:193–205.
17. Coste A, Gilain L, Roger G, Sebbagh G, Lenoir G, Manach Y, Peynegre R. Endoscopic and CT-scan evaluation of rhinosinusitis in cystic fibrosis. Rhinology 1995; 33:152–156.
18. Pownell PH, Minoli JJ, Rohrich RJ. Diagnostic nasal endoscopy. Plast Reconstr Surg 1997; 99:1451–1458.
19. Georgitis JW, Druce HM, Goldstein S, Meltzer EO, Okuda M, Selner JC, Schumacher MJ. Rhinopharyngolaryngoscopy. J Allergy Clin Immunol 1993; 91:961–962.
20. White PS, Maclennan AC, Connolly AAP, Crowther J, Bingham BJ. Analysis of CT scanning referrals for chronic rhinosinusitis. J Laryngol Otol 1996; 110:641–643.
21. Katz RM, Friedman S, Diament M, Siegel SC, Rachelefsky GS, Spector SL, Rohr AS, Schoettler J, Dorris A. Allergy Proc 1995; 16: 123–127.
22. Casellanos J, Axelrod D. Flexible fiberoptic rhinoscopy in the diagnosis of sinusitis. J Allergy Clin Immunol 1989; 83:91–94.
23. Bonifazi F, Bilo B, Antoniceli L, Bonetti MG. Rhinopharyngoscopy, computed tomography and magnetic resonance imaging. Allergy 1997; 52(suppl 33):28–31.
24. Filiaci F, Masieri S, Zambetti G, Orlando MP. Nasal hypersensitivity in purulent middle ear effusion. Allergol Immunopathol (Madr) 1997; 25:914.

11

Diagnostic Assessment of Otitis Media

Phillip H. Kaleida and Philip Fireman
University of Pittsburgh School of Medicine and Children's Hospital of Pittsburgh, Pittsburgh, Pennsylvania

I. INTRODUCTION

Otitis media (OM) is one of the most common conditions encountered by clinicians who deliver health care to children. From 1986 to 1987 alone, 31 million physician office visits in the United States were related to OM, with an estimated annual cost of at least $3.5 billion (1). Klein (2), citing a survey conducted by the Centers for Disease Control and Prevention (CDC), also noted the high occurrence of OM. It was the principal diagnosis for 24.5 million office visits in 1990. Moreover, in a recent report that analyzed data for both 1981 and 1988, Lanphear and colleagues (3) asserted that the prevalence of recurrent OM increased.

Otitis media varies in clinical expression, both in duration (from acute to chronic middle ear inflammation) and in intensity (from markedly symptomatic to asymptomatic). Acute OM (AOM, or suppurative OM) manifests as a concurrent or subsequent, frequently suppurative, middle ear inflammation that typically evolves from an upper respiratory tract infection (URI). Fever, otalgia, or both often accompany AOM. Recurrent AOM is present when a patient experiences repeated episodes of this acute process. Otitis media with effusion (OME, also referred to as serous OM, secretory OM, or nonsuppurative OM) refers to usually asymptomatic inflammation of the middle ear accompanied by fluid. It develops concurrently or follows URI. Both AOM and OME can cause hearing loss, which is usually conductive in nature and temporary in duration. Chronic OME refers to OME in which the effusion persists longer than 12 weeks.

Because most patients with OM have concomitant nasal inflammation, it is helpful to decide whether this inflammation (rhinitis) is infectious or allergic in nature. The differentiation between infection and perennial rhinitis can be difficult. Coexisting fever, malaise, acutely profuse or purulent rhinorrhea, pharyngitis, or exposure to family members or other individuals with similar acute symptoms would suggest infection. Recurrent or prolonged rhinitis with sneezing and pruritus of eyes, ears, nose, and throat suggests allergic rhinoconjunctivitis. Other allergic conditions associated with allergic rhinitis include atopic dermatitis, asthma, and a family history of allergic respiratory disease (4).

Risk factors for developing OM include URI, day care attendance, young age (the first 5–6 years after birth), and male gender (2). Some studies, but not others, have also implicated bottle-feeding of infants (i.e., breast-feeding may reduce risk) and passive exposure to tobacco smoke (5). Additionally, allergic rhinitis has been implicated as a potential risk factor in children with a history of OME and hearing loss of more than 5 months' duration (6). An individual patient's history and physical examination should help to distinguish the subgroup of children with recurrent or chronic OM for whom a suspicion of allergic rhinitis is high.

Despite the high prevalence of OM, accurate diagnosis of middle ear disease is often difficult and cannot rely entirely on the history or the general physical examination alone. Moreover, diagnosis tends to be most difficult in infants and young children, the group with the highest prevalence of OM. The U.S. Public Health Service's Agency for Health Care Policy and Research and the American Academy of Pediatrics both consider pneumatic otoscopy to be the preferred method for diagnosing middle ear effusion (7,8). In the Agency's Clinical Practice Guideline on OME in young children, otoscopy without insufflation is not recommended. This guideline also discusses tympanometry and audiometry as additional options during the diagnostic evaluation, and it recommends audiometry when bilateral OME has been present for at least 3 months (9).

This chapter will address the key elements of pneumatic otoscopy, including a helpful mnemonic for diagnosing and teaching. Tympanometry, audiometry (both behavioral and objective testing), and acoustic reflectometry are adjunctive tests that also will be discussed. This chapter will review these diagnostic methods as they apply to children, the population primarily affected by OM.

II. PREPARATION FOR OTOSCOPIC EXAMINATION

Before the otoscopist can perform examination or instrumentation of the ear, he or she must position the child properly. Cooperative and older children may be examined while they are sitting or lying alone on the examination table. Other children may be able to be examined while sitting unrestrained on a parent's lap. Younger children often need assistance. Such children can be examined in a sitting position, facing forward, on the parent's lap while being held against the parent's chest and shoulders. In this way the parent can control movement of the child's upper extremities and head with his or her arms and movement of the child's lower extremities with his or her knees. Mildly uncooperative younger children also may be able to be examined while the parent holds the child so that his or her head is facing first one and then the other shoulder of the parent. When a child is too uncooperative for these maneuvers, he or she may need to be restrained on the examination table. Such an infant can be examined in either the prone or supine position, with his or her head steadied against the table. Two adults should help to restrain the child, one holding the child's head and upper extremities and the other holding the child's buttocks and lower extremities. In this way, the examiner is free to stand between the adults to perform an examination, or a procedure, or both.

Once the child has been positioned properly, the otoscopist may need to remove obstructing cerumen from the external auditory canal. Usual methods of cerumen removal include the use of a curette or cotton-tipped applicator, gentle suction, use of cerumenolytics, and lavage with a dental irrigator or ear syringe. There are several key principles involved in the mechanical removal of cerumen by a blunt ear curette. First, a suitable curette should be selected. For infants and younger children, a size "00" or "0" is often needed. Second, the child must be adequately restrained to avoid instrument trauma. A common error is failure of the otoscopist to seek assistance for this purpose. Finally, the examiner should remove cerumen under direct visualization through either an operating head or the partially opened lens of a pneumatic head of an otoscope. A cotton-tipped applicator, either wet or dry, can be used to swab the ear canal. The otoscopist should be confident of the integrity of the tympanic membrane before using cerumenolytic otic drops, a dental irrigator, or an ear syringe. Additionally, when using the irrigator, the clinician should use warm water (37°C) and begin with the lowest water pressure settings.

After completing these preparations, the otoscopist is ready to examine the ear. Use of otoscopes, such as the Welch Allyn Model 20200 Pneumatic Otoscope (Welch Allyn, Skaneateles Falls, New York 13153-0220), is preferred.

III. THE "COMPLETES" MNEMONIC

Use of the "COMPLETES" mnemonic may facilitate one's own diagnostic examination and may prove to be a useful adjunct in instructing others how to perform pneumatic otoscopy (10). This mnemonic reminds the otoscopist to consider certain essential elements of the ear examination (Table 1). The **C** stands for the color of the tympanic membrane; **O**, for other conditions; **M**, for mobility; **P**, for position; **L**, for lighting; **E**, for entire surface; **T**, for translucency; **E**, for external ear; and **S**, for (pneumatic) seal. The mnemonic is intended primarily to remind otoscopists, particularly novices, of the specific tympanic membrane characteristics and other findings that should be assessed when determining the presence or absence of middle ear effusion. It does not specify the order of examination, because often the external ear is assessed first and the degree of tympanic membrane mobility is assessed last. The components of this mnemonic are described below.

C (*color*). The color of the tympanic membrane ranges from "pearly gray" to white, pale yellow, amber, pink, red, or blue. With the exception of pearly gray, each is usually suggestive of disease. However, a mild degree of injection, or even a pink hue, in an otherwise normal tympanic membrane, may be noted when a child is crying or after cerumen has been mechanically removed. An inexperienced otoscopist may sometimes confuse such mild injection, often localized to the region of the malleus, with early AOM without effusion.

A diffusely red, bulging eardrum is typical of AOM. Diffuse erythema of the tympanic membrane in AOM is not universal, however, as is illustrated by the predominantly pale yellow color of the tympanic membrane (see Fig. 11.1, color insert).

O (*other conditions*). When examining the tympanic membrane, one also searches for fluid levels, bubbles, perforations, otorrhea, bullae, tympanosclerosis, atrophic areas, retraction pockets, and cholesteatomas.

Figure 11.1 (color insert) also demonstrates air-fluid (pus) levels. Figure 11.2 (color insert) shows prominent tympanosclerosis and an atrophic area.

Cholesteatoma is uncommon in the general population, but it is important to recognize. It may appear as an intratympanic cyst, greasy-appearing white debris, or as a mass with or without an apparent perforation of the tympanic

Table 1 The "COMPLETES" Mnemonic

Color	Gray
	White
	Pale yellow
	Amber
	Pink
	Red
	Blue
Other conditions	Fluid level
	Bubbles
	Perforation
	Otorrhea
	Bullae
	Tympanosclerosis
	Atrophic area
	Retraction pocket
	Cholesteatoma
Mobility	4+, 3+, 2+, 1+, 0
	Hypermobile
Position	Full/bulging
	Neutral
	Retracted
Lighting	Halogen light source
	Fully charged battery
Entire surface	Anterior superior quadrant
	Anterior inferior quadrant
	Posterior superior quadrant
	Posterior inferior quadrant
Translucency	Translucent
	Opacified
External auditory canal and auricle	Deformed
	Displaced
	Inflamed
	Foreign body
Seal	Airtight pneumatic system
	Large enough speculum

Source: Ref 10.

membrane. Cholesteatoma may also present as chronic otorrhea, an important consideration when evaluating persistently draining ears. A clinician should consider cholesteatoma in the differential diagnosis whenever he or she observes a white mass at otoscopy and should promptly refer the patient to an otolaryngologist.

M (*mobility*). To assess the degree of mobility adequately, the otoscopist must first achieve an airtight seal. To do so, one should use the largest speculum that fits comfortably into the cartilaginous portion of the external auditory canal. Gentle intermittent pressure is then applied to the rubber pneumatic bulb. Use of a speculum that is too small may not permit satisfactory visualization of the tympanic membrane. In addition, such a speculum may contact the bony portion of the canal, causing pain (11).

Except in the presence of an obvious fluid level or bubbles, the degree of mobility is usually the single most significant physical finding in determining the presence or absence of a middle ear effusion. Mobility is conventionally categorized as 4+, 3+, 2+, 1+, none, or hypermobile, where 4+ represents normal mobility, and 3+, 2+, and 1+ represent decreasing degrees of mobility. One should observe the response of the tympanic membrane to both positive and negative pressure introduced by the intermittent squeezing and releasing of the pneumatic bulb. For example, when an eardrum is retracted, there may be greater mobility with negative pressure than with positive pressure. Middle ear effusion is the most common cause of impaired mobility of the tympanic membrane.

P (*position*). The position of the tympanic membrane ranges from full (or bulging) to neutral to retracted (in varying degrees). When the eardrum is retracted, the malleus may appear foreshortened and the lateral process may be prominent. In such cases, it may be helpful to break the pneumatic seal, compress the bulb, reinsert the speculum, and then release the bulb. This maneuver may cause a return of the eardrum toward the neutral position, facilitating assessment of mobility.

L (*lighting*). Before examining the child, it is important to confirm that the otoscope is functioning optimally. A bright (halogen) light source with a satisfactorily charged battery should provide proper illumination. If good illumination is not provided, the tympanic membrane may appear dull, discolored, or both, thus making the task of correct diagnosis even more difficult.

E (*entire surface*). It is important to attempt to visualize the entire surface of the tympanic membrane. Some of the most concerning problems, such as cholesteatomas and retraction pockets, can occur in the pars flaccida or the posterior-superior portion of the pars tensa. These areas of the eardrum may not ordinarily come into view unless the otoscopist makes an active effort to visualize them.

It is conventional to divide the tympanic membrane into four quadrants, each created by drawing an imaginary line through the long axis of the malleus and another intersecting perpendicular line through the umbo. These four quadrants are the anterior-superior, anterior-inferior, posterior-superior, and posterior-inferior. Such a designation may help to standardize localization of particular eardrum findings and thus facilitate verbal and written communication regarding them.

T (*translucency*). The otoscopist also should assess the translucency of the tympanic membrane, which may be described dichotomously as either translucent or opacified. Opacification of the eardrum suggests a greater likelihood of an abnormality (most often a middle ear effusion).

E (*external ear*). Examination of both the auricle and the external auditory canal should not be overlooked. The otoscopist should look for the presence of any deformity or displacement of the auricle, inflammation of the external auditory canal, foreign body, otorrhea, or other abnormal conditions.

S (*seal*). The last letter in the ''COMPLETES'' mnemonic, **S**, stands for (pneumatic) seal, as a reminder to the clinician to ensure an airtight seal within the external auditory canal during otoscopy. Before placing the speculum into the canal, the examiner should periodically assess the pneumatic system for an air leak. One way to accomplish this is to place a finger over the tip of the speculum and then squeeze the rubber bulb. Resistance to airflow should be encountered. Once the otoscopist actually inserts the speculum into the external auditory canal, it is essential to obtain a hermetic seal unless the tympanic membrane is not intact. A common error in the assessment of mobility, often leading to false-positive diagnoses, is the failure to obtain this airtight seal. Such failure is often attributable to the use of an inappropriately small speculum, a failure to insert the speculum far enough into the external auditory canal, or the presence of an air leak in the system. For many children, a 4-mm speculum will suffice. If an airtight seal is not achievable with standard specula, the use of a larger, soft-tipped speculum may prove helpful.

IV. "COMPT" AND THE DIAGNOSIS OF AOM AND OME

By using ''COMPT,'' a shortened version of the previous mnemonic, one can still pursue a systematic approach for the diagnosis of OM. The otoscopist examines the tympanic membrane for **C**olor, **O**ther conditions, **M**obility, **P**osition, and **T**ranslucency. As shown in Table 2, the presence of a pearly gray color (**C**), no other conditions (**O**), 4+ (or sometimes 3+) mobility (**M**), neutral position (**P**) and translucent appearance (**T**) suggests a low likelihood of middle ear effusion.

The presence of a red or pale yellow color (**C**), sometimes accompanied by a pus level, new-onset otorrhea through either a perforation or a tympanostomy tube, or bullae (**O**), decreased mobility (**M**), full or bulging position (**P**), and

Table 2 "COMPT" and the Diagnosis of Otitis Media

	Normal	AOM	OME
Color	Pearly gray	Red, pale yellow	Amber, blue
Other conditions	None	Fluid (pus) Perforation with otorrhea (new) Bullae	Fluid level Bubbles
Mobility	4+	0–3+	0–3+
Position	Neutral	Full, bulging	Retracted Neutral
Translucency	Translucent	Opacified	Opacified

Table does not include all possible findings or combinations of findings.
Source: Ref. 10.

opacification (**T**) suggests the diagnosis of AOM. Figure 11.3 (color insert) displays AOM presenting as bullous myringitis.

On the other hand, the presence of an amber or blue color (**C**), sometimes accompanied by a fluid level or bubbles (**O**), decreased mobility (**M**), retracted or neutral position (**P**), and opacification (**T**) suggests the diagnosis of OME. Figure 11.4 (color insert) displays an amber, retracted tympanic membrane typically seen in OME.

Finally, it is worth noting that there is frequently overlap in the clinical presentation of AOM and OME (12). Therefore, an individual child's physical findings are interpreted most meaningfully when combined with his or her history of present illness and past medical history (e.g., underlying medical conditions or history of recurrent or chronic OM). As noted previously, URI precedes or accompanies both AOM and OME in the majority of cases. The development of otalgia (ear rubbing or irritability in younger children), fever, or both suggests the diagnosis of AOM. It should be noted, however, that irritability is nonspecific and can be present with a URI that is not complicated by AOM. Similarly, fever also occurs in uncomplicated URI, but it is not present in all cases of AOM. On the other hand, OME is commonly asymptomatic, except when accompanied by perceived hearing loss. Hearing loss may be difficult for parents to appreciate and may be displayed only by apparent inattention or by increased television or radio volume.

V. TYMPANOMETRY

Tympanometry is a test that assesses tympanic membrane compliance (immittance) and middle ear pressure, and it has become an important diagnostic aid for the identification or confirmation of middle ear effusion. The tympanogram is the graphic display obtained by the use of an acoustic immittance instrument, which was formerly called an electroacoustic impedance bridge. Tympanometry varies the external auditory canal air pressure through a rubber seal that occludes the external auditory canal to create an airtight seal. Varying the applied canal air pressure from +200 to −400 or even −600 daPa alters the stiffness (position) of the tympanic membrane (Fig. 5). The abscissa of the tympanogram records air pressure in daPa (1 daPa equals 1.02 mm of water) and the ordinate of the tympanogram records tympanic membrane compliance. Tympanic membrane compliance is maximal when air pressure on both sides of the eardrum is equal. The normal tympanogram usually peaks at 0 daPa. If pressure within the middle ear is negative, the peak of the graph will lie in the negative pressure zone of

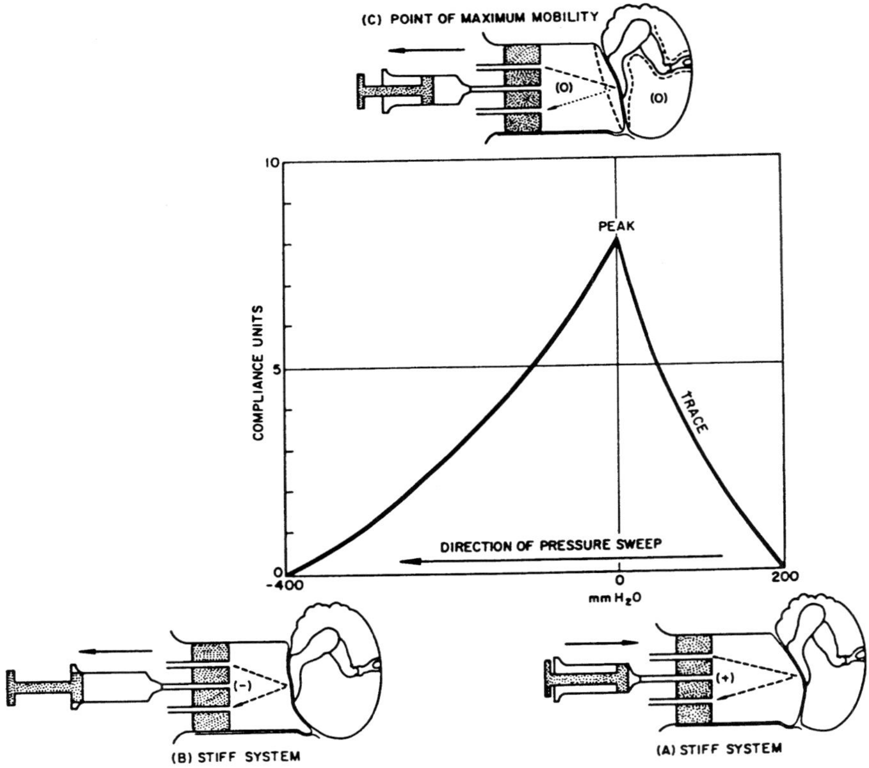

Figure 5 Tympanogram tracing. *daPa units now commonly used rather than mm H_2O (1 daPa equals 1.02 mm H_2O). (From Ref. 11.)

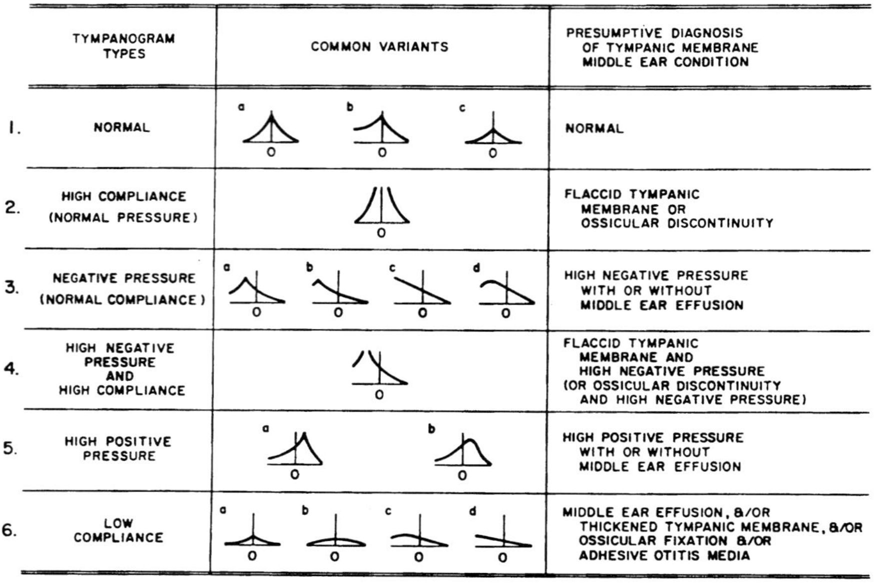

	TYMPANOGRAM TYPES	COMMON VARIANTS	PRESUMPTIVE DIAGNOSIS OF TYMPANIC MEMBRANE MIDDLE EAR CONDITION
1.	NORMAL	a 0, b 0, c 0	NORMAL
2.	HIGH COMPLIANCE (NORMAL PRESSURE)	0	FLACCID TYMPANIC MEMBRANE OR OSSICULAR DISCONTINUITY
3.	NEGATIVE PRESSURE (NORMAL COMPLIANCE)	a 0, b 0, c 0, d 0	HIGH NEGATIVE PRESSURE WITH OR WITHOUT MIDDLE EAR EFFUSION
4.	HIGH NEGATIVE PRESSURE AND HIGH COMPLIANCE	0	FLACCID TYMPANIC MEMBRANE AND HIGH NEGATIVE PRESSURE (OR OSSICULAR DISCONTINUITY AND HIGH NEGATIVE PRESSURE)
5.	HIGH POSITIVE PRESSURE	a 0, b 0	HIGH POSITIVE PRESSURE WITH OR WITHOUT MIDDLE EAR EFFUSION
6.	LOW COMPLIANCE	a 0, b 0, c 0, d 0	MIDDLE EAR EFFUSION, &/OR THICKENED TYMPANIC MEMBRANE, &/OR OSSICULAR FIXATION &/OR ADHESIVE OTITIS MEDIA

Figure 6 Tympanogram types and variants related to clinical findings. (From Ref. 11.)

the tympanogram. Thus, the peak of the tracing along the longitudinal axis is an indirect indication of the middle ear pressure. The height of the tympanogram is also evaluated because decreased tympanic membrane compliance (increased stiffness) will be manifest as a lower or absent peak.

Tympanometry offers a good means of identifying or confirming middle ear effusion, but it is not perfect. Figure 6 shows some of the types of tympanogram tracings that are seen in a variety of middle ear/tympanic membrane abnormalities. Normal variants with a high probability of no effusion are shown in panel 1. Panel 2 shows a graph that could be seen with a flaccid tympanic membrane. Negative pressure variants are shown in panel 3. Of these, the tympanogram with the sharp peak in 3a is less likely to have an effusion and the tympanogram with the blunted peak in 3d is more likely to have an effusion. The tympanograms with positive pressure in panel 5 can be seen in AOM, particularly variant 5b. All of the tympanogram variants shown in panel 6 are usually associated with a higher probability of a middle ear effusion, especially variants 6b, 6c, and 6d (13). Specific schemas are also available for classifying tympanograms that predict the probability of middle ear effusion (14,15).

Although pneumatic otoscopy and tympanometry essentially measure the same thing—tympanic membrane mobility or compliance—the strengths of one test can offset the weaknesses of the other. For example, pneumatic otoscopy gives a qualitative measure of tympanic membrane mobility, whereas tympanometry gives a quantitative measure of this variable. An algorithm based on the complementary nature of otoscopy and tympanometry has been constructed for the diagnosis of otitis media with effusion (16). Performing pneumatic otoscopy before or after tympanometry provides valuable information about ear anatomy and tympanic membrane mobility, facilitating interpretation of tympanometric results. For example, impacted cerumen, a foreign body, tympanic membrane perforation, medial canal stenosis, or improper placement of the instrument tip on the canal wall can cause false-positive tympanometry results (abnormal tympanograms in the absence of effusion). Accordingly, the Agency for Health Care Policy and Research Guideline recommends pneumatic otoscopy as the primary diagnostic test and tympanometry as an optional confirmatory test (17).

VI. ACOUSTIC REFLECTOMETRY

Acoustic reflectometry has been proposed as another adjunctive method for determining the presence or absence of middle ear effusion. In acoustic reflectometry, a device emits an 80-dB spectrum of sound into the external ear canal and then processes the sum of the resultant sound energy (18). Units range from 0–9. In infants and children more than 3 months of age, a numeric value of 6 or more is generally considered to be highly predictive of middle ear effusion (18). The procedure does not require an airtight seal in the external ear canal. Attention to proper technique, however, is essential because the device is very sensitive to user variability (18). The Clinical Practice Guidelines of the Agency for Health Care Policy and Research make "no recommendation" regarding the use of acoustic reflectometry as a screening or diagnostic test for OME (19). In a report published in 1994, Combs cites several studies and asserts that "acoustic reflectometry has been validated as an accurate method of testing for middle ear effusion in children and infants more than 3 months of age" (18). Others also note, however, that its validity and reliability is highly dependent on the way the test is performed (20). For these reasons, additional information is needed to clarify the role of acoustic reflectometry in the detection of middle ear effusion.

VII. ASSESSMENT OF HEARING

Hearing loss is the most prevalent complication and morbid outcome of OM, and one or more intra-aural complications or sequelae may cause it. Assessment of hearing in infants and children is not an accurate method for identifying the presence of middle ear effusion, but it can be valuable in determining the effect of middle ear disease on hearing function. Hearing assessment is also important in clinical decision making, particularly regarding the management of recurrent OM and chronic OME. For example, individual patients with OM should undergo evaluation if their hearing loss is suspected to be moderate to severe, persistent, sensorineural, or accompanied by other symptoms or signs. The Agency for Health Care Policy and Research Guideline recommends a hearing evaluation for children with persistent bilateral OME lasting for 3 months or more. The Guidelines consider earlier testing to be optional (21). To varying degrees, a fluctuating or persistent hearing deficit is frequently associated with otitis media. The audiogram usually reveals mild-to-moderate conductive hearing loss. When OME is present, the average air conduction threshold is 27-dB hearing level (22). Although unusual, sensorineural deficits may occur. Hearing loss may result from irreversible changes secondary to recurrent or chronic OM (e.g., adhesive otitis, tympanosclerosis, or ossicular discontinuity). Children younger than 2 years of age are the group at highest risk for middle ear effusion and associated hearing loss. In these patients, standard audiometric assessment may be difficult to perform. Nonetheless, properly trained and experienced audiologists can assess auditory function in children as young as 6 months of age (23).

All infants and children should have their hearing evaluated when recurrent OM or chronic bilateral middle ear effusion is present. The type of hearing loss (i.e., conductive, sensorineural, or both) and its degree will have a bearing on the selection and timing of the various management options available to the clinician. In general, there are two methods by which to evaluate hearing in children: behavioral and objective (nonbehavioral). The child's age, ability to cooperate, and level of cognitive function usually dictate the tests that are selected.

A. Behavioral Hearing Tests

Conventional audiometry, which requires a response such as raising one's hand, is usually reserved for children 5 years of age and older. Skilled audiologists can use it for certain younger children, depending on the cooperation and abilities of the child. The assessment should include pure-tone and speech audiometry to determine air and bone conduction thresholds to ascertain the type and degree of hearing loss for each ear.

Play audiometry can be used to assess the hearing of children 2 years of age and older and can occasionally be used in younger children. Play audiometry requires a child to display a conditioned response (such as putting a bead in a bottle) when he or she hears a sound. This interests the young child, and the test is usually conducted in the form of ''play.'' The assessment can provide information regarding both speech and pure-tone stimuli and can determine the degree of hearing loss for the individual ear. In addition, play audiometry can provide threshold information on both air and bone conduction and can determine whether a loss is conductive, sensorineural, or both.

Visual reinforcement audiometry (VRA) also involves the presentation of a stimulus sound and the observation of a child's conditioned head-turn response. The response, however, is rewarded by visual reinforcement, such as a blinking light, an illuminated picture or toy, or an animated toy that is located above the loudspeaker through which the stimulus is presented. The test is most successful for assessing infants aged 6 months to 2 years of age.

Behavioral observation audiometry (BOA) is a technique used for testing neonates and young infants. The examiner presents a stimulus sound and observes the child's associated behavioral response (startle, eye blink, eye widening, slight head turn, or arm and leg movement). It does not require conditioning. Simple noisemakers, such as rattles, squeak toys, and bells are common stimulus devices used in the office setting, but test booths in audiology centers use calibrated stimuli.

B. Objective (Nonbehavioral) Tests

The auditory brainstem response (ABR) is currently the best and most widely used method of the objective techniques available to assess hearing. It is a test that is relatively independent of the child's behavioral response and is used to evaluate infants and children for whom information on behavioral hearing tests is either unobtainable or unreliable.

Because excessive muscle activity can interfere with the test, the child must be completely relaxed or asleep. Natural sleep can be facilitated in babies up to about 6 months of age by feeding them immediately prior to the test. Children 7 years of age or older can lie quietly for the procedure. Infants and children between these ages, however, typically require sedation.

The ABR test can be valuable in identifying a conductive hearing loss associated with chronic middle ear effusion, especially in the young infant. However, the technique does not assess the perceptual event called "hearing." The ABR reflects auditory neural electric responses that are adequately correlated to behavioral hearing thresholds, but a normal result on the ABR only suggests that the auditory system up to the midbrain level is responsive to the stimulus used. It does not guarantee a normal behavioral response to sound.

In cases of middle ear impairment, the entire series of ABR waves is delayed by a length of time commensurate with the degree of attendant conductive hearing loss, and measurement of the latency of wave I provides a better index of middle ear impairment (24). The consistent nature of the ABR in young infants makes it particularly useful in the evaluation of hearing when chronic OME is present in this age group.

VIII. SUMMARY

Accurate diagnosis of OM is important but often difficult. To enhance the likelihood of accurate diagnosis, pneumatic otoscopy is the preferred method of examination generally available to clinicians. Findings by pneumatic otoscopy should be coupled with the presence or absence of symptoms and signs to delineate a diagnosis of AOM or OME. Tympanometry can be a useful adjunct in the clinical assessment of middle ear effusion. Audiometry is particularly important for patients with recurrent or chronic middle ear disease.

IX. SALIENT POINTS

1. Otitis media represents a spectrum of diseases that typically evolves from URI.
2. Other risk factors for developing OM include day care attendance, young age, male gender, perhaps bottle-feeding and passive exposure to tobacco smoke, and allergic rhinitis.
3. Careful clinical history and physical examination can help to distinguish AOM from OME and infectious rhinitis from allergic rhinitis.
4. Assessment of the degree of tympanic membrane mobility is *key* in determining the likelihood of middle ear effusion. Therefore, pneumatic otoscopy is strongly recommended as a routine part of the diagnostic evaluation of the ear.
5. Use of the COMPLETES mnemonic may prove helpful in diagnosing and teaching about OM.
6. Whenever a clinician observes a white mass at otoscopy, he or she should consider cholesteatoma in the differential diagnosis and should promptly refer the patient to an otolaryngologist.
7. Tympanometry is a useful adjunctive tool and diagnostic aid in the identification or confirmation of middle ear effusion.
8. Audiometry can be valuable in determining the effect of middle ear disease on hearing function, and it is important in clinical decision-making regarding the management of recurrent OM and chronic OME.
9. Children of any age can undergo assessment of the auditory system. Therefore, referral to a specialist should not be delayed if concerns regarding hearing are either suspected or apparent.

ACKNOWLEDGMENTS

The authors express gratitude to Clyde G. Smith, M.Sc., and Melanie G. Gettemy, M.A., for reviewing portions of this manuscript.

REFERENCES

1. Stool SE, Field MJ. The impact of otitis media. Pediatr Infect Dis J 1989; 8:S11–S14.
2. Klein JO. Lessons from recent studies on the epidemiology of otitis media. Pediatr Infect Dis J 1994; 13:1031–1034.
3. Lanphear BP, Byrd RS, Auinger P, Hall CB. Increasing prevalence of recurrent otitis media among children in the United States. Pediatrics 1997; 99:468.
4. Fireman P. Otitis media. In: Fireman P, Slavin RG, eds. Atlas of Allergies. 2nd ed. Baltimore: Mosby-Wolfe, 1996:179.
5. Agency for Health Care Policy and Research. Clinical Practice Guideline (No. 12): Otitis Media with Effusion in Young Children. U.S. Department of Health and Human Services, Public Health Service, Rockville, MD, July 1994, pp. 37–39.
6. Caffarelli C, Savini E, Giordano S, Gianlupi G, Cavagni G. Atopy in children with otitis media with effusion. Clin Exp Allergy 1998; 28:591–596.
7. Agency for Health Care Policy and Research. Clinical Practice Guideline (No. 12): Otitis Media with Effusion in Young Children. U.S. Department of Health and Human Services, Public Health Service, Rockville, MD, July 1994, pp. 30–32.
8. Clark G. New otitis media guidelines released. AAP News. American Academy of Pediatrics, Elk Grove Village, IL, July 1994, pp. 1,8,25.
9. Agency for Health Care Policy and Research. Clinical Practice Guideline (No. 12): Otitis Media with Effusion in Young Children. U.S. Department of Health and Human Services, Public Health Service, Rockville, MD, July 1994, pp. 32–36.
10. Kaleida PH. The COMPLETES exam for otitis. Contemp Pediatr 1997; 14:93–101.
11. Bluestone CD, Klein JO. Otitis Media in Infants and Children. 2nd ed. Philadelphia: WB Saunders, 1995:92–93.
12. Paradise JL. On classifying otitis media as suppurative or nonsuppurative, with a suggested clinical schema. J Pediatr 1987; 111:948–951.
13. Bluestone CD, Klein JO. Otitis Media in Infants and Children. 2nd ed. Philadelphia: WB Saunders, 1995:103–115.
14. Paradise JL, Smith CG, Bluestone CD. Tympanometric detection of middle ear effusion in infants and young children. Pediatrics 1976; 58:198–210.
15. Smith CG, Paradise JL, Young TI. Modified schema for classifying positive-pressure tympanograms. Pediatrics 1982; 69:351–354.
16. Cantekin EI, Bluestone CB, Fria TJ, Stool SE, Beery QC, Sabo DL. Identification of otitis media with effusion in children. Ann Otol Rhinol Laryngol 1980; 89:190–195.
17. Agency for Health Care Policy and Research. Clinical Practice Guideline (No. 12): Otitis Media with Effusion in Young Children. U.S. Department of Health and Human Services, Public Health Service, Rockville, MD, July 1994, pp. 30–34.
18. Combs JT. The diagnosis of otitis media: new techniques. Pediatr Infect Dis J 1994; 13:1039–1046.
19. Agency for Health Care Policy and Research. Clinical Practice Guideline (No. 12): Otitis Media with Effusion in Young Children. U.S. Department of Health and Human Services, Public Health Service, Rockville, MD, July 1994, pp. 34–35.
20. Van Cauwenberge PB, Dhooge I, Downs MP, Feagans LV, Gates GA, Karma P, Margolis RH, Marchisio P, Passali D, Renvall U, Stewart IA. Diagnosis and screen-

ing. In: Lim DJ, ed. Recent Advances in Otitis Media: Report of the Sixth Research Conference. St. Louis, MO: Annals Publishing Company, 1998; 107(Suppl. 174): 62.

21. Agency for Health Care Policy and Research. Clinical Practice Guideline (No. 12): Otitis Media with Effusion in Young Children. U.S. Department of Health and Human Services, Public Health Service, Rockville, MD, July 1994, pp. 35–36.
22. Fria TJ, Cantekin EI, Eichler JA. Hearing activity of children with otitis media with effusion. Arch Otolaryngol Head Neck Surg 1985; 111:10–16.
23. Bluestone CD, Klein JO. Otitis Media in Infants and Children. 2nd ed. Philadelphia: WB Saunders, 1995:117–122.
24. Fria, TJ, Sabo DL. Auditory brainstem responses in children with otitis media with effusion. Ann Otol Rhinol Laryngol 1980; 89(68):200–206.

ADDITIONAL READING

1. Cavanaugh RM. Pneumatic otoscopy in healthy full-term infants. Pediatrics 1987; 79: 520–523.
2. Cavanaugh RM. Obtaining a seal with otic specula: must we rely on an air of uncertainty? Pediatrics 1991; 87:114–116.
3. Clarke LR, Wiederhold ML, Gates GA. Quantitation of pneumatic otoscopy. Otolaryngol Head Neck Surg 1987; 96:119–124.
4. Eavey RD, Stool SE, Peckham GJ, Mitchell LR. How to examine the ear of the neonate. Clin Pediatr 1976; 15:338–341.
5. Kaleida PH, Stool SE. Assessment of otoscopists' accuracy regarding middle-ear effusion. AJDC 1992; 146:433–435.

12

Imaging of the Upper Airway and Sinuses

John A. Arrington
University of South Florida College of Medicine,
Tampa, Florida

I. INTRODUCTION

The diagnosis and treatment of inflammatory sinonasal disease has improved during the past 10–15 years. Understanding the normal mucociliary drainage of the paranasal sinuses and physiology of the sinonasal cavity and advances in the endoscopic evaluation of the sinonasal region has led to this improvement and to the evolution of functional endoscopic sinus surgery (FESS). The development of FESS and the need for a more detailed evaluation of the anatomy of the sinonasal cavity spurred the advancement of computed tomography (CT) of the nasal cavity and sinuses.

The clinician treating sinus disease needs a basic understanding of the pathology of inflammatory and infectious sinus disease, of the CT anatomy, and of FESS. A detailed description of the anatomy of the ostiomeatal complex (OMC) and the nasal cavity and paranasal sinuses is beyond the scope of this chapter, which has been written for the practicing physician. It is not intended to give an exhaustive list or detailed description of all pathological processes that can affect the sinonasal region, but it concentrates on the critical findings of the most common entities.

The key to the correct diagnosis and treatment of upper airway obstruction is the clinical evaluation. No advances or expertise in imaging can make up for a lack of understanding of clinical concepts. It is helpful to have a multidisciplinary approach to upper airway disease, with close communication among the subspecialties of allergy/immunology, otolaryngology, and radiology. The imaging component is critical to the overall care of these patients; however, it is important not to place too much importance or significance on these findings. Anatomical variants, mild mucosal thickening and small retention cysts are common CT findings, but may be normal variants and not clinically significant.

Imaging defines the anatomical location of abnormalities of the sinonasal region and helps categorize them; however, the importance of the CT findings can only be determined clinically. Imaging cannot result in a clinical or tissue diagnosis. For example, an early or small sinonasal carcinoma can mimic the findings of benign inflammatory disease (nasal polyposis or mucocele). Allergic and infectious sinusitis can coexist, and the CT appearance of these two diseases can be similar. This chapter will review the most common and expected sinusitis, nasal polyposis, and nasal carcinoma.

II. IMAGING OVERVIEW

Clinicians treating patients with sinusitis should be comfortable reviewing imaging studies. This requires an understanding of the following: anatomy of the ostiomeatal complex and paranasal sinuses, goals and limitations of imaging, findings of allergic and infectious sinusitis, patterns that help distinguish between inflammatory and neoplastic etiologies, and common complications of sinusitis.

Imaging modalities used for upper airway obstruction include radiographs, CT, and magnetic resonance imaging (MRI). Computed tomography is the mainstay of sinonasal cavity imaging because of its capacity to show detailed bony architecture, subtle osseous changes, and soft tissue abnormalities. The superior bone detail obtained with CT permits optimum evaluation of the ostiomeatal complex and osseous changes such as osteitis, osteomyelitis, or bone destruction. Computed tomography adequately displays the soft tissue component of both benign and malignant sinonasal disease.

Radiographs of the paranasal sinus are usually ordered either as a full sinus x-ray series, or limited to a Waters view. Screening CT of the sinuses has replaced radiographs in most institutions. Whereas mucosal abnormalities and air-fluid levels can be demonstrated on radiographs, the CT is more sensitive to detect minimal or mild mucosal disease as well as air-fluid levels. Computed tomography is superior to plain films in evaluating the bony walls of the sinus, because CT is more sensitive to detect mild bone thickening or early bone erosion. Whereas the bony anatomy of the ostiomeatal complex is best defined by coronal CT, if the clinical question is simply whether there is fluid in the maxillary sinus, a Waters view is the most cost effective study.

Magnetic resonance imaging is best viewed as a problem solver for complicated CT cases. The additional information gained with MRI includes the multiplanar anatomical display of benign and malignant soft tissue masses, evaluation of intracranial extension of sinonasal carcinomas, and estimation of the extent of tumor in the nasal cavity. Although the CT best defines and delineates bony destruction of the skull base, the contrast-enhanced MRI with multiplanar

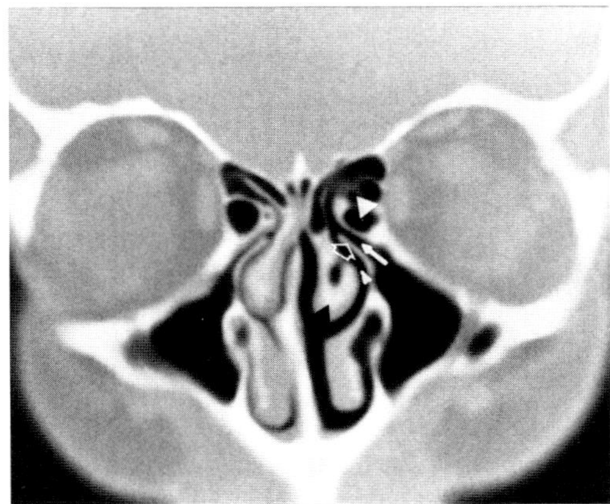

Case 1 Normal anatomy. Coronal CT scan demonstrates marked asymmetry of the right and left nasal airway and ostiomeatal complex. The right middle meatus and nasal airways are much smaller in comparison to the left, with some slight mucosal thickening in the infundibulum. The normal anatomy on the left is marked: ethmoidal bulla (*white arrowhead*), infundibulum of the left maxillary sinus (*white arrow*), uncinate process (*open white arrowhead*), middle turbinate (*black arrowhead*), middle meatus (*small white arrowhead*).

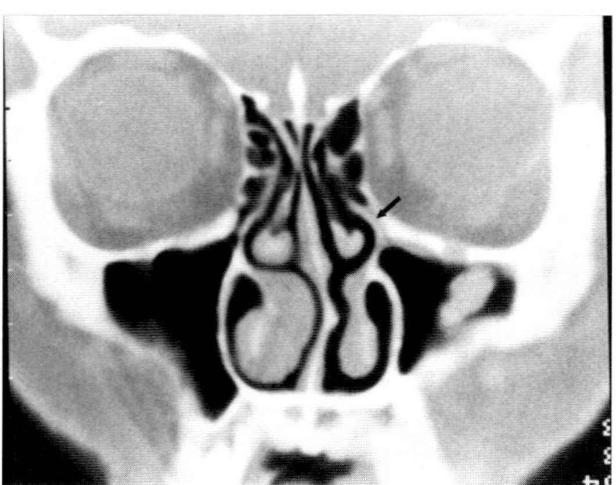

Case 2 Minimal mucosal disease. Coronal CT scan at the level of the ostiomeatal complex demonstrates soft tissue filling the infundibulum of the left maxillary sinus (*black arrow*). The infundibulum on the right is symmetrically narrow but is aerated. The middle meatus is well aerated bilaterally.

imaging is very helpful to stage the intracranial extension of the neoplasm. Magnetic resonance imaging can also be helpful to distinguish between carcinoma and inflamed mucosa in the sinonasal cavity. Therefore, otolaryngologists often obtain presurgical MRI studies as well as CT scans for patients with suspected sinonasal carcinoma to evaluate the tumor in the sagittal, coronal, and axial planes, to delineate any intracranial extension or subtle dural involvement and to estimate the extent of the tumor in the sinonasal cavity.

A basic understanding by the clinician of MR signal characteristics is necessary. Fluid on MRI typically has low signal intensity or grayness on T1-weighted images and high signal intensity or whiteness on T2-weighted images. Any process that increases water content will increase the signal on T2-weighted images. Inflamed or polypoid mucosa, retention cysts, secretions, and pus usually are high signal (white) on T2-weighted MRI images. When there is obstruction of a sinus, there can be signal changes in the secretions as they become inspissated. This is illustrated by case 18, in which the obstructed secretions in the right maxillary sinus show whiteness or increased signal. The fluid should have the same signal intensity (gray) as seen in the sphenoid sinus. Although not always reliable, neoplasms on T2-weighted images usually have low signal intensity (gray) as compared to the normal high signal intensity (white) of inflamed or thickened mucosa. Primary carcinomas of the sinonasal cavity, including squamous cell carcinoma, adenocarcinoma, sinonasal undifferentiated carcinoma, rhabdomyosarcoma, and lymphoma, all tend to have intermediate or low signal intensity on the T2-weighted images, whereas polypoid mucosa tends to have high signal intensity due to the increased or high water content of the inflamed mucosa.

This is illustrated in case 13 on the T2-weighted MR image. The squamous cell carcinoma is filling most of the maxillary sinus with extension into the nasal cavity and is seen as intermediate or gray signal intensity. There is inflamed mucosa along the lateral wall of the maxillary sinus, seen as increased signal or whiteness. The MRI can add additional information in selected cases about soft tissue processes. For example, review the axial MRI and axial CT in case 18. The medial wall of the right maxillary sinus is thinned and remodeled, bowing into the maxillary sinus. The thinned bony wall cannot be identified on the MRI, but is seen on CT. Different signal characteristics of the inverting papilloma and obstructive sinusitis are seen on the MRI.

Computed tomography in the coronal plane is the mainstay of imaging for upper airway obstruction and sinonasal disease. The small and detailed bony architecture of the nasal cavity and paranasal sinuses can best be visualized with CT and cannot be adequately evaluated with radiographs or MRI. Most radiology departments offer both limited coronal and axial sinus CT. A coronal scan is primarily indicated to define the anatomy of the ostiomeatal complex and to evaluate polypoid mucosal disease. It is cost competitive with the full sinus X-ray series. A limited axial CT scan is used for a follow-up, to help determine and document resolution, recurrence, or chronicity of a preexisting problem.

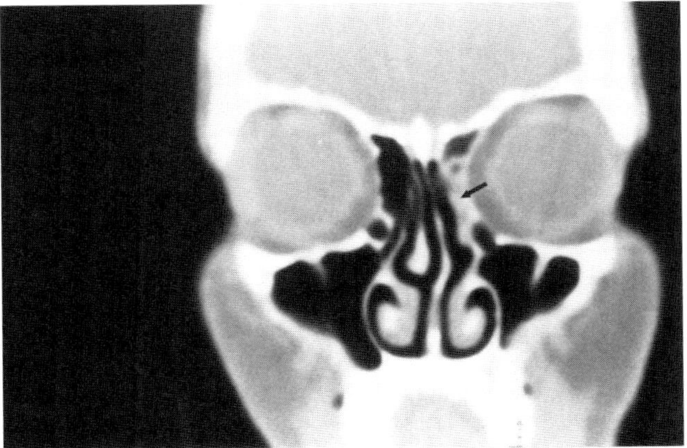

Case 3 Fibrosis with adhesions. Coronal CT scan at the level of the OCM demonstrates the left middle meatus to be adherent to the infundibulum with scar tissue in the left middle meatus. The complex of scar tissue, middle turbinate, and uncinate process is denoted by the black arrow.

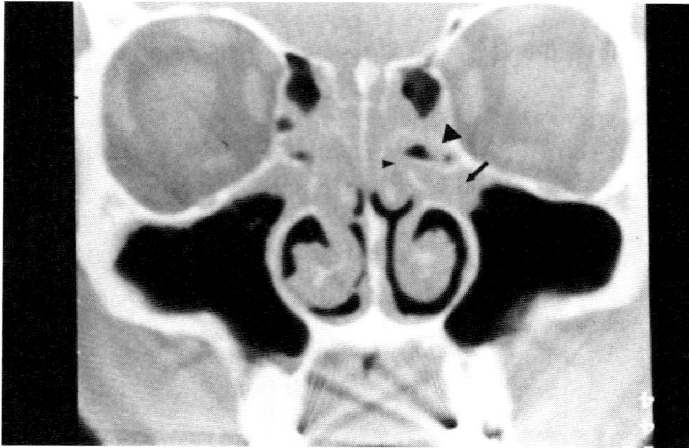

Case 4 Mild nasal polyposis. Coronal CT scan at the level of the OCM demonstrates symmetrical anterior ethmoidal air-cell disease and nasal polyposis involving the superior nasal cavity filling the middle meatus (*small black arrowhead*) and infundibulum of the left maxillary sinus (*black arrow*). Mucosal thickening within the left ethmoid bulla is also noted (*large black arrowhead*).

A. Ostiomeatal Complex

Although a detailed knowledge of the anatomy of the nasal airway and paranasal sinuses is mandatory for the radiologist, the clinician needs a basic understanding of the anatomy of the ostiomeatal complex (case 1). The clinician should be familiar with the following airways or passages: ostium of the maxillary sinus, infundibulum, middle meatus, and sphenoethmoid recess. The clinician should also be familiar with the following bony landmarks: nasal septum, middle turbinate, uncinate process, and ethmoidal bulla. Nasal septal deviation is a very fre-

---

Case 5 Unilateral anterior sinusitis. Coronal CT scans **(a, b)**, demonstrate complete opacification of the right maxillary sinus (*large arrow*), anterior ethmoidal air cells (*arrowhead*), and the nasal cavity including the middle meatus (*small arrow*). Scan a, which is more anterior, demonstrates the anterior ethmoidal air cell disease. Scan b, which is more posterior, demonstrates redundant or polypoid mucosa extending from the right maxillary antrum into the middle meatus (*open black arrowhead*). After treatment with antibiotics and nasal steroids, a 6-week follow-up CT scan **(c)** demonstrates complete resolution of the mucosal thickening and nasal polyposis. The bony architecture and detail of the ostiomeatal complex on the right is now well visualized.

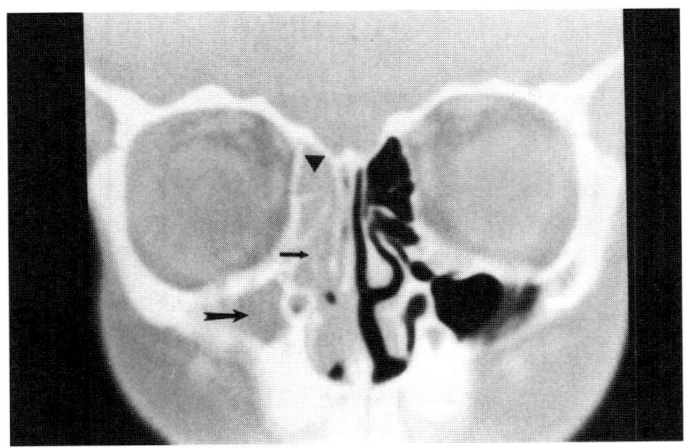

a

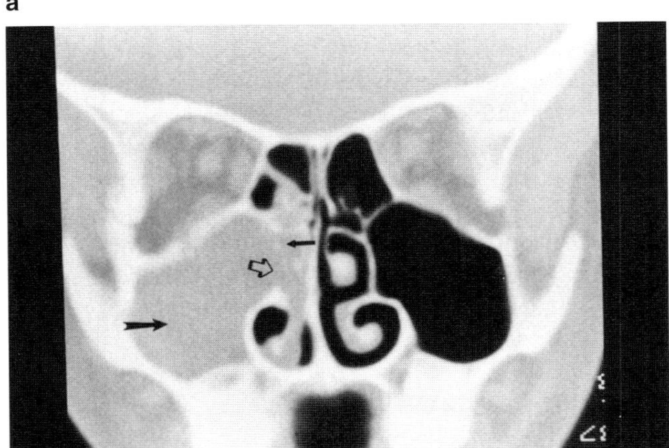

b

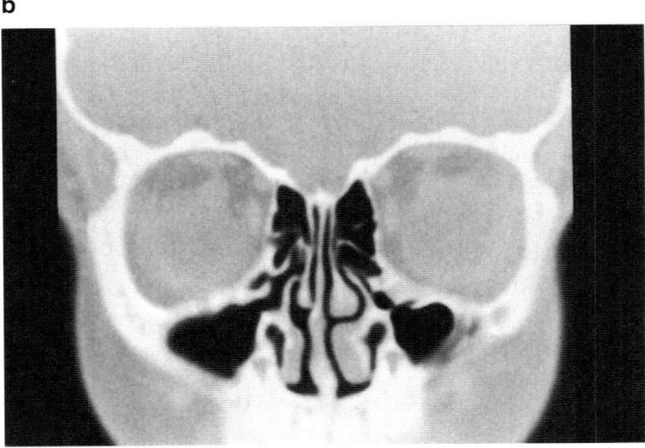

c

quent anatomical variant, which may include a septal spur. The middle and inferior turbinates are easily visible in all patients. However, the superior turbinate is very difficult to visualize in most CTs of the nasal cavity. Any lateral deviation or expansion of the middle turbinate with aeration (concha bullosa) can narrow the middle meatus.

The uncinate process can be deviated superiorly or laterally and can occlude the drainage of the maxillary sinus. It also can contain an ethmoidal air cell that can narrow both the infundibulum and the middle meatus. The ethmoidal bulla is the ethmoidal air cell at the level of the uncinate process or hiatus semilunaris. Anatomical variation in the size of this air cell can lead to expansion and narrowing of the hiatus semilunaris and infundibulum. The frontal sinus, anterior ethmoidal air cells, and maxillary sinuses all drain into the middle meatus. The frontal sinus drains into the middle meatus by way of the frontal recess. The anterior ethmoidal air cells have separate ostia that drain into the middle meatus. The maxillary sinus drains into the middle meatus through the ostium and infundibulum. Therefore, anatomical variants, mucosal disease, or soft tissue nasal masses that occlude the middle meatus can result in obstructive sinusitis affecting the frontal and maxillary sinuses and the anterior ethmoidal air cells.

The posterior ethmoid and sphenoid sinuses drain into the sphenoethmoid recess. The sphenoid sinus drains through an anterior wall ostium and the posterior ethmoid air cells have separate ostia. Any soft tissue mass or abnormality in the sphenoethmoid recess can obstruct the sphenoid sinus as well as the posterior ethmoidal air cells. The sphenoethmoid recess is occluded with soft tissue in case 14.

III. ACUTE AND CHRONIC SINUSITIS

The presence of an air-fluid level is considered to be one of the radiographic hallmarks of acute sinusitis. However, it is important to note that an air-fluid level is not pathognomonic of acute sinusitis. It can also be seen with trauma and in patients who have had their maxillary sinus lavaged. A CT is superior to radiographs to determine whether there is fluid in a sinus. A patient can have acute sinusitis without an air-fluid level noted on imaging studies. Imaging may demonstrate only smooth or irregular mucosal thickening of a sinus, which either can be present with active sinusitis or a nonspecific finding.

It is not always possible to distinguish between acute and chronic sinusitis radiographically. Mucosal thickening may be present with both acute and chronic sinusitis. An air-fluid level usually indicates acute sinusitis; however, such a finding is not present in all cases of acute sinusitis.

Chronic sinusitis represents either persistent or recurrent disease. Osteitis is seen as a thickening of the bony walls of the paranasal sinus and is best appreci-

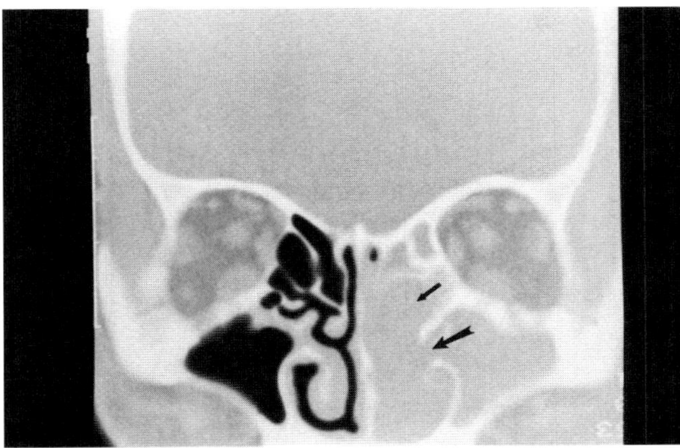

a

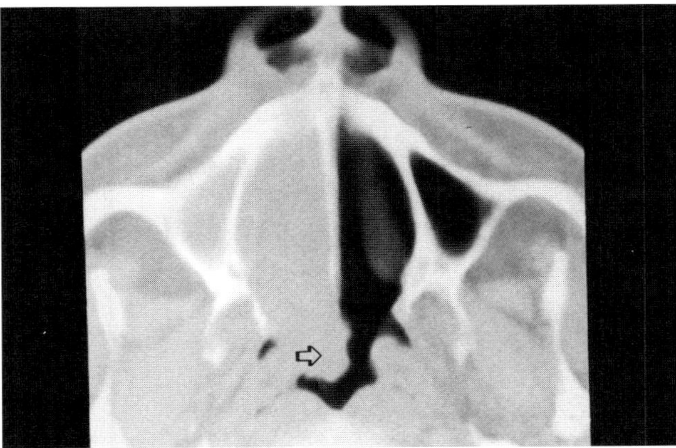

b

Case 6 Unilateral sinusitis with nasal polyposis. Coronal (**a**) and axial (**b**) CT images demonstrate extensive unilateral anterior sinus disease involving the ethmoidal air cells and maxillary sinus, as well as soft tissue density filling the entire nasal cavity, consistent with polyposis. The coronal scan demonstrates hyperplastic or polypoid mucosa extending from the ethmoidal air cell (*small arrow*) and the maxillary sinus (*large arrow*) into the nasal cavity. The axial image demonstrates complete filling of the nasal cavity by the polypoid mucosa, which extends into the nasopharynx posteriorly (*open arrowhead*).

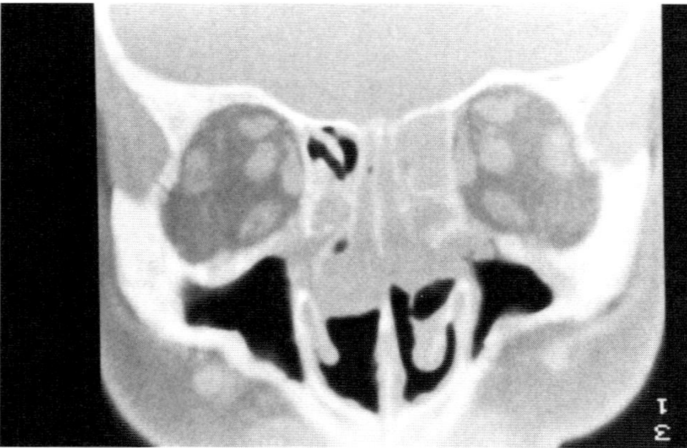

Case 7 Ethmoidal sinusitis with polyposis. Coronal CT at the level of the ostiomeatal complex demonstrates near-complete opacification and maxillary sinus, and a soft tissue density filling the entire nasal cavity consists of polyposis. No significant inflammatory changes are noted in the maxillary sinuses.

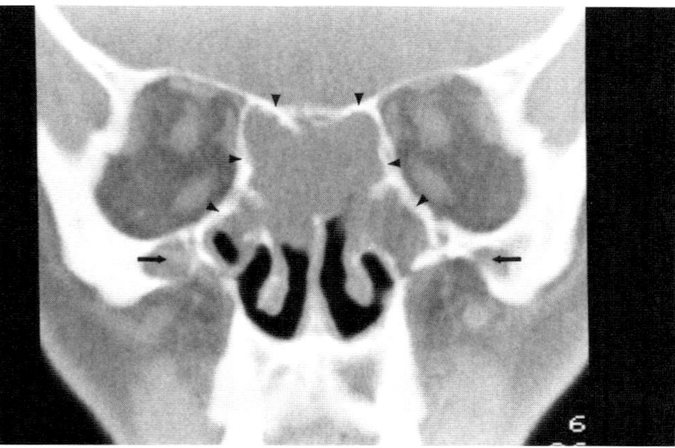

Case 8 Chronic ethmoid sinusitis with polyposis. Coronal CT scan at the level of the ostiomeatal complex demonstrates extensive soft tissue density filling the ethmoid bed. The patient had prior ethmoidectomy. There are also inflammatory changes of the maxillary sinuses. There is bony thickening of the lamina papyracea and cribriform plate, as well as the inferior orbital rim from chronic osteitis (*black arrowheads*). The maxillary sinuses have decreased volume and size from the chronic sinusitis (*black arrow*).

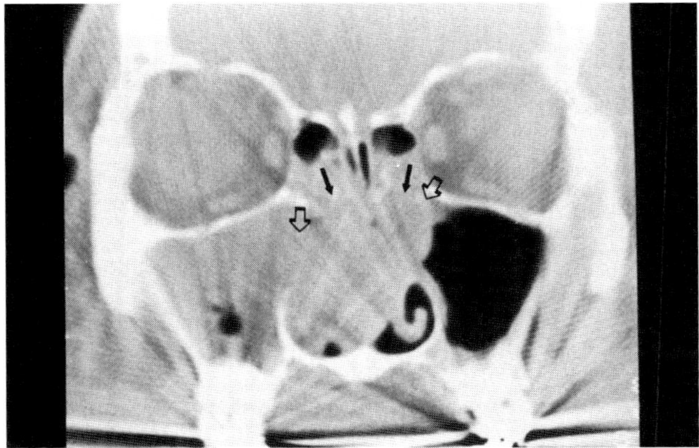

Case 9 Extensive nasal polyposis. Coronal CT at the level of the maxillary sinus and anterior ethmoidal air cells demonstrates extensive nasal soft tissue mass and right maxillary sinus opacification. There is extensive soft tissue filling the nasal cavity consistent with hyperplastic or polypoid mucosa. There is also extensive anterior ethmoidal and maxillary sinus disease. Note the confluent soft tissue extending from the maxillary sinuses (*open black arrowhead*) and the ethmoidal air cells (*black arrow*), which represents redundant or hyperplastic sinus mucosa prolapsing or extending into the nasal cavity.

ated on CT. It is a response to the chronically inflamed mucosa. The severity of the osteitis is related to the length of infection or the frequency of recurrence. In the maxillary sinus, severe osteitis and mucosal scarring can lead to a decrease in the size or volume of a sinus.

IV. FUNGAL SINUSITIS

Fungal sinusitis has a wide spectrum of clinical and imaging findings. The clinician must always be on the lookout for the possibility of a fungal infection, especially in the immunocompromised patient. Early diagnosis is critical in immunocompromised patients because mycotic infections can have an extremely fulminant course and may quickly extend from the paranasal sinus into the orbit, cavernous sinus, and brain.

The imaging findings of early fungal infection are nonspecific and include inflamed nasal and sinus mucosa. The mucoperiosteal thickening may be smooth or nodular. Air-fluid levels are rare with mycotic infections. As the infection progresses, bony walls of the sinus can thicken, but this also is a nonspecific finding frequently seen with chronic sinusitis. There are radiographic findings,

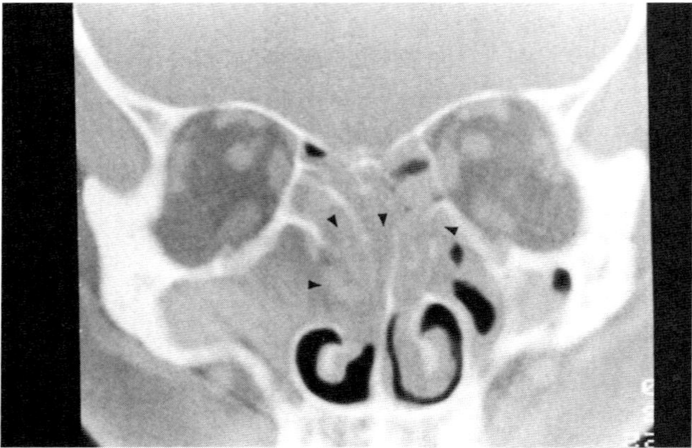

Case 10 Extensive pansinusitis and nasal polyposis. Coronal CT scan at the level of the ostiomeatal complex demonstrates extensive soft tissue changes with soft tissue density or masses filling the right maxillary and ethmoidal air cells with near complete opacification of the left maxillary sinus. There is associated soft tissue density or mass within both right and left nasal cavities. Note the extensive confluent soft tissue density between the nasal polyposis and the hyperplastic or redundant sinus mucosa (*small black arrowheads*).

however, that are red flags for the presence of mycotic infection. Bony changes such as expansion, remodeling, or erosion of a sinus raises the possibility of a fungal infection. These bony changes can also be seen with bacterial infections, mucoceles, or pyomucoceles. Atypical CT density and an atypical MRI signal also raise the possibility of fungal sinusitis. Inflamed mucosa typically follows water signal characteristics on MRI studies. Inflamed mucosa results in a decreased signal (gray) on T1- and increased signal (white) on T2-weighed MR images due to the increased water content of the inflamed mucosa. Increased case density within a sinus cavity on noncontrast CT scans (Case 14) is atypical and raises the possibility of a mycotic infection. Atypical mucosal signal changes include increased signal (white) or very decreased signal (black) on T2-weighted images as well as very decreased signal (black) on T2-weighted images. These CT and MRI findings are due to the presence of trace elements and heavy metals (calcium, iron, manganese, and magnesium) that are essential to fungal metabolism. These findings, however, are also nonspecific and can be seen with dystrophic calcification and inspissated secretions. Although there are no pathognomonic imaging findings of fungal infection, bony erosion and atypical CT density or MRI signal in the paranasal sinus must be viewed as red flags and should be considered evidence of a mycotic infection until ruled out clinically. The immunocompromised patient must be treated differently. Even the most minimal

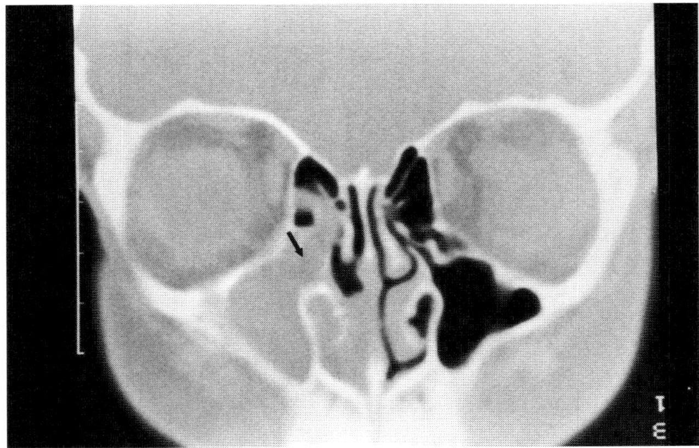

a

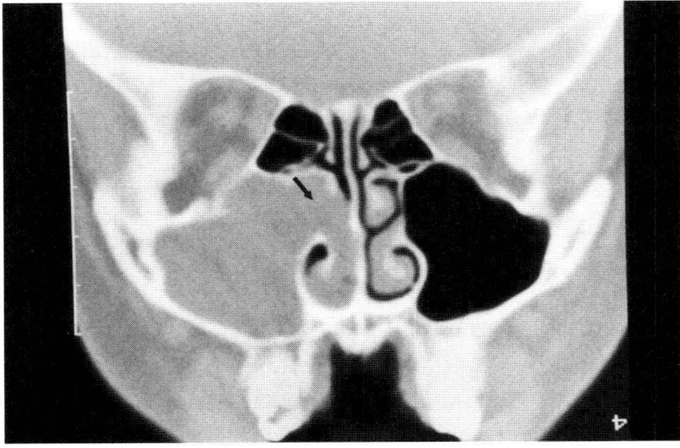

b

Case 11 Antrachoanal polyp. Coronal CT scans **(a, b)** were obtained at the level of the OCM **(a)** and posterior to the OCM **(b)**. These scans demonstrate complete opacification of the right maxillary sinus with extension of the soft tissue mass into the right nasal cavity consistent with an antrachoanal polyp.

changes of bone erosion or atypical imaging findings must alert the radiologist and clinician to the possibility of a mycotic infection.

A. Complications of Sinusitis

The complications of sinusitis essentially represent the extension of the infection beyond the sinus mucosa. An abbreviated list includes osteomyelitis, orbital in-

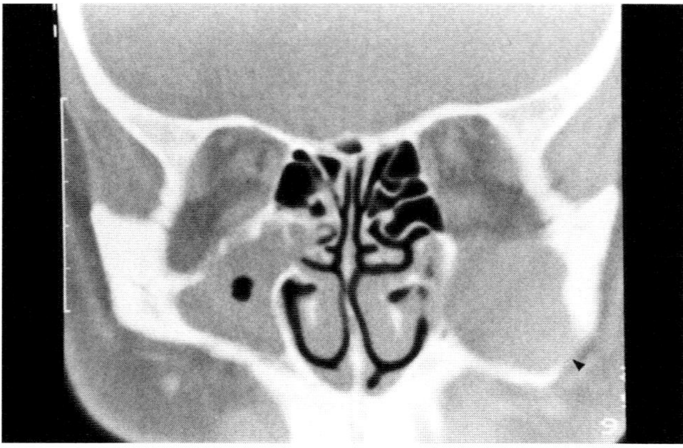

a

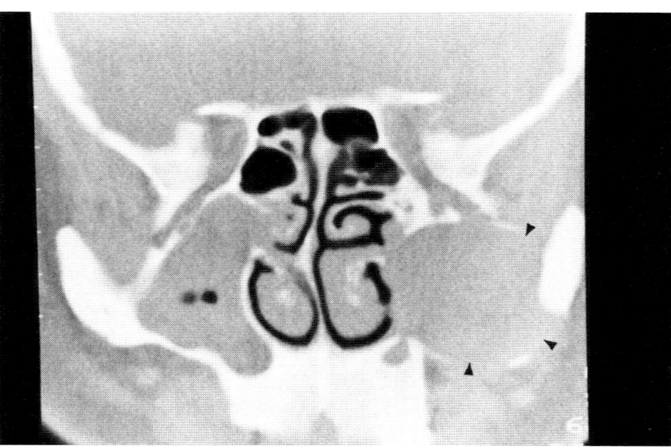

b

Case 12 Sinusitis with mucocele. Coronal CT scan **(a, b)** demonstrates bilateral maxillary sinus disease with some inflammatory soft tissue changes in the ostiomeatal complex, greater on the right. The expansion and bony erosion (*black arrowheads*) of the walls of the left maxillary sinus represents a mucocele.

Case 13 Squamous cell carcinoma of the maxillary sinus. Consecutive coronal sinus CT scans **(a, b)** demonstrate complete opacification of the maxillary sinuses with soft tissue extending into the nasal cavity. There is mild anterior ethmoidal air cell disease. There is bony erosion of the floor of the right orbit (*arrowheads*). A T2-weighted coronal MRI **(c)** demonstrates a difference in signal intensities between inflamed mucosa and carcinoma. The squamous cell carcinoma is gray or has lower signal intensity (*large arrow*) in comparison to the high signal intensity or white inflamed mucosa (*small arrow*).

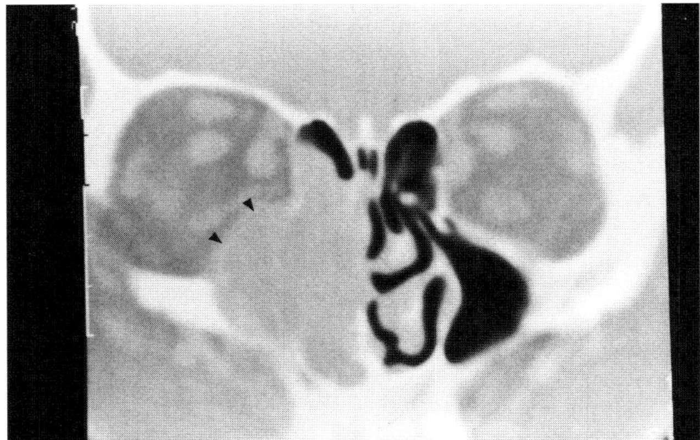

a

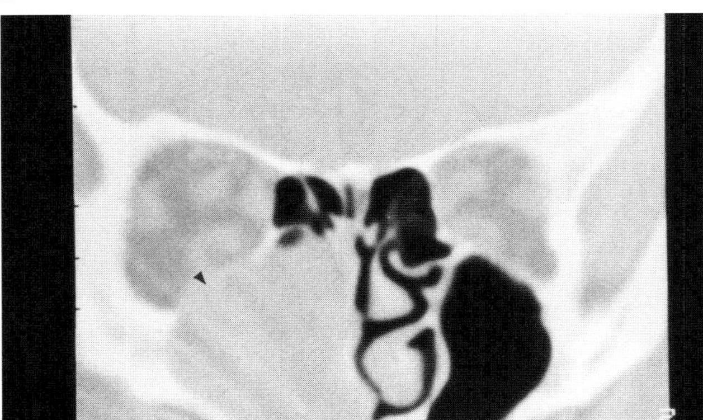

b

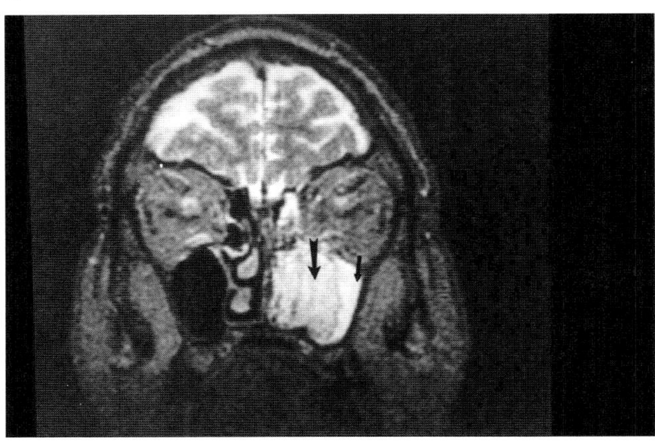

c

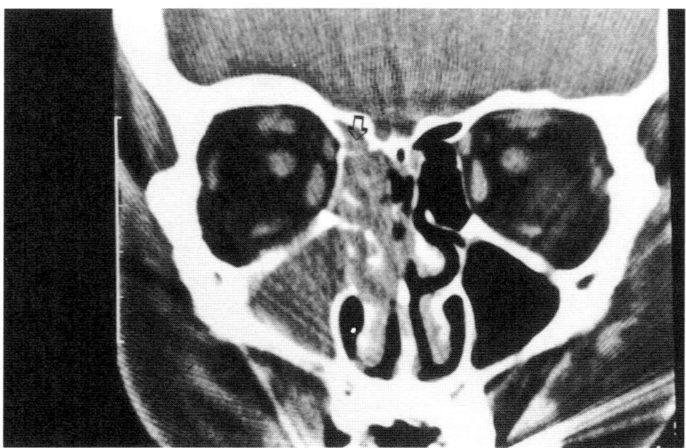

a

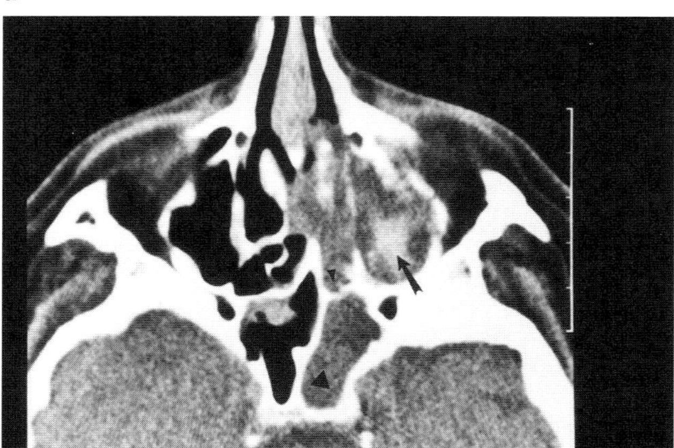

b

Case 14 Aspergillus sinusitis. Coronal CT scan at the level of the ostiomeatal complex (**a**) demonstrates extensive anterior sinus disease. There is opacification of the right frontal sinus and frontal recess (*open arrowhead*), and opacification of anterior ethmoidal air cells in the right maxillary sinus and associated nasal soft tissue inflammation. The axial scan (**b**) demonstrates involvement of the sphenoid sinus (*large arrowhead*), and an abnormal soft tissue density filling the sphenoethmoidal recess (*small arrowhead*). Increased density is noted in the maxillary sinus (*black arrow*) indicating the *Aspergillus* superinfection.

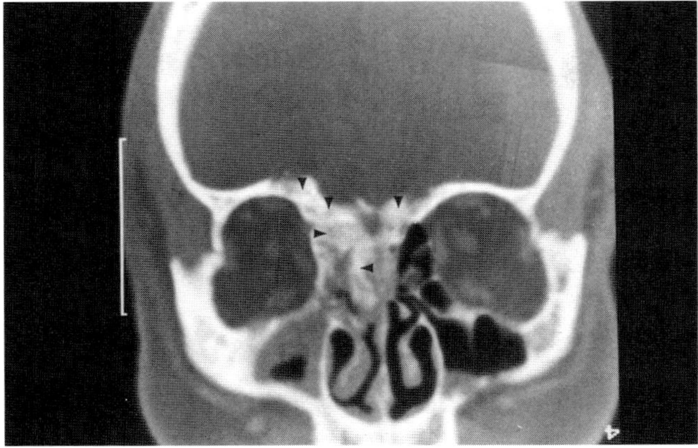

Case 15 Invasive meningioma. Coronal noncontrast CT scan demonstrates extensive bony changes of the anterior cranial fossa and right nasal cavity with hyperostosis of the roof of the right orbit, cribriform plate, lamina papyracea, and right middle turbinate (*arrowheads*). There is associated abnormal soft tissue density extending from the subfrontal intracranial region through the cribriform plate into the superior nasal cavity.

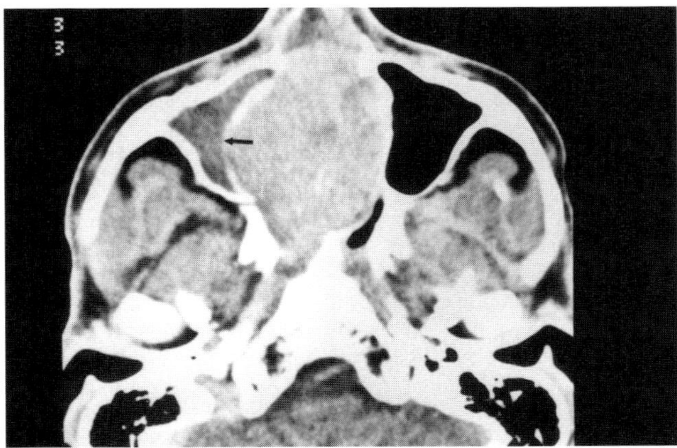

Case 16 Rhabdomyosarcoma. Axial CT scan at the level of the inferior maxillary sinus and nasal cavity demonstrates a large soft tissue mass filling the nasal cavity, with more extensive soft tissue on the right extending posteriorly and anteriorly. There is associated obstructive sinusitis of the right maxillary sinus with bony remodeling of the medial wall of the right maxillary sinus (*arrow*).

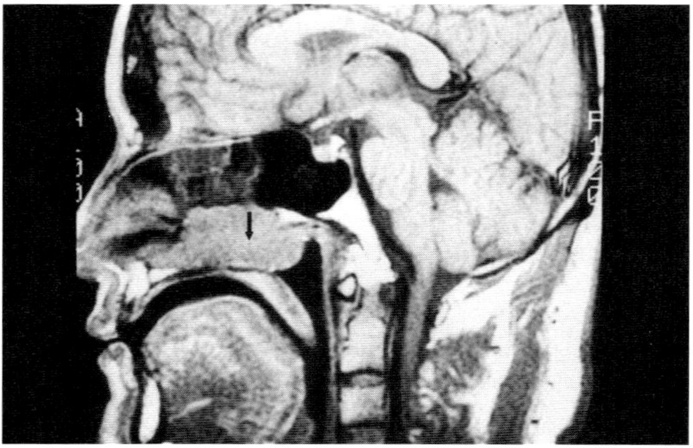

a

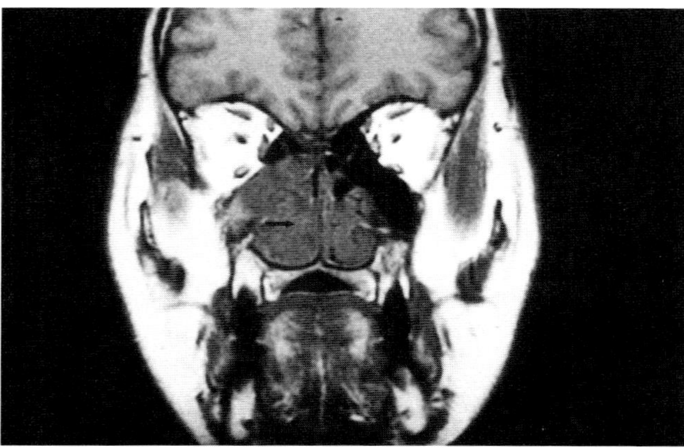

b

Case 17 Lymphoma. T1-weighted sagittal (**a**) and coronal (**b**) MRI images demonstrate a right-sided nasal mass (*arrow*) with associated soft tissue mass or opacification of the right maxillary sinus and some ethmoidal air cells. The nasal mass represents a lymphoma with associated sinusitis of the right maxillary and some ethmoidal air cells.

fection (cellulitis or abscess), and intracranial infection (meningitis, subdural abscess, cerebritis, and cerebral abscess). Clinicians must be sensitive to the onset of orbital or intracranial symptoms in their sinusitis patients. If orbital or intracranial symptoms are present, imaging of the orbit or brain is indicated. When imaging a sinusitis patient with suspected orbital complications, CT is superior to MRI. Computed tomography is necessary to evaluate for subtle or significant bone erosion and adequately demonstrates intraorbital extension of infection or abscess. When intracranial extension is suspected, MRI is the superior modality. It is more sensitive in the evaluation of venous thrombosis and cavernous sinus thrombosis and far superior to CT in the evaluation of meningeal and subtle subdural pathology. Meningitis that is seen as smooth or nodular meningeal enhancement on MRI cannot be easily identified with CT. Also, small and early subdural empyemas are better demonstrated with MRI than CT. Patients with intracranial extension demonstrated on MRI may also need a CT scan to adequately evaluate the bony wall of a sinus and to determine clearly the extent of any bone destruction.

V. IMAGING SPECTRUM OF MUCOSAL DISEASE

Complete opacification of a sinus can result from mucosal thickening, hyperplastic or polypoid mucosa, secretions, fluid, benign or malignant mass, or a combination of these findings.

Cases 1 and 2 illustrate that only slight or minimal mucosal thickening can occlude the drainage pathways of the sinus or airway. In case 1, with only minimal mucosal thickening in the infundibulum, there is marked narrowing of the right infundibulum. There is some nasal septal deviation to the right and lateral deviation of the right middle turbinate, which also causes marked narrowing of the right middle meatus. Therefore, with only two slight anatomical variants (septal deviation and middle turbinate deviation) and minimal mucosal thickening, there is significant asymmetry in the size or aeration of the ostiomeatal complex.

With mucosal thickening, there may be apposition of mucosa surfaces. Mucosal apposition in the infundibulum is illustrated in case 2. In this case, mucosal thickening completely occludes the infundibulum and ostium of the left maxillary sinus, blocking its normal drainage. Secondary ostia of the maxillary sinus are common variants but are difficult to visualize with imaging. With chronic recurrent inflammatory disease in the middle meatus, scarring and granulation tissue can occur, and adhesions between mucosal surfaces can develop. Case 3 demonstrates a confluence of the infundibulum, scarred mucosa, and middle turbinate on the left occluding the left middle meatus and the left infundibulum. A normal right uncinate process and middle turbinate and a normally aerated right infundibulum and right middle meatus are seen.

When imaging the paranasal sinuses, the major focus is on the ostiomeatal complex, nasal airways, and the paranasal sinuses. However, one must always evaluate carefully the nasal septum for abnormalities, which can present with nasal obstruction. Septal defects that can be seen with cocaine abuse are readily identified on CT. Case 19 demonstrates the low attenuation appearance of a septal abscess in a patient without sinusitis.

VI. IMAGING OF POLYPS

As the mucosa becomes inflamed, it is seen as a soft tissue density on CT. When the mucosa becomes redundant or polypoid, it appears more mass-like on CT. Case 4 demonstrates mild-to-moderate-size nasal polyps with abnormal soft tissue filling the superior nasal cavity, the middle meatus, and the nasal airway between the nasal septum and middle turbinate. There is mucosal disease in the infundibulum of both right and left maxillary sinuses and the ethmoidal air cells. Cases 5 through 11 demonstrate progressively worse or more extensive inflammatory sinonasal disease with more extensive nasal polyposis. The nasal polyposis is usually the result of inflamed, hyperplastic, or redundant nasal mucosa. However, with extensive inflammatory changes in the paranasal sinus, the hyperplastic or redundant mucosa can extend from the sinus into the nasal cavity. Polyps usually originate from the anterior ethmoidal air cells. The bony architecture and detail of the nasal cavity and ostiomeatal complex become very poorly defined as nasal mucosal thickening or polyps increase in size. Compare cases 1 and 2 to cases 4 through 10. Note that in case 4, with minimal nasal polyps, there is very poor visualization of the middle turbinate, and the uncinate process cannot be seen. Also, the bony septa of the ethmoidal air cells are not well visualized. In cases 6, 7, 9, and 10, even larger bony structures, such as the nasal septum and medial wall of the maxillary sinus, appear incomplete or indistinct. The lack of visualization or apparent bony erosion of these structures is due to demineralization of these osseous structures from pressure caused by the polyps. In case 5, on the pretreatment scans a and b, the middle turbinate and infundibulum of the right maxillary sinus cannot be clearly identified; however, on the posttreatment scan c, the uncinate process and middle turbinate are visualized. Note that the infundibulum of the right maxillary sinus appears larger than the left on the posttreatment scan c. Cases 7 and 8 have a similar appearance. In case 7, the normal bony septae of the ethmoidal air cells are poorly visualized due to bony demineralization from the extensive polyps or hypertrophied nasal mucosa. The patient in case 8 had a prior ethmoidectomy with surgical removal of the normal septations of the ethmoid air cells.

VII. IMAGING OF BENIGN AND MALIGNANT SOFT TISSUE AND OSSEOUS CHANGES

Long-standing inflammatory changes of the mucosa of a sinus can cause chronic osteitis or thickening of the bony walls of the sinus. This is due to the chronic inflammation of the mucoperiosteum. With severe chronic sinusitis, the maxillary sinuses can become quite small and lose volume due to a combination of the osteitis and mucosal scarring. This is illustrated in case 8. Osteitis is also illus-

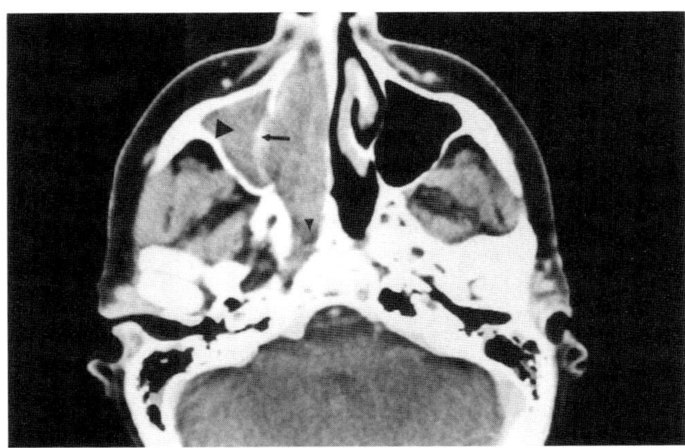

a

b

Case 18 Inverting papilloma. Axial CT scan **(a)** and axial T1-weighted MRI **(b)** demonstrates a right-sided nasal mass that is extending the full length of the nasal cavity and into the sphenoethmoid recess and superior nasopharynx (*small arrowheads*). There is associated obstructive sinusitis of the right maxillary sinus (*large arrowhead*) and sphenoid (*large arrow*) sinus. Note the bowing or bony remodeling of the medial wall of the right maxillary sinus (*small arrow*).

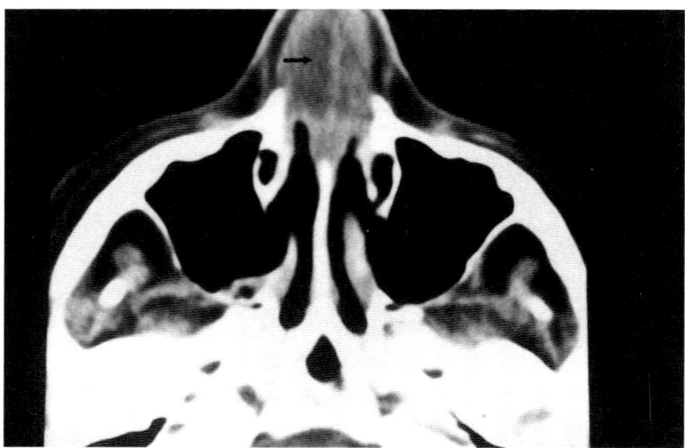

Case 19 Septal abscess. Axial CT scan at the level of the nasal septum and mid-maxillary sinus demonstrates a soft tissue mass in the anterior nasal cavity (*arrowhead*), which is slightly larger on the right with low attenuation on the CT scan representing fluid (*arrow*).

trated in case 8, with bony thickening of the cribriform plate and skull base and the medial and inferior walls of the orbits. The osteitis involves both the right and left maxillary sinuses symmetrically.

In rare cases, osteitis can be confused with an invasive cribriform plate meningioma. This is illustrated in case 15, in which a meningioma extends from the subfrontal intracranial space through the cribriform plate and into the superior nasal cavity. The meningioma has caused a hyperostosis response by the skull base and cribriform plate and the middle turbinate.

Symmetrical pansinusitis with or without nasal polyps is the usual expectation when imaging allergic sinusitis. Cases 4 and 10 are the more common and expected appearance for mild (case 4) and extensive (case 10) allergic rhinitis and polyposis. However, unilateral sinusitis and nasal polyposis can occur, as illustrated in cases 5 and 6. Case 5 shows resolution of the inflammatory and hyperplastic changes with 6 weeks of treatment. When nasal polyps are unilateral, the appearance mimics both benign (inverting papilloma or angiofibroma) or malignant nasal masses (squamous cell carcinoma, sinonasal undifferentiating carcinoma, or lymphoma). The axial CT findings in cases 6, 16, and 18 are very similar except for the size of the soft tissue mass. Note that in all three cases, there is bowing of the medial wall of the maxillary sinus and obstructive sinusitis in the ipsilateral maxillary sinus. Carcinoma cannot be excluded, even when there is a more benign appearance to the bony changes (remodeling or pressure erosion). All three cases denote some bowing and bony remodeling of the maxillary sinus without gross bony destruction, and the diagnosis varies from polyposis to inverting papilloma to rhabdomyosarcoma.

This point is also illustrated in comparing cases 12 and 13. Case 12 illustrates mucocele formation of the left maxillary sinus, whereas case 13 represents a squamous cell carcinoma of the right maxillary sinus. In both cases, there is a soft tissue mass filling the maxillary sinus with bony changes. The mucocele has expanded the maxillary sinus, and there is thinning of much of the sinus wall and bony destruction or bony defects as noted. In the case of the squamous cell carcinoma, there is also expansion of the sinus with bony destruction of the floor of the right orbit. In these two cases, both a benign and a malignant process have similar CT appearance. Therefore, it is important never to rely solely on a CT appearance to distinguish a benign from malignant process. Whenever bone destruction or bone erosion is present, carcinoma should be considered. Carcinoma and inflammatory sinus disease can, and frequently do, coexist. If the process completely clears with treatment, as seen in case 5, then biopsy can be avoided. To reiterate, any suspicious CT finding must be followed up until resolution to completely rule out a neoplasm.

VIII. SUMMARY

Before imaging the sinusitis patient, the clinican needs to establish diagnostic goals and be aware of the limitations of imaging. When reviewing imaging studies of the paranasal sinuses, the clinican needs a basic understanding of the anatomy of the ostiomeatal complex and sinonasal cavity, the common anatomical variants, and the typical appearances of inflammatory, infectious, and neoplastic etiologies.

IX. SALIENT POINTS

1. The anatomy of the OMC can only be adequately evaluated with CT in the coronal plane and in the absence of mucosal disease.
2. Infectious sinusitis tends to be localized because the infection develops in an obstructed sinus.
3. Allergic sinusitis tends to be symmetrical and diffuse because of its systemic basis.
4. Imaging cannot always distinguish between infectious and allergic sinusitis because they can coexist.
5. A single CT scan cannot distinguish between acute and chronic sinusitis; follow-up scans are necessary to document persistent or recurrent disease.

6. The imaging finding of osteitis indicates that the inflammatory changes are chronic.
7. Fungal sinusitis must be considered when bone erosion or atypical CT density/MR signal is present in a sinus.
8. Both benign and malignant etiologies can result in bone erosion.
9. Benign and malignant nasal tumors may result in obstructive sinusitis and mimic inflammatory sinonasal disease on CT.
10. Doctors treat patients, not CT scans.

13

Diagnostic Tests for Type IV or Delayed Hypersensitivity Reactions

David E. Cohen, Ronald R. Brancaccio, and Nicholas A. Soter
New York University School of Medicine, New York, New York

I. INTRODUCTION

Contact dermatitis accounts for more than 90% of all occupational skin diseases and is one of the most important occupational illnesses affecting American workers (1). Contact dermatitis comprises two distinct inflammatory processes caused by adverse exposure of the skin: irritant and allergic contact dermatitis. These syndromes have indistinguishable clinical characteristics. Classically, erythema (redness), induration (thickening and firmness), lichenification (accentuation of skin folds), scaling (flaking), and vesiculation (blistering) are present on areas directly contacted by the chemical agent. Histologically there is a mixed-cell inflammatory infiltrate of lymphocytes and eosinophils and the hallmark finding of spongiosis, epidermal intercellular edema. These histopathological features are not sufficient to differentiate allergic from irritant contact dermatitis, atopic dermatitis, and many other eczematous dermatitides, although there are subtle differences in the inflammatory responses (2). Because their etiology is different, the two syndromes are presented separately.

II. IRRITANT CONTACT DERMATITIS

Irritant dermatitis is intrinsically a nonimmune-related response caused by the direct action of an agent on the skin. It accounts for the majority of cases of contact dermatitis. Variables such as concentration, pH, temperature, duration, repetitiveness of contact, and occlusion influence the appearance of the eruption. Strong acids, bases, solvents, and unstable or reactive chemicals rank high among the many possible human irritants.

Strongly noxious substances such as those with extreme pH can produce an immediate, irreversible, and potentially scarring dermatitis after a single exposure. This acute irritant phenomenon is akin to a chemical burn and has been described as an ''etching'' reaction (3). More commonly, repeated exposures are necessary to elicit clinically noticeable changes. Such repeated exposures eventually result in either an eczematous dermatitis with clinical and histopathological changes similar to allergic contact dermatitis or a fissured, thickened eruption without a substantial inflammatory component. Chemicals inducing the latter reaction are known as marginal irritants.

Because the thresholds for irritant reactions vary greatly from person to person, a genetic component to the response has been considered. Monozygotic twins have shown greater concordance than dizygotic twins in their reactions to irritant chemicals such as sodium lauryl sulfate and benzalkonium chloride (4). Whereas young individuals with fair complexions appear to be more sensitive to irritant chemicals, gender/sex does not appear to be a significant factor (15). Attempts to predict the relative irritancy of substances based upon their chemical relatedness to other irritants have been unsuccessful.

Mechanisms for the pathophysiology of irritant dermatitis are different and depend on its multiple etiologies (6). Direct corrosives, protein solvents, oxidizing and reducing agents, and dehydrating agents act as irritants by disrupting the keratin ultrastructure or by directly injuring critical cellular macromolecules or organelles. Marginal irritants require multiple variables to create disease and may not be capable of producing reactions under all circumstances. Tetradecanoylphorbol acetate (the major active ingredient of croton oil, a potent irritant) induced a tenfold increase in prostaglandin E_2 (PGE_2) in cultured human keratinocytes, whereas ethylphenyl propriolate induced no change in PGE_2 (7). Langerhans cells (LC), which are the skin's major antigen-presenting cells, are not increased after provocation with croton oil on guinea pig skin (8). Intercellular adhesion molecule-1 (ICAM-1), which is upregulated in allergic contact dermatitis, may not be substantially affected in irritant dermatitis (9). Irritant contact dermatitis does not occur as a result of immunological mechanisms involving the recognition of antigen-presenting cells by activated T lymphocytes. Epidermal cell secretion of inflammatory mediators, such as interleukin-6 (IL-6) and tumor necrosis factor-alpha (TNF-alpha), appear to play an important role in lymphocyte recruitment (10).

No single testing method has been successful in determining the irritancy potential of specific chemicals. The tests involve either a single or repeated application of the same material to the skin. The use of animals in testing of potentially irritant chemicals is based on a variety of epicutaneous methods, and they have been used for decades. Both intact and abraded skin of albino rabbits is tested to various materials under occluded patches. The patches are removed in 24 hours, and the tested areas of the skin are evaluated at this time and again in 1 to 3 days.

The repeat insult patch test and the cumulative irritancy test, which are used primarily in humans, are occlusive patch tests in which chemicals are repeatedly placed on the same location for a 2- to 4-week period (11,12). The chamber scarification test modifies the aforementioned tests by abrading the skin to expose the upper dermis (13). The tests are interpreted by overt clinical changes, such as erythema and induration at the site of challenge with a potential irritant.

Transepidermal water loss, which is elevated in dermatitis, can be measured with an evaporometer (14). Currently, there is no test that can be used to correlate a specific chemical with a clinically apparent irritant dermatitis. Irritant reactions observed in patch tests, which are traditionally used for the evaluation of allergic contact dermatitis, may not be used to infer irritancy in the clinical setting.

III. CHEMICAL BURNS

Extremely corrosive and reactive chemicals may produce immediate coagulative necrosis that results in severe tissue damage. This is distinct from irritant dermatitis because the lesion is the direct result of the chemical insult and does not rely heavily on secondary inflammation.

IV. ALLERGIC CONTACT DERMATITIS

Allergic contact dermatitis represents delayed-type or cell-mediated hypersensitivity (15). Because this is a true allergy, only minute quantities of material are necessary to elicit clinical reactions. This is distinct from irritant contact dermatitis, in which the intensity of the reaction is proportional to the dose applied. An estimated 20% of all contact dermatitis is allergic in nature. Currently more than 3000 chemicals have been described as potential allergens (16). For allergic contact dermatitis to occur, one must first be sensitized to the potential allergen. Subsequent contact elicits the clinical and pathological findings. Genetic control of allergic contact dermatitis was demonstrated as early as the 1940s (17). Recent work has linked the presence of specific human leukocyte antigen (HLA) alleles to allergy to nickel, chromium, and cobalt (18). Thus, to mount an immune reaction, one must be genetically able to become sensitized, have a sufficient contact with a sensitizing chemical, and then have repeated contact later.

In general, low-molecular-weight electrophilic or hydrophilic chemicals (haptens) are responsible for causing allergic contact dermatitis. Haptens, which are not complete allergens, must link with epidermal carrier proteins to form a complete allergen (19). Current evidence suggests that these binding proteins are probably cell surface molecules on the LC, most likely Class II antigens encoded by genes of the HLA-DR locus (20).

The hapten/carrier protein complex is incorporated into the cytoplasm of an LC for intracellular processing (21). The LC subsequently migrates to a regional lymph node to present the processed antigen to CD4 T-cells. An LC bearing HLA-DR antigen and the hapten on its surface presents this bundle to a T-cell, which also must bear an antigen-specific receptor (CD3-Ti) and the cell surface molecule CD4. During antigen presentation, the LC produces IL-1, which directly stimulates the T-cell to produce IL-2 and interferon gamma. This cascade produces proliferation of T-cells specifically sensitized to that antigen. The subsequent recruitment of activated T-cells leads to the epidermal changes pathognomonic for contact dermatitis (22). Keratinocytes themselves are capable of producing a legion of cytokines, including IL-1 and IL-2, and of expressing HLA-DR antigen under certain circumstances. Hence, the keratinocyte is vital in the amplification process during the sensitization and elicitation phases of allergic contact dermatitis (23). After sensitization occurs, contact with the identical antigen initiates a similar but more rapid immunological cascade.

Contact dermatitis may occur after skin exposure to allergens routinely encountered. Table 1 lists frequent allergens based on common exposure patterns. Typical nonoccupational sources of exposure include the use of topical medications, personal hygiene products, rubber materials, textiles, cosmetics, glues, pesticides, and plastics. Contact with uncommon allergens occurs frequently in the workplace. Table 2 lists the frequency of reactivity of the 12 most common allergens in a group of 3120 individuals in whom patch tests were evaluated by the North American Contact Dermatitis Group (24). Review of the chemicals listed in Tables 1 and 2 indicates that causes of allergic contact dermatitis are ubiquitous in the products that touch human skin regularly. Some allergens, however, such

Table 1 Frequent Allergens Based on Common Exposure Patterns

Antibiotics
Bacitracin
Neomycin
Therapeutics
Benzocaine
Corticosteroids
Personal Hygiene Products/Cosmetics
Benzalkonium chloride
Ethylenediamine
Lanolin
p-Phenylenediamine
Propylene glycol
Benzophenones
Fragrances
Plants and Trees
Abietic acid
Pentadecylcatechols
Balsam of Peru
Sesquiterpene lactone
Rosin (colophony)
Tuliposide A
Glues and Bonding Agents
Acrylic monomers
Bisphenol A
Cyanocrylates
Epoxy resins
Formaldehyde
p-(t-butyl)formaldehyde resin
Toluene sulfonamide resins
Urea formaldehyde resins
Metals
Beryllium
Chromium
Cobalt
Gold
Mercury
Nickel
Palladium
Preservatives
Formaldehyde
Methylchloroisothiazolinone/Methylisothiazolinone
Quaternium-15
Imidazolidinyl
Diazolidinyl urea
DMDM hydantoin
Bromonitropropane
Rubber Products
Mercaptobenzothiazole
Carbamates
Hydroquinone
Sulfonamides
Thioureas
Thiurams
Antiseptics
Chlorhexidine
Chloroxylenol
Glutaraldehyde
Hexachlorophene
Mercurials
Thimerosal (merthiolate)
Leather
Formaldehyde
Potassium dichromate
Glutaraldehyde
Paper Products
Abietic acid
Dyes
Formaldehyde
Rosin (colophony)

Table 2 Common Contact Allergens by Frequency of Reactivity

Allergen	Reactivity Rate (%)
Nickel sulfate	14.3
Fragrance mix	14.0
Neomycin sulfate	11.6
Balsam of Peru	10.4
Thimerosal	10.4
Formaldehyde	9.2
Quaternium 15	9.2
Bacitracin	9.1
Cobalt chloride	8.0
Thiuram mix	6.8
Paraphenylenediamine	6.8
Carba mix	5.7

Source: Ref. 24.

as nickel, chromium, cobalt, and some food flavorings are ingested in foods. In cases in which an individual has a contact sensitivity to an agent that is parenterally and orally administered, a generalized skin eruption with associated symptoms such as headache, malaise, and arthralgia may occur. Skin changes that occur in the setting of systemic contact dermatitis include a flare at the site of a previous contact dermatitis to the same substance, vesicular hand eruptions, and an eczematous eruption in flexural areas. Pink-to-dark violet eruptions around the buttocks and genitalia have been termed the ''baboon syndrome.'' Systemic contact dermatitis may produce a delayed-type hypersensitivity reaction or deposition of immunoglobulins and complement proteins in the skin (25).

Cross-reactions between chemicals may occur if they share similar functional groups critical to the formation of complete allergens (hapten plus carrier protein). Failure to recognize the potential cross-reactions may cause difficulties in controlling allergic contact dermatitis. Avoidance of known allergens alone may result in continued exposure to potentially cross-reacting substances. For example, a patient allergic to formaldehyde may need to avoid chemicals known to donate formaldehyde molecules in their function as preservatives. They include quaternium 15, DMDM hydantoin, diazolidinyl urea, imidazolidinyl urea, and bromonitropropane.

A. Methodology

As with irritant dermatitis, animals have been used to determine the allergenicity of chemicals with the hope of correlating the data to humans. The Draize test is an intradermal test in which the induction of sensitization is accomplished by 10 intracutaneous injections of a specific test material. Subsequent challenges are graded by their clinical appearance. The guinea pig maximization test attempts to induce allergy by serial intradermal injections of an agent with the addition of Freund's complete adjuvant, which is an immune enhancer consisting of mycobacterial proteins. Subsequent challenge reactions with the agent alone under an occluded chamber are graded clinically.

Variations of the aforementioned animal tests are performed on humans before their introduction into consumer products. These tests have been used successfully to predict the allergenicity of strongly sensitizing substances in human beings. However, weaker allergens are often not discovered until they reach a large human population.

Determining the cause of a contact dermatitis requires a careful evaluation of possible chemical exposures, history of the illness, and the distribution of lesions. This evaluation will raise suspicion of groups or classes of allergens but will be insufficient to identify the specific offending chemical. Proper identification of the purported allergen is of paramount importance, inasmuch as without strict avoidance, the dermatitis will continue. Diagnostic patch testing has been used for almost 100 years (26). Since its introduction, little has changed in either the procedure or its usefulness (27).

Standardized concentrations of allergens dissolved or suspended in petrolatum or water are placed on aluminum chambers (Finn chambers) adhering to acrylic tape. Most allergens are commercially available, and the concentrations have been tested in a sufficiently large population to establish a nonirritancy threshold. A premixed test series uses allergens dispersed in a cellulose gel matrix adhered to a polyester film. Distributed as T.R.U.E. TEST® (Glaxo Dermatology Research, Triangle Park, NC), this series containing 23 allergens and one control is similar with regard to its allergen content to the Allergen Patch Test Kit® (Hermal Laboratories, Inc., Reinbek, Germany). In the United States, the Food and Drug Administration regulates the sale and distribution of patch test materials. Tables 3 and 4 describe the currently approved test series available in the United States.

The utility of a standard allergen series as the sole screening tool in the diagnosis of allergic contact dermatitis has been examined, and it has limited usage (28). Only 23% of 732 patients with positive patch tests reacted exclusively to one or more allergens in the standard series. When clinical relevance was considered, the percentage of patients completely evaluated by the standard series was further lowered to 15.7%. Testing to a series at least as comprehensive as the North American Contact Dermatitis Group Series (Table 5) is strongly recommended. Patch testing to additional allergens is encouraged and may be accomplished by preparing allergens in the office, with the assistance of a pharmacist or chemist, or obtaining them through commercial sources in other countries.

The T.R.U.E. TEST is a ready-to-use patch test system and requires application to the patient's back. Because the number of allergens in this system is limited to 23, additional testing must be performed with the use of standardized

Table 3 T.R.U.E. TEST® Allergen Series

1. Nickel sulfate	13. P-tert-butyl phenol formaldehyde resin
2. Wood alcohol	14. Paraben mix
3. Neomycin sulfate	15. Carba mix
4. Potassium dichromate	16. Black rubber mix
5. Caine mix	17. Cl + ME isothiazolone
6. Fragrance mix	18. Quaternium-15
7. Colophony	19. Mercaptobenzothiazole
8. Epoxy mix	20. P-phenylenediamine
9. Control	21. Formaldehyde
10. Balsam of Peru	22. Mercapto mix
11. Ethylenediamine dihydrochloride	23. Thimerosal
12. Cobalt chloride	24. Thiuram mix

concentrations of allergens and patch test chambers. The Allergen Patch Test Kit is composed of 20 allergens loaded in syringes for ease of application to a patch test chamber. The Finn Chambers (Epitest Ltd., Tuusula, Finland) on Scanpor tape (Norgesplaster Aksjeselskap, Vennesia, Norway) are the most commonly used patch test chambers, but other systems such as the IQ chambers (Chemotechnique Diagnostics AB, Malmö, Sweden) are available. Before filling the chambers, the tape strips should be labeled, as this is necessary to identify the location of the allergens in the future. Finn chambers are filled with standardized concentrations and quantities of allergens. In general, a 5-mm ribbon of allergen in petrolatum is placed in the chamber. Allergens in water or alcohol are applied with a dropper on a 5-mm diameter filter paper insert.

The mass of allergen per unit area of skin is the correct measure of the dermal dose of the allergen, and not the allergen concentration (29). In the exam-

Table 4 United States Standard Allergen Series (Allergen Patch Test Kit®)

1. Benzocaine 5% pet	11. Formaldehyde 1% aq
2. Mercaptobenzothiazole 1% pet	12. Ethylenediamine dihydrochloride 1% pet
3. Colophony 20% pet	13. Epoxy resin 1% pet
4. P-phenylenediamine 1% pet	14. Quaternium-15 2% pet
5. Imidazolidinyl urea 2% aq	15. P-tert-butyl phenol formaldehyde resin 1% pet
6. Cinnamic aldehyde 1% pet	16. Mercapto mix 1% pet
7. Lanolin alcohol 30% pet	17. Black rubber mix 0.6%/IPPD 0.1% pet
8. Carba mix 3% pet	18. Potassium dichromate 0.25% pet
9. Neomycin sulfate 20% pet	19. Balsam of Peru 25% pet
10. Thiuram mix 1% pet	20. Nickel sulfate 2.5% pet

Abbreviations: pet, petrolatum; *aq*, aqueous.

Table 5 North American Contact Dermatitis Group's Current Standard Series

1. Benzocaine 5% pet	27. Paraben mix 12% pet
2. Mercaptobenzothiazole 1% pet	28. Methyldibromo glutaronitrile/ phenoxyethanol 1% pet
3. Colophony 20% pet	29. Fragrance mix 8% pet
4. P-phenylenediamine 1% pet	30. Glutaraldehyde 0.2% pet
5. Imidazolidinyl urea 2% aq	31. 2-bromo-2-nitropropane-1,3-diol 0.5% pet
6. Cinnamic aldehyde 1% pet	32. Sesquiterpene lactone mix 0.1% pet
7. Lanolin alcohol 30% pet	33. Thimerosal 0.1% pet
8. Carba mix 3% pet	34. Propylene glycol 10% aq
9. Neomycin sulfate 20% pet	35. Methylchloroisothiazolinone/ methylisothiazoline 100 ppm pet
10. Thiuram mix 1% pet	36. Chloroxylenol (PCMX) 1% pet
11. Formaldehyde 1% aq	37. DMDM hydantoin 1% aq
12. Ethylenediamine dihydrochloride 1% pet	38. Diazolidinyl urea 1% aq
13. Epoxy resin 1% pet	39. Ethyleneurea melamine formaldehyde 5% pet
14. Quaternium-15 2% pet	40. Phenoxyethanol 1% pet
15. P-tert-butyl phenol formaldehyde resin 1% pet	41. BHA 2% pet
16. Mercapto mix 1% pet	42. Glutaraldehyde 1% pet
17. Black rubber mix 0.6%/IPPD 0.1% pet	43. BHT 2% pet
18. Potassium dichromate 0.25% pet	44. Ethyl acrylate 0.1% pet
19. Balsam of Peru 25% pet	45. Glycerol thioglycolate 1% pet
20. Nickel sulfate 2.5% pet	46. Toluene sulphonamide formaldehyde resin 10% pet
21. Diazolidinyl urea 1% pet	47. Methyl methacrylate 2% pet
22. DMDM hydantoin 1% pet	48. Cobalt chloride 1% pet
23. Imidazolidinyl urea 2% pet	49. Tixocortol-21-pivalate 1% pet
24. Bacitracin 20% pet	50. Budesonide 0.1% pet
25. Mixed dialkyl thioureas 1% pet	
26. Methylchloroisothiazolinone/ methylisothiazolinone 100 ppm aq	

Abbreviations: pet, petrolatum; *aq*, aqueous.

ple of an allergen in petrolatum, the difference between a 4-mm ribbon and an 8-mm ribbon with the same concentration of allergen will result in markedly different dermal delivery doses. The increase in the dose delivered has been shown to improve sensitivity; however, standardization has been tested using this established 5-mm ribbon. Exceeding this amount may result in false-positive or irritant reactions. The T.R.U.E. TEST system serves to overcome this technical dilemma by providing the exact dosage of allergen in a fixed surface area.

Either system should be placed on the upper back and secured with hypo-allergenic tape. Allergens should be applied when the patient is sitting upright, and the midline should not be used (Fig. 1). The test sites should not be cleansed with soaps or solvents before application. Shaving the back may be necessary.

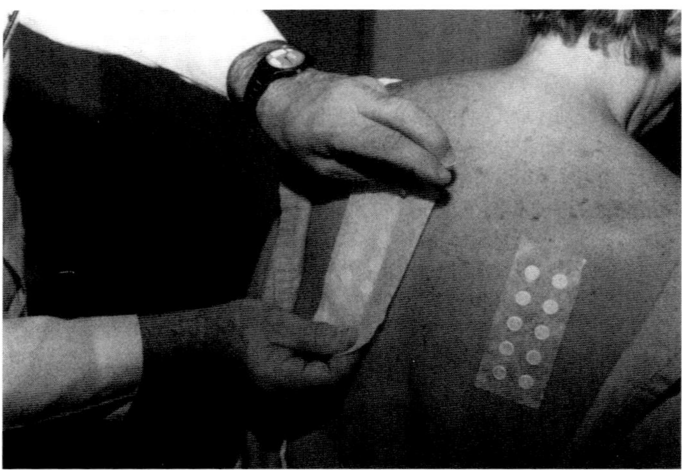

Figure 1 Correct placement of allergens on the back.

The upper back is the preferred site for testing, as allergen concentrations and vehicles have been designed based on this test site. Patients should be instructed regarding certain physical and medical restrictions before the test begins. The use of immunosuppresive medications, such as systemic corticosteroids, antimetabolites, and antirejection medications will inhibit the ability of the test to evoke an allergic reaction. It is advisable to discontinue these medications at least 1 week before testing. Recent sunburns and potent topical corticosteroids may result in false-negative readings. Systemic antihistamines are permitted, as they do not appear to influence the ability to elicit reactions in this setting. Tests should only be applied to skin that appears normal; if active dermatitis is present at or near the test site, false-positive reactions may occur.

Although infrequent, adverse reactions to patch testing may occur. The most common include: irritant reactions, postinflammatory pigmentary changes, persistence of a patch test reaction, ectopic flares of dermatitis elsewhere on the skin, or active sensitization to a tested allergen. Anaphylactoid reactions, although extremely rare, have occured with ammonium persulfate and bacitracin (30).

Test chambers should remain dry because moisture may loosen the test strips and lessen contact time with the skin. Hence, showering, swimming, and sweat-inducing activities should be avoided. Patients return for patch test removal and an initial reading after 48 hours. Supplementary tape and patch test strips should be removed, and each chamber marked with indelible ink or a surgical marking pen (Fig. 2). The back should be allowed to air dry for 20 minutes once the patches are removed. This allows pressure indentation and possible physical

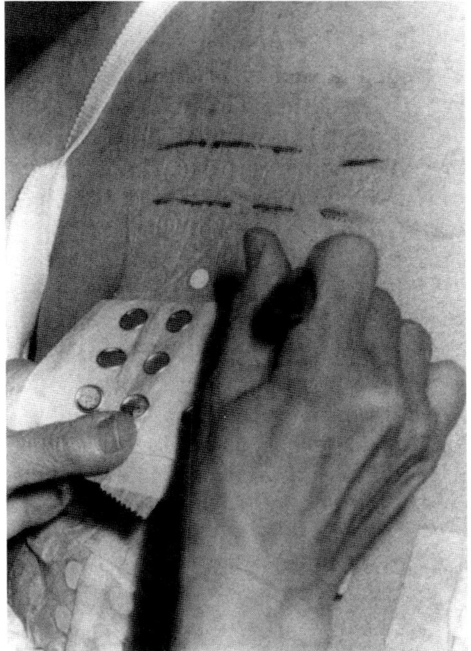

Figure 2 Removal of patch tests.

urticaria from the chambers and tape to disperse. An initial interpretation of the tests should be performed at this time. Patients should return for a final reading in 24–96 hours. Delayed positive patch test responses are found in 35% of patients, emphasizing the need for two separate readings (31).

The patch tests are graded based on the severity of the inflammatory response using a scoring system referred to as the ''patch test reading morphology codes.'' These scores are numbered 1 through 6. A 1+ positive reaction has erythema with edema or papules; a 2+ reaction is a stronger response with erythema, edema, papules, and vesicles (Fig. 3); a 3+ reaction is an extreme positive response that spreads beyond the patch test site; a score of 4 signifies a doubtful reaction with only macular erythema. These responses are the most difficult to interpret, as the difference morphologically between a weak positive and weak irritant reaction may be negligible. Evaluation of this response over time, such as at the delayed or second reading, is the best means of distinguishing between the two. Irritant reactions (a score of 5) are usually sharply demarcated, with a shiny, glazed, or cigarette paper appearance generally confined to the area cov-

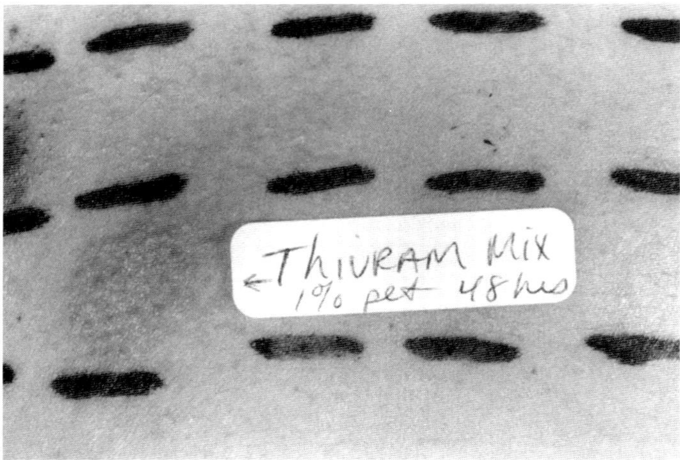

Figure 3 A 2+ reaction to thiuram mix.

ered by the chamber. These reactions do not evolve or spread but rather fade by the second reading in many cases. The use of nonstandardized allergens or an irritating concentration of a test substance can lead to irritant or false-positive patch test reactions. Conversely, allergic patch test reactions are red, raised, palpable, vesicular, or spreading reactions that usually increase in intensity and persist for 3 or more days. A reading value of 6 indicates a negative reading.

Repeated open application test (ROAT) with the product containing the suspected allergen can also be useful. Skin care products or topical medications are applied uncovered to the volar surface of the forearm twice a day for 1 week. Such use tests are helpful in determining the relevance of positive reactions. Patch or use testing with unknown substances such as chemicals from occupational sources should be avoided.

False-positive patch test reactions can occur in a state of skin hyperirritability known as the excited skin syndrome or angry back (32). Multiple, positive, patch tests develop, most of which can be demonstrated to be negative on retesting at a later date. This reaction pattern is more likely to occur in the presence of a strong positive patch test response. Judging the importance or relevance of multiple positive patch tests must be done cautiously and may require retesting.

The correlation of a positive patch test to a patient's eczematous dermatitis is referred to as assigning clinical relevance. This relationship may be difficult because an in-depth knowledge of allergen sources is required to counsel patients. A patch test reaction is considered clinically relevant if a clear temporal relationship between the onset and distribution of the dermatitis can be correlated with exposure to the allergen. Investigations into personal hygiene products, cosmetics, and occupational and environmental contacts are necessary to make relevance conclusions. Some allergens may explain previous contact dermatitis or have no known relevance. Educating the patient to avoid the offending allergen and providing alternative products will enhance the clinical outcome.

Negative patch tests usually can be interpreted as the patient not being allergic to the tested chemicals. However, dermatitis may be allergic in nature in the setting of a negative patch test, particularly if the allergen battery was too limited or inappropriately directed. False-negative reactions also can occur if the allergen is not tested in the proper concentration or vehicle. If the patch tests are negative and clinical suspicion of allergic contact dermatitis remains high, a search for the allergen should continue with patch testing to other substances that are relevant to the patient's situation.

V. ALLERGIC PHOTOCONTACT DERMATITIS

A thorough history is the most important area of the evaluation of the patient with allergic photocontact dermatitis. However, not all patients who are photosensitive can directly relate their problem to ultraviolet radiation. A detailed medication history, including both systemic and topical preparations should be obtained. Topical products, such as sunscreens, soaps, cosmetics, and perfumes, are some of the most common causes of allergic photocontact dermatitis. Questions concerning the occupational history may uncover exposure to chemicals that are known photosensitizers in the workplace (Table 6). The occupational history also

Table 6 Occupational Photodermatoses

Occupation	Photosensitizer	Photodermatosis
Bartenders	Lime (furocoumarin)	Phototoxic contact dermatitis
Cement workers, lithographers, tanning industry	Chromium	Photoallergic contact dermatitis
Dye manufacturing	Anthroquinone dyes	Photoallergic and phototoxic contact dermatitis
Handlers of carrots, celery, dill, fennel, figs, parsley, parsnips	Furocoumarins	Phototoxic contact dermatitis
Nurses, pharmacists	Phenothiazines	Photoallergic and phototoxic contact dermatitis
Roofers	Coal tar pitch	Phototoxic contact dermatitis
Ultraviolet-cured ink manufacturing	Dimethyl aminobenzoate	Phototoxic contact dermatitis

should include potential exposure to artificial light sources, such as welding arcs, lasers, germicidal lamps, mercury vapor lamps, and sunlamps. Phototoxic contact dermatitis is a nonimmune response caused by the interaction of ultraviolet radiation and chemicals. It is recognized as an enhanced sunburn reaction.

In a patient with allergic photocontact dermatitis, the lesions are usually confined to exposed areas. Commonly involved sites include the face, posterior aspect of the neck, ears, ''V'' area of the chest, dorsa of the hands, and extensor aspects of the forearms. The most striking feature is the sparing of characteristic areas, which include the upper eyelids, submental area, posterior auricular area upper lip, web spaces of the fingers, and creases within folds of skin. In contrast, areas characteristically spared in a photoallergic contact dermatitis would be involved in an airborne contact dermatitis. A photoallergic contact dermatitis secondary to cosmetics or perfumes may follow the pattern of application.

If the history and physical examination suggest the possibility of a photoallergic contact dermatitis, photopatch tests should be performed. Photopatch tests are expensive and time consuming and should be performed only if there is adequate clinical suspicion.

Photopatch testing may produce false-negative or false-positive results. In a survey of 2041 positive photopatch test results, only 108 were considered to be secondary to photoallergy and possibly clinically relevant (33). The poor specificity of photopatch tests also was demonstrated in a study in which only 14 of the 27 patients with photoallergic contact reactions were considered to have relevant reactions (34).

One of the greatest variations in photopatch test procedures in different medical centers is the photoallergens used. Because the photoallergic patient often is unable to implicate a specific substance as the cause of photoallergic contact dermatitis, testing is performed with a variety of photoallergens. When a specific photoallergen is suspected, testing is also performed with that substance.

The photoallergens used at our medical center include the North American Contact Dermatitis Group photopatch test series and the New York University Skin and Cancer Unit photopatch test/sunscreen sensitivity series (Table 7). This combination provides most of the usually described photoallergens as well as sunscreen ingredients, plants, and pesticides. Because the action spectrum of almost all photoallergens is in the ultraviolet A (UVA) (320-400 nm) range, this is the only radiation used in photopatch testing.

Although there is no standard procedure for photopatch testing, the procedure used at our medical center will be outlined to provide a general framework. Four visits are required with this protocol. The first three are on consecutive days, and the fourth is up to 1 week after the initial visit. On day 1, the minimal erythema dose (MED) test to UVA is performed. The MED is the least amount of UVA radiation that elicits a uniform pink response in the site exposed. Also during this visit, duplicate sets of photoallergens are applied to the back and then

Table 7 New York University Skin and Cancer Unit Photoallergen Series

Antigens	Concentration
Octyl methoxycinnamate	7.5% pet
Sulisobenzone (BZP-4)	10% pet
Cinoxate	1% pet
Thiourea (thiocarbamide)	0.1% pet
Dichlorophen	1% pet
Triclosan	2% pet
Hexachlorophene	1% pet
Chlorhexidine diacetate	0.5% aq
Sandalwood oil	2% pet
Chlorpromazine hydrochloride	0.1% pet
Musk ambrette	1% pet
Para-aminobenzoic acid (PABA)	5% etoh
Petrolatum control	
Tribromosalicylanilide	1% pet
Octyl dimethyl PABA	5% etoh
Oxybenzone (BZP-3)	3% pet
Promethazine	1% pet
Bithionol (Thiobis-dichlorophenol)	1% pet
Musk ambrette	1% etoh
Fenticlor (thiobis-chlorophenol)	1% pet
Menthyl anthranilate	5% pet
6-Methylocoumarine	1% pet
Diphenhydramine hydrochloride	1% pet
Trichlorocarbanilide	1% pet
Sulfanilamide	1% pet
3-(4-methylbenzyliden)-camphor (Eusolex 6300)	2% pet
1-(4-Isopropylphenyl)-3-P-phenyl-1,3-propandione (Eusolex 8020)	2% pet
Plants	
Chamomilla romana	1% pet
Diallyldisulfide	1% pet
Amica montana	0.5% pet
Taraxacum officinale	2.5% pet
Achillea millefolium	1% pet
Propolis	10% pet
Chrysanthemum cinerariaefolium	1% pet
Sesquiterpene lactone mix	0.1% pet
a-Methylene-g-butyrolactone	0.01% pet
Tanacetum vulgare	1% pet
Alantolactone	0.1% pet
Lichen acid mix	0.3% pet

Table 7 Continued

Pesticides	Concentration
Captan	0.1% pet
Zineb	1% pet
Capatafol	0.1% pet
Maneb	1% pet
Folpet	0.1% pet
Pyrethrum	2% pet
Benomyl	0.1% pet
Ziram	1% pet

Abbreviations: pet, petrolatum; *aq*, aqueous; *etoh*, alcohol.

covered by opaque tape. On day 2, before irradiation of one set of photoallergens, the MED-A is quantified. In patients with a normal MED-A, one set of photoallergens is exposed to 10 J/cm^2 of UVA while the duplicate set remains covered. If the MED-A is abnormal, the exposure is 50% of the MED-A. On day 3, both the irradiated and nonirradiated test sites are evaluated and the responses are graded. Up to 1 week after the initial visit, the patch and photopatch test sites are evaluated for delayed reactions.

A positive response at the irradiated site in the absence of a response at the nonirradiated site indicates a photoallergic contact dermatitis, whereas positive responses of equal intensity and duration at both the irradiated and nonirradiated sites indicate an allergic contact dermatitis. The presence of both allergic contact dermatitis and photocontact dermatitis is indicated by positive responses at both irradiated and nonirradiated sites in which the response at the irradiated site is more pronounced or persists for a longer period than that of the nonirradiated site. Differentiation of irritant and allergic reactions is often not possible. In severe irritant responses, well-defined erythema that resolves promptly may be observed. Allergic responses are more commonly eczematous, with poorly defined borders and slower resolution.

VI. CONCLUSION

Although it is a biological assay with inherent problems, patch testing has demonstrated both reliability and reproducibility. Reliability is defined as a test's ability to give consistent results when performed on the same individual. A reliability of 82% was demonstrated when 128 patients were rechallenged with allergens that were previously positive (35). Another approach to evaluating reliability is to examine concordance of patch test reactions on different parts of the back. Variable results have been obtained by different investigators, but confirm the reproducibility of the test.

Patch testing remains the best method of confirming the diagnosis of allergic contact dermatitis. The cost effectiveness of patch testing was examined and found to be more economical than the cost of either repeated patient office visits or medications (36). Patch testing is safe and effective and should be considered in the evaluation of the patient with a suspected allergic contact dermatitis.

VII. SALIENT POINTS

1. Contact dermatitis accounts for more than 90% of all occupational skin diseases and is one of the most important occupational illnesses affecting American workers.
2. Approximately 20% of all contact dermatitis is allergic in nature and more than 3000 chemicals have been described as potential allergens.
3. Low-molecular-weight electrophilic or hydrophilic chemicals (haptens) are responsible for causing allergic contact dermatitis.
4. Patch testing remains the standard diagnostic tool for allergic contact dermatitis.
5. A standard allergen series as the sole screening tool is of limited value in the diagnosis of allergic contact dermatitis.
6. The use of immunosuppressive medications, such as systemic corticosteroids, antimetabolites, and antirejection medications, will inhibit the ability of the patch test to elicit an allergic reaction. Systemic antihistamines are permitted, as they do not appear to influence patch testing adversely.
7. The correlation of a positive patch test to a patient's eczematous dermatitis assigns clinical relevance. Establishing clinical relevance may be difficult inasmuch as an in-depth knowledge of allergen sources is required to counsel patients.
8. Topical products, such as sunscreens, soaps, cosmetics, and perfumes, are some of the most common causes of allergic photocontact dermatitis.
9. The action spectrum of most photoallergens is in the UVA (320–400 nm) range, and UVA is the only radiation used in photopatch testing.
10. Nickel, fragrances, topical antibiotics, and preservatives are the most common contact allergens in the United States.

REFERENCES

1. American Academy of Dermatology. Proceedings of the National Conference on Environmental Hazards to the Skin, Washington, DC, 1994.
2. Mihm MC, Soter NA, Dvorak HF, and Austen KF. The structure of normal skin and the morphology of atopic eczema. J Invest Dermatol 1976;67:305–312.
3. Bjornberg A. Irritant dermatitis. In: Maibach H I ed. Occupational and Industrial Dermatology. 2d ed. Chicago: Year Book Medical Publishers, Inc., 1987:15–21.
4. Holst R, Moller H. One hundred twin pairs patch tested with primary irritants. Br J Dermatol 1975; 93:145–149.
5. Bjornberg A. Skin reactions to primary irritants in men and women. Acta Dermatol Venereol 1975; 55:191–194.
6. Patrick E, Burkhalter A, Maibach HI. Recent investigations of mechanisms of chemically induced skin irritation in laboratory mice. J Invest Dermatol 1987; 88:124s–131s.
7. Bloom E, Goldyne M, Maibach HI, Tammi R, Polansky J. In vitro effects of irritants using human skin cell and organ culture models. J Invest Dermatol 1987; 88:478.
8. Kanauchi H, Furakawa F, Imamura S. Evaluation of ATPase-positive Langerhans' cells in skin lesions of lupus erythematosus and experimentally induced inflammations. Arch Dermatol Res 1989; 281:327–332.
9. Vejlsgaard GL, Ralfkiaer E, Avnstorp C, Czajkowski M, Marlin SD, Rothlein R. Kinetics and characterization of intercellular adhesion molecule-1 (ICAM-1) expression on keratinocytes in various inflammatory skin lesions and malignant cutaneous lymphomas. J Am Acad Dermatol 1989; 20:782–790.
10. Oxholm A. Epidermal expression of interleukin-6 and tumor necrosis factor-alpha in normal and immunoinflammatory skin state in humans. APMIS Suppl 1992; 24:1–32.
11. Shelanski HV, Shelanski MV. A new technique of human patch tests. Proc Sci Sect Toilet Goods Assoc 1953; 19:46.
12. Patrick E, Maibach HI. Predictive skin irritation tests in animals and humans in dermatotoxicology. In: Marzulli FN, Maibach HI, eds. Dermatotoxicology. 4th ed. New York: Hemisphere Publishing Corp., 1991:211–212.
13. Frosch PJ, Kligman AM. The chamber scarification test for irritancy. Contact Dermatitis 1976; 2:314–324.
14. Lammintausta K, Maibach HI, Wilson D. Susceptibility to cumulative and acute irritant dermatitis. An experimental approach in human volunteers. Contact Dermatitis 1988; 19:84–90.
15. Landsteiner K, Jacobs J. Studies on the sensitization of animals with simple chemical compounds: II. J Exp Med 1935; 61:625–639.
16. de Groot, Anton C. Unwanted Effects of Cosmetics and Drugs Used in Dermatology. New York: Elsevier, 1994.
17. Chase MW. Inheritance in guinea pigs of the susceptibility to skin sensitization with simple chemical compounds. J Exp Med 1941; 73:711–726.
18. Emtestam L, Zetterquist H, Olerup O. HLA-DR, -DQ, and -DP alleles in nickel, chromium, and/or cobalt-sensitive individuals: genomic analysis based on restriction fragment length polymorphisms. J Invest Dermatol 1993; 100:271–274.

19. Baer RL. The mechanism of allergic contact hypersensitivity. In: Fisher AA (ed.) Contact Dermatitis. 3rd ed. Philadelphia: Lea and Febiger, 1986: 1–8.
20. Reinherz EL, Meuer SC, Schlossman SF. The delineation of antigen receptors on human T lymphocytes. Immunol Today 1983; 4:5–9.
21. Hanau D, Fabre M, Lepoittevin JP, Stampf JL, Grosshans E, Benezra C. Adsorptive pinocytosis, disappearance of membranous ATPase activity and appearance of Langerhans granules are observable in Langerhans cells during the first 24 hours following epicutaneous application of DNCB in guinea pigs. J Invest Dermatol 1985; 84: 434.
22. Belsito DV. The rise and fall of allergic contact dermatitis. Am J Contact Dermat 1997; 8:1–6.
23. Baer RL. Allergic contact dermatitis: a historical view of its mechanism. Am J Contact Dermat 1990; 1:7–12.
24. Marks JG, Belsito DV, DeLeo VA, Fowler JF Jr, Fransway AF, Maibach HI, Mathias CG, Nethercott JR, Rietschel RL, Sherertz EF, Storrs FJ, Taylor JS. North American Contact Dermatitis Group patch test results for the detection of delayed-type hypersensitivity to topical allergens. J Am Acad Dermatol 1998; 38:911–918.
25. Menne T, Veien N, Sjolin KE, and Maibach HI. Systemic contact dermatitis. Am J Contact Dermat 1994; 5:1–12.
26. Jadassohn J. Zur Kenntnis der medikamentossen Dermatosen. In: Jarish A, Neisser A, eds. Verhandlungen der Deutschen Dermatolgishen Gasellschaft. V. Kongress, 1895; 103–129.
27. Sulzberger MB. Dermatologic Allergy. Baltimore: Charles C Thomas, 1940; 87–128.
28. Cohen DE, Brancaccio R, Andersen D, Belsito DV. Utility of a standard allergen series alone in the evaluation of allergic contact dermatitis: a retrospective study of 732 patients. J Am Acad Dermatol 1997; 36:914–918.
29. Fowler J, Finley B. Quantity of allergen per unit area is more important than concentration for effective testing. Am J Contact Dermat 1995; 6:157–159.
30. Rouge G, Strannegard O. Anaphylactic shock elicited by topical administration of bacitracin. Arch Dermatol 1969; 100:450.
31. Rietschel RL, Adams RM, Maibach HI. The case for patch test readings beyond day 2. J Am Acad Dermatol 1988; 18:42–45.
32. Mitchell JC. The angry back syndrome: eczema creates eczema. Contact Dermatitis 1975; 1:193–194.
33. Holzle E, Neumann N, Hausen B, Przybilla B, Schauder S, Honigsmann H, Bircher A, Plewig G. Photopatch testing: the 5-year experience of the German, Austrian, and Swiss Photopatch Test Group. J Am Acad Dermatol 1991; 25:59–68.
34. Menz J, Muller SA, Connolly SM. Photopatch testing: a six-year experience. J Am Acad Dermatol 1988; 18:1044–1047.
35. Belsito DV, Storrs FJ, Taylor JS. Reproducibility of patch tests: a United States multicenter study. Am J Contact Dermat 1992; 3:193–200.
36. Rietschel RL. Is patch testing cost-effective? J Am Acad Dermatol 1989; 21:885–887.

14

Controversial and Unproven Diagnostic Tests for Allergic and Immunologic Diseases

Abba I. Terr
Stanford University Medical Center, Stanford, California

I. INTRODUCTION

A variety of unproven procedures to diagnose allergic and immunological diseases and specific allergic sensitivities are currently marketed to both physicians and the general public. Some of them are based on false premises about disease pathogenesis, others on empirical and anecdotal experiences that have not been validated. Their use must be discouraged, because an incorrect diagnosis of disease based on these tests leads to inappropriate therapies, including unnecessary restrictions of diet and environmental exposures as well as the use of ineffective medications. Furthermore, a patient who wrongly believes that he or she suffers from allergy or an inadequate immune system because of a faulty test risks unnecessary restrictions and fears.

An incorrect diagnosis of allergy also can result from the inappropriate use of procedures that detect and quantitate specific antibodies. It is incumbent upon the clinician to understand the physiological significance of any test that measures the presence of antibodies in the patient's serum and to use the result in the context of the patient's clinical history and examination findings.

The ''tests'' discussed here include those that are unsuitable for allergy diagnosis for one of several reasons. Some of the tests are based on an unproven or disproven theory of allergic or immunological disease. Others are derived from acceptable testing techniques, but they are methodologically flawed. Some are legitimate tests that are appropriate for use in other conditions, but they cannot be used to diagnose allergy. Some of the procedures described here have no diagnostic validity for any medical condition at all.

Many of these controversial and unproven methods have certain features in common. They are often used to diagnose food allergy, especially in patients who complain of nonspecific symptoms without objective signs of allergic disease. Some of them are advertised directly to the public. In all cases, their proponents have not subjected them to the scrutiny of clinical trials using appropriate controls and rigorous methodology to establish efficacy and safety before introducing them into clinical practice. In some instances, particularly when a questionable test has gained considerable popularity, other investigators have taken on this responsibility. Too often, however, a procedure is not abandoned or reexamined by its proponents in response to negative studies reported by others.

The methodology of these unproven tests is often poorly described, enabling their practitioners to modify the test in ways that make the procedure difficult if not impossible to reproduce. Some of the tests are based on claims that they can diagnose a variety of conditions that have no allergic or immunological basis.

These unconventional tests have particular appeal to nonconventional or so-called ''alternative'' practitioners with no particular training, expertise, or experience in dealing with allergic patients. Many of these practitioners subject their patients to a palette of several of these unproven methods.

The tests described here, including those that are bizarre to even the most unsophisticated observer, appeal to certain patients who are attracted to unscientific health care theories and practices. In some cases a diagnosis of allergy is claimed to be possible using techniques derived from such practices as acupuncture and chiropractic. Some of them are part of the testing and treatment options of physicians who subscribe to the controversial and still-unproven concept of multiple chemical sensitivities or environmental illness, because the underlying concept of this condition precludes any reliance on conventional methodology.

The testing procedures discussed here have been reviewed extensively elsewhere (1–7). Most of these diagnostic procedures have been the subjects of position statements by professional medical (8–10) and governmental (11–13) organizations. Some have been specifically excluded from Medicare coverage by the United States Health Care Financing Administration (12,13).

II. CYTOTOXIC TEST

In 1956, well before the discovery that antibodies responsible for atopic diseases belong to a unique class of immunoglobulin known now as IgE, an in vitro ''test'' called the cytotoxic test was devised to assist in the diagnosis of allergy, especially allergy to foods (14). It is a simple procedure in which the buffy coat from a drop of the patient's blood is placed on a microscope slide coated with a dried extract of the food or other allergen, secured with a cover slip, and then observed microscopically for alteration in the appearance of the white blood cells. The test is based on the theory that allergy results in ''toxicity'' to leukocytes.

Documented food allergy, that is clinical reactions to foods that can be reproduced by deliberate controlled exposures in a double-blind protocol, are consistent with an immunological mechanism in which the patient's food-specific IgE antibodies react with the ingested food to produce immediate reactions consistent with the effects of mast cell mediators that are released to act on certain target organs. Immediate food allergy most often manifests in skin reactions, especially urticaria, and gastrointestinal symptomatology arising from gut muscle contraction and excessive glandular secretion. Since there is no evidence for any disease in which allergy to a food involves a cytotoxic mechanism, there is no theoretical basis for the cytotoxic test. Immunologically mediated delayed food allergy has long been postulated, but to date this cannot be reproduced by double-blind, placebo-controlled food challenges (15). Furthermore, no form of immunological cytotoxicity, whether mediated by complement activation, cytotoxic T-cells, or natural killer (NK) cells, has ever been shown to be diagnosed by the leukocyte cytotoxicity test as described here.

The cytotoxic test has never been standardized, and it remains to be seen whether the leukocyte ''changes'' presumably observed in this test are not artifacts attributed to the effects of pH, temperature, osmolarity, time of incubation, or an in vitro toxic effect of the food extract used in the test. In practice, a sample of the patient's blood is tested to a panel of 100 or more individual foods. The feasibility of microscopic visual inspection of this many fresh blood cell specimens in which a sufficient number of leukocytes must be located, correctly identified, and subjectively rated for degrees of morphological alterations must be seriously questioned. Several studies have failed to document that cytotoxic testing has any validity for diagnosing allergy (16–18).

III. PROVOCATION–NEUTRALIZATION

Deliberate provocation of an allergic reaction by exposure of the patient to a small, measured quantity of the allergen to evoke an objective response that can be quantitated is a process that is an essential part of the clinical practice of allergy and clinical research. It is requisite in studies defining the mechanism of allergy in humans and in some phases of therapeutic trials. The essential features of a diagnostic provocative challenge allergy test are listed in Table 1.

Before the advent of in vitro methods for detecting circulating IgE antibodies to specific allergens, prick and intradermal skin testing was the only available diagnostic procedure for routine use in practice, and it continues to be the standard by which other specific testing is measured. It is a provocative test in the sense that the patient's skin is provoked locally to produce an objective, visible wheal and erythema that can be quantitated and are reproducible. The result is a localized area of inflammation entirely consistent with the known mechanism of IgE-mediated atopic or anaphylactic forms of human allergy. Inhalation provocation is an accepted method of testing in which a small quantity of allergen is delivered in a measured dose into the bronchial tree while the patient's response is monitored and quantitated by spirometry or plethysmography. The test is not necessary for routine diagnosis, but it is useful for certain unusual clinical presentations and for research purposes. It is the definitive procedure for identifying and studying the biphasic feature of the atopic reaction as it affects asthma. It is consistent with the recognized pathophysiology of allergic asthma and is the means by

Table 1 Essential Features of Provocative Testing for Allergy

1. Use of an objective endpoint measure consistent with the disease under test
2. Endpoint quantitated to establish a dose-response
3. Inclusion of a negative control to assess nonspecific reactivity
4. Double-blind, placebo-controlled protocol for studying subjective symptoms
5. Latent period between allergen administration and test result measurement consistent with known mechanism of the disease being tested
6. Test procedure consistent with known or suspected mechanism of the disease being tested
7. Test validation by comparison with other accepted disease manifestations in adequate numbers of patients and nondiseased controls

which its mechanism has been studied. A corresponding provocative allergen challenge technique is available for studying rhinitis by measuring objective changes in nasal airway resistance, but the procedure is much less frequently used. The skin patch test for delayed allergic contact dermatitis is performed by applying the test allergen to unbroken skin for 48 hours to elicit the skin inflammation characteristic of the disease but restricted to the test site.

These provocative allergy testing methods are all based on protocols that test for objective evidence of allergic inflammation. Oral food allergen challenge has been invaluable for assessing the numerous self-reported adverse effects that patients suspect are food-related. These may be exacerbations of respiratory symptoms, skin reactions, and gastrointestinal complaints. Because of the subjective nature of many adverse responses to foods and the potential for bias in a provocative test that has the patient ingest the food in a form that can be recognized, the correct procedure used for diagnosis and study is the double-blind, placebo-controlled method in which both the food and the placebo are disguised as contents of opaque capsules (15).

A controversial and unproven procedure called provocation-neutralization must be carefully distinguished from the types of acceptable provocation testing described above. It is performed by using intradermal, subcutaneous, or sublingual administration of allergens or other substances, followed by the patient's self-reporting of subjective ''symptoms or complaints'' beginning immediately after test dose application and ending 10 minutes later (19–21).

There is no limit to the number, severity, or nature of the provoked symptoms constituting a ''positive'' result. The testing proceeds in serial fashion with increasing doses of allergen until the patient again achieves a positive test result.

Provocation-neutralization testing differs from conventional allergy testing in several important ways. The items tested are not necessarily those elicited or suspected by the history, and allergy is diagnosed to any item giving a ''positive'' result whether the patient experiences any symptoms on ordinary exposure to that item. There are no standardized criteria for a positive test; these are left up to the discretion of the tester. Vague or nonspecific symptoms that do not correspond with the history are nevertheless considered as ''positive.'' Negative control tests are not included. Symptom recording begins immediately after challenge and concludes 10 minutes later, an arbitrary period that has not been evaluated as meaningful, and no provision is made for carryover of symptoms from one test to the next.

The serial increases (or decreases) in dosage are fivefold, but the volume of solution injected varies for no obvious reason from 0.01–0.05 mL. The neutralization component of the test consists of additional challenges with the same allergen immediately after a positive result is elicited. These additional tests are given at either a lower or higher concentration than previously, and they are intended to ''neutralize'' the reaction, that is to elicit no symptoms. When a particular test is negative, the dose for that test is prescribed as the concentration of vaccine to be used by the patient for immediate therapeutic neutralization as the need arises in the future (22).

There is no physiological explanation for allergy symptom neutralization as used in this fashion. Proponents of the procedure have postulated various immunological scenarios that are unproven and unlikely, such as generation of instantaneous antibody formation or dissolution of presumed pathogenic immune complexes (21,23), but no plausible theory, except for suggestion, is satisfactory to explain the as-yet undocumented neutralization of symptoms.

The procedure has evolved from anecdotal experiences. A number of attempts at clinical trials to investigate diagnostic efficacy of provocation-neutralization have been published. Results are mixed, because many of them suffer from methodologic flaws (24–28). The most rigorous of these showed that sublingual provocation-neutralization using food vaccines yielded negative results when compared to placebo in double-blind testing (29).

IV. ELECTRODERMAL DIAGNOSIS

A procedure called electrodermal or electro-acupuncture allergy testing, an offshoot of acupuncture, has been used in Europe for decades and recently, to a limited extent, in the United States (30,31). It features the use of equipment that is impressive to patients because of its seeming ''high-tech'' appearance.

Electrodermal diagnosis is predicated on the unfounded belief that an allergic reaction changes the electrical potential of the skin. The procedure is performed by applying an electric potential to the skin and observing for a change in electrical resistance in the presence of an allergen. In actual practice, the test vaccines of allergen are enclosed in vials that are supposedly inserted into the electric circuit. Various points on the skin corresponding to acupuncture points are touched with a metal probe. Different areas of the skin are said to possess information about different allergic manifestations and different allergens. A printout of the results given to the patient at the completion of the testing session reinforces the impression of a truly state-of-the-art methodology. In fact the entire procedure lacks any scientific basis, and no proper study has ever verified the results with any objective measure of allergic disease.

Electrodermal allergy testing is not approved by the Food and Drug Administration for use as a medical device in the United States.

V. APPLIED KINESIOLOGY

Testing the patient's muscle strength is used by certain ''alternative'' practitioners, especially chiropractors, presumably to diagnose various medical conditions. The practitioner applies manual force to an extremity and, by a subjective sense of the amount of his or her own effort required to move certain muscle groups against the patient's force to resist. Any number of diseases, including allergy, can allegedly be ''diagnosed'' (32).

The procedure for determining allergy, usually to foods, is to place a sample of the food in a container on the patient's chest while the patient is lying supine, or the patient may hold the container in hand. A perceived lessening of muscle strength while the container (not the food itself) is in contact with the body constitutes a positive test for allergy to that food. There is not the remotest connection between such a procedure and any conceivable theory of allergy that has any scientific validity. No form of allergy to food nor any other allergen has been described that involves altering the function of striated musculature. The idea that the test is done with the allergen separated by its container from the patient's body during the testing clearly precludes any rational explanation. Nevertheless, proponents of applied kinesiology use such mystical terms as ''energy field'' and ''liver stress'' to explain the results. The procedure does, however, appeal to many naive individuals who probably perceive the benefit because of the personal, physical touch of the tester, thereby accepting the results as valid. Persons who unnecessarily fear the prospect of needles or injections involved in allergy testing are prime targets for applied kinesiology practitioners.

Some variations in this basic procedure are even more bizarre. For example, testing of infants is done by surrogate testing of a parent or unrelated relative. The adult is tested first in the fashion described above, and then again while carrying the infant or holding a child's hand. Any ''difference'' reported by the tester is attributed to the child's allergy.

Claims for efficacy or even reproducibility of applied kinesiology are anecdotal only. There is a single, published study using a blinded protocol in which 20 subjects were ''tested'' to multiple foods. The results were found to be random and not reproducible (32).

VI. PULSE TEST

A theory propounded many years ago that allergy alters the pulse rate (33) led to a simple diagnostic test in which the patient's pulse is monitored for a change in rate when the patient is exposed to an allergen (34). Surprisingly, the ''test'' is still used and recommended even today by some alternative practitioners, and even more surprisingly, some patients accept the results.

The test dose of allergen can be applied by injection, ingestion, inhalation, or by any other route. The time interval preceding and during pulse measurement has never been standardized. A change of 10 beats per minute is accepted by proponents of this procedure, but there is a difference of opinion as to whether an increase, decrease, either, or both is acceptable as a positive response.

The simplicity and ready availability of pulse measurement as a ‘‘test’’ for allergy could lead to misdiagnosis on a large scale, but it is likely that most patients would easily discern that the test is worthless, even though the few practitioners who subscribe to it do not. The theory of the procedure has no support in our current understanding of allergy pathogenesis, and there are no clinical studies on diagnostic efficacy.

VII. BLOOD CHEMICAL ANALYSIS

Testing blood serum—and sometimes samples of urine, stool, hair, erythrocytes and fat—by quantitative analysis for many different environmental chemicals, metals, foods, drugs, vitamins, amino acids, and allergens is part of the diagnostic workup for so-called ‘‘multiple chemical sensitivities’’ or ‘‘environmental illness.’’ The unsupported theories of this condition postulate that almost any of these substances can be toxic to the immune system, leading to a state of subjective sensitivity to the environment (35). These theories also conclude that the presence of environmental chemicals within the body, even in minute quantities, is evidence of such a disease.

The analytical methods used for these determinations are often reliable and sensitive for this purpose, but to date there has been no evidence that the exceedingly low concentrations of such chemicals reported in patients suspected of having environmental illness are significantly different from asymptomatic individuals (3).

VIII. IgG ANTIBODIES

The various immunological bases for allergic diseases in humans are now well accepted, and these established mechanisms serve as the foundation for tests to identify specific sensitivities to the clinically relevant allergen or allergens in each patient. Immunoglobulin E antibodies react with allergens to trigger release of mast cell or basophil-derived mediators in the atopic diseases and in anaphylaxis. Specific sensitivities are detected by the presence of IgE antibodies in the patient’s serum using the radioallergosorbent test (RAST) or the enzyme-linked immunosorbent assay (ELISA) technology. Alternatively, the presence of these antibodies in tissue is determined by skin testing in which allergen introduced into the skin activates skin mast cell-fixed IgE antibodies to release mediators resulting in an immediate skin test reaction of erythema and whealing. Serum sickness and some forms of hypersensitivity pneumonitis are mediated by IgG (and probably IgM) antibodies that activate the complement cascade to generate complement-derived proinflammatory factors. In these cases, identification of the specific antibody requires one of many standard procedures, such as the precipitin-in-gel reaction. Although in vitro immune precipitation requires a large quantity of circulating antibody, high-dose in vivo antibody appears to be a necessary (although not sufficient by itself) criterion for pathogenesis of these diseases. Detection of specific precipitins—in conjunction with the clinical evidence of exposure to the allergen and the disease manifestations—is the appropriate test. Since allergic contact dermatitis is mediated by specifically sensitized effector T-cells, so the delayed skin patch test, which identifies localized skin contact inflammation after approximately 48 hours of continuous exposure is a well-validated method for detecting the causal allergen in that disease.

Unfortunately, the correct matching of test method with clinical allergic disease is not always followed in practice. The RAST and ELISA technologies are especially useful when antibody-mediated disease occurs, even though the concentration of antibody in the patient's serum is exceedingly low, as is the case in IgE-mediated allergy. Either test also can be used to detect similarly low concentrations of specific antibodies of other classes, such as IgG. As a result, some laboratories offer testing of IgG antibodies to common atopic allergens, especially foods and airborne molds, by these or similar techniques. Low levels of these IgG antibodies, and undoubtedly IgG antibodies to other environmental proteins, can be found normally, but they have yet to be shown to cause disease. Some clinicians erroneously attribute diagnostic significance to these antibodies in atopy, and others claim that IgG antibodies to foods and molds cause a variety of nonspecific symptoms.

IX. IMMUNE COMPLEXES

Some commercial medical laboratories offer a test to detect and quantitate circulating immune complexes containing food antigens, and some clinicians use the presence of such complexes as evidence for allergy to that food.

These laboratories use one of several two-step incubation methods using a solid-phase immunosorbent to detect the presence of both the specific food antigen and the antibody isotype (IgG, IgA, or IgE) in the immune complex captured from the test serum (36–38). The methodology is based on sound principles, and the tests are technically feasible. In fact, immune complexes do circulate in normal children and adults, and these may increase in amount after ingestion of the food (37–39). Furthermore, preliminary studies by several investigators have shown that, compared to normal controls, significantly larger amounts of such immune complexes show up in the circulation after ingestion of the food in some patients with either intestinal malabsorption or atopy (39–41). However, the quantity of circulating food immune complexes has not been shown to correlate with a food-specific allergic reaction and is therefore not useful in diagnosis (41). Diagnosing food allergy by this test may result in both unnecessary dietary food restrictions and a failure to detect the presence of an anaphylactic food allergy.

By analogy with serum sickness caused by the injection of heterologous serum or a drug such as penicillin, it might be postulated that circulating food immune complexes induce a similar disease with a chronic course because of the continued exposure to the food. To date, however, such a scenario is theoretical only, and there exists no proven pathogenic role for food immune complexes, regardless of the isotype of the antibody in the complex.

X. OTHER IMMUNOLOGIC TESTS

The modern diagnostic clinical immunology laboratory is equipped to provide accurate and reproducible quantitative measurements of circulating antibodies of any isotype (immunoglobulin class) to almost any antigen, including autoantigens. Total levels of immunoglobulins and each of the components of the complement system, as well as functional testing of various portions of the complement cascade, also can be done. Quantitative counting of leukocytes bearing one or more surface markers known as clusters of differentiation (CD markers) and lymphocyte and neutrophil functional analyses are also available to the clinician. Each of these tests has a place in aiding the diagnosis of current or past infections, immune deficiencies, autoimmune diseases, and neoplasms of the immune system.

The current availability of these powerful tools makes them just as available for misuse. Inappropriate reliance on these tests to diagnose controversial forms of allergy or other presumed immunological diseases is as detrimental to the patient's interests and well being as is the use of unproven methods discussed in this chapter.

XI. SERIAL ENDPOINT TITRATION

Standard clinical practice among allergists in the United States includes skin testing for detection of specific allergen sensitivities in IgE-mediated diseases. Some allergists supplement this practice with in vitro IgE antibody testing in selected cases, whereas others use in vitro testing exclusively. Although skin testing procedures vary, the usual practice for detecting specific sensitivities in atopy is by the initial prick testing of suspected allergens, followed by the more sensitive intradermal test for those allergens that failed to react by prick testing.

Although the preliminary prick (percutaneous) procedure is not done by allergists in Great Britain, its use reduces the risk of a systemic reaction. Intradermal testing uses a standard concentration of allergen for each of the common environmental allergen vaccines. Diagnostic intradermal testing in cases of anaphylactic sensitivity to the Hymenoptera insect venoms or drugs is typically done by a tenfold serial dilution method (after establishing that a preliminary prick test is negative), because of the occasional patient with exquisite sensitivity. The initial concentration is low enough to exclude a positive skin test and risk of anaphylaxis in virtually all such patients.

The endpoint titration method commonly attributed to Rinkel uses fivefold serially increasing concentrations of allergen intradermally in all patients with suspected atopic allergy (42–44). The method uses the ''endpoint'' established by the test as the indicator of both an optimal dose to initiate immunotherapy and the maintenance dose believed to achieve the best results for this type of treatment. The endpoint is defined as the concentration of allergen used in testing that initiates a progressive increase in wheal diameter of 2 mm or greater by subsequently higher fivefold test concentrations. The use of this concentration of antigen to calculate the starting and maintaining therapeutic injection dosages is arbitrary and not based on empirical or other data.

The skin endpoint titration method relies solely on the appearance of a wheal at the skin test site, ignoring the presence or absence of a surrounding wheal. A skin test wheal without erythema does not indicate an IgE reaction, but is often a sign of nonspecific irritation that is especially likely to result from crude vaccines of dust or molds. Quantitating the test result by wheal diameter is acceptable only if accompanied by significant erythema; to ignore the latter leads to false-positive results and an incorrect diagnosis of allergy where it does not exist.

A series of trials to test the efficacy of the endpoint method as an indication of immunotherapy dosing reveals that Rinkel's method is too conservative in estimating a safe starting dose, thereby prolonging the period of dose buildup for many patients (45). It is also not capable of determining an ''optimal'' dose for treatment (46).

XII. SALIENT POINTS

1. There is no scientific basis for unconventional theories and unproven diagnostic methods in allergic diseases.
2. Results obtained by unproven diagnostic methods are not reproducible.
3. Results from these tests are subject to variations at the whim of the practitioner.
4. Some diagnostic tests are not specific to allergy.

5. Legitimate tests can be misused to diagnose allergic disease.
6. Patients with suspected food allergy appear to be especially susceptible to acceptance of these unproven tests and controversial theories.
7. Clinicians need to be knowledgeable about controversial tests so that they may advise patients appropriately.

REFERENCES

1. Golbert TM. A review of controversial diagnostic and therapeutic techniques employed in allergy. J Allergy Clin Immunol 1975; 56: 170.
2. Grieco MH. Controversial practices in allergy. JAMA 1982; 247:3105.
3. Terr AI. Unconventional theories and unproven methods in allergy. In: Middleton E, Reed CE, Ellis EF, Adkinson NF, Yunginger JW, Busse WW, eds. Allergy: Principles and Practice. 5th ed. St Louis: Mosby, 1998:1235.
4. David TJ. Unorthodox allergy procedures. Arch Dis Child 1987; 62:1060.
5. California Medical Association Scientific Task Force on Clinical Ecology. Clinical ecology: a critical appraisal. West J Med 1986; 144:239.
6. Van Arsdel PP, Larsen EB. Review: diagnostic tests for patients with suspected allergic disease: utility and limitations. Ann Intern Med 1989; 110:304.
7. Goldberg BJ, Kaplan MS. Controversial concepts and techniques in the diagnosis and management of food allergies. Immunol Allergy Clin North Am 1991; 11:863.
8. American Academy of Allergy and Immunology. Position statements: clinical ecology. J Allergy Clin Immunol 1986; 78:269.
9. American Academy of Allergy and Immunology. Position statements: measurement of circulating IgG and IgE food-immune complexes. J Allergy Clin Immunol 1988; 81:758.
10. American College of Physicians. Position paper: allergy testing. Ann Intern Med 1989; 10:318.
11. National Center for Health Care Technology. Technology: summary of assessments. JAMA 1981; 246:1499.
12. Health Care Financing Administration. Availability of compliance policy guide for cytotoxic testing for allergic diseases. Fed Register 1985; 50:14025.
13. Health Care Financing Administration. Medicare program: exclusion of certain food allergy tests and treatments from Medicare coverage. Fed Register 1990; 55:35466.
14. Black AP. A new diagnostic method in allergic disease. Pediatrics 1956; 17:716.
15. Bock SA, Sampson HA, Atkins FM, Zeiger RS, Lehrer S, Sachs M, Bush RK, Metcalfe DD. Double-blind, placebo-controlled food challenge (DBPCFC) as an office procedure: a manual. J Allergy Clin Immunol 1988; 82:986–997.
16. Lieberman P, Crawford L, Bjelland J, Connell B, Rice M. Controlled study of the cytotoxic food test. JAMA 1974; 231:728.
17. Benson TE, Arkins JA. Cytotoxic testing for food allergy: evaluations of reproducibility and correlations. J Allergy Clin Immunol 1976; 58:471.
18. Lehman CW. The leukocytotoxic food allergy test: a study of reliability and reproducibility. Effect of diet and sublingual food drops on this test. Ann Allergy 1980; 45:150.

19. Willoughby JW. Provocative food test technique. Ann Allergy 1965; 23:543.
20. Lee CH, Williams RT, Binkley EL. Provocative testing and treatment for foods. Arch Otolaryngol 1969; 90:87.
21. Morris DL. Use of sublingual antigen in diagnosis and treatment of food allergy. Ann Allergy 1971; 27:289.
22. Kailin EW, Collier R. ''Relieving'' therapy for antigen exposure. JAMA 1971; 217:78.
23. Dolowitz DA. Theories of allergy brought up to date. Ann Allergy 1974; 32:183.
24. Breneman JD, Crook WC, Deamer W, Exline L, Gerrard JW, Heiner D, Hurst A, Leney FL. Report of the food allergy committee on the sublingual method of provocation testing. Ann Allergy 1973; 31:382.
25. Rea WJ, Podell RN, Williams M, Fenyves E, Spague DE, Johnson AR. Elimination of oral food challenge reaction by injection of food extract. Arch Otolaryngol 1984; 110:248.
26. Draper LW. Food testing in allergy: intradermal provocation vs. deliberate feeding. Arch Otolaryngol 1972; 96:196.
27. Crawford LV, Lieberman P, Harfi HA, Hale HR, Nelson H, Selner J, Wittig H, Postman M, Zietz A. A double-blind study of subcutaneous food testing. J Allergy Clin Immunol 1976; 57:236.
28. Caplin I. Report of the committee on provocative food testing. Ann Allergy 1973; 31:375.
29. Jewett DL, Fein G, Greenberg MH. Double-blind study of symptom provocation to determine food sensitivity. N Engl J Med 1990; 323:429.
30. Voll R. The phenomenon of medicine testing in electroacupuncture according to Voll. Am J Acupunct 1980; 8:87.
31. Tsuei JJ, Lehman CW, Lam FMK, Zhu DAH. A food allergy study utilizing the EAV acupuncture technique. Am J Acupunct 1984; 12:105.
32. Garrow JS. Kinesiology and food allergy. BMJ 1988; 296:1573.
33. Coca AF. Familial Nonreaginic Food Allergy. 3rd ed. Springfield, IL: Charles C Thomas, 1953.
34. Coca AF. The Pulse Test. New York: L. Stuart, 1956.
35. Sparks PJ, Daniell W, Black DW, Kipen HM, Altman LC, Simon GE, Terr AL. Multiple chemical sensitivity syndrome: a clinical perspective. I. Case definition, theories of pathogenesis, and research needs. J Occup Med 1994; 36:718.
36. Inganas M, Johansson SGO, Dannaeus A. A method for estimation of circulating immune complexes after oral challenge with ovalbumin. Clin Allergy 1980; 10:293.
37. Haddad ZH, Vetter M, Friedman J. Detection and kinetics of antigen-specific IgE and IgG immune complexes after oral challenge with ovalbumin. Ann Allergy 1983; 51:255.
38. Leary HL, Halsey JF. An assay to measure antigen-specific immune complexes in food allergy patients. J Allergy Clin Immunol 1984; 74:190.
39. Paganelli R, Atherton DJ, Levinsky RJ. The differences between normal and milk allergic subjects in their immune response after milk ingestion. Arch Dis Child 1983; 68:201.
40. Cunningham-Rundels C, Brandeis WE, Good RA, Day NK. Bovine proteins and the formation of circulating immune complexes in selective IgA deficiency. J Clin Invest 1979; 64:272.
41. Sheffer AL, Lieberman PL, Aaronson DW, Position statement: measurement of cir-

culating IgG and IgE food-immune complexes. J Allergy Clin Immunol 1988; 81: 758.

42. Rinkel HJ, Lee CH, Brown DW, Jr. The diagnosis of food allergy. Arch Otolaryngol 1963; 79:71.
43. Williams RI. Skin titration: testing and treatment. Otolaryngol Clin North Am 1971; 3:507.
44. Willoughby JW. Serial dilution titration skin tests in inhalant allergy. A clinical quantitative assessment of biologic skin reactivity to allergenic extracts. Otolaryngol Clin North Am 1974; 7:579.
45. Van Metre TE, Adkinson NF, Lichtenstein LM. A controlled study of the effectiveness of the Rinkel method of immunotherapy for ragweed pollen hay fever. J Allergy Clin Immunol 1980; 65:288.
46. Van Metre TE. Critique of controversial and unproven procedures for diagnosis and therapy of allergy disorders. Pediatr Clin North Am 1983; 30:807.

Index

About the Editors

Stephen F. Kemp is Assistant Professor of Medicine and Pediatrics, Founding Codirector of the Division of Allergy and Immunology, Department of Medicine, and Medical Codirector of the Adult Asthma Services Pharmaceutical Care Clinic at the University of Mississippi Medical Center, Jackson, and was the Founding Chief of the Allergy and Immunology Section, Medical Service, G.V. (Sonny) Montgomery Veterans Affairs Medical Center, Jackson, Mississippi. He is the author, coauthor, editor, or coeditor of over 50 research papers, editorials, book chapters, Internet CME articles, audio tapes, and abstracts. Dr. Kemp is a Fellow of the American Academy of Allergy, Asthma, and Immunology; the American College of Allergy, Asthma, and Immunology; and the American College of Physicians–American Society of Internal Medicine, and a member of numerous other societies. He received the B.A. degree (1983) from Duke University, Durham, North Carolina, the B.S. degree (1986) from Virginia Commonwealth University, Richmond, and the M.D. degree (1990) from the Medical College of Virginia, Virginia Commonwealth University, Richmond.

Richard F. Lockey is Professor of Medicine, Pediatrics, and Public Health, the Joy McCann Culverhouse Professor in Allergy and Immunology, and Director of the Division of Allergy and Immunology, University of South Florida College of Medicine, Tampa. Additionally, he is Chief of the Section of Allergy and Immunology, James A. Haley Veterans' Hospital, Tampa, Florida. He is the editor or coeditor of five books, including *Allergens and Allergen Immunotherapy, Second Edition, Revised and Expanded* (Marcel Dekker, Inc.), and the author or coauthor of more than 500 monographs, experimental papers, reviews, book chapters, and abstracts. A Past President and Fellow of the American Academy of Allergy, Asthma, and Immunology, and a Fellow of the American College of the Physicians–American Society of Internal Medicine, Dr. Lockey is a member of several societies, including the American Thoracic Society, the Clinical Immunology Society, and the American Medical Association, and is on the board of the International Association of Allergology and Clinical Immunology. He received the B.S. degree (1961) from Haverford College, Pennsylvania, the M.S. degree (1972) from the University of Michigan, Ann Arbor, and the M.D. degree (1965) from Temple University School of Medicine, Philadelphia, Pennsylvania.